Lippincott Fast Facts for

NCLEX-RN®

Second Edition

Rebecca A. Cox-Davenport, PhD, RN
Assistant Professor of Nursing
Wilson College
Chambersburg, Pennsylvania

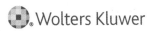

. Wolters Kluwer

Philadelphia • Baltimore • New York • London
Buenos Aires • Hong Kong • Sydney • Tokyo

Senior Digital Product Manager: Renee A. Gagliardi
Associate Content Strategist: Bernadette Enneg
Clinical Development Editor: Beverly Ann Tscheschlog, MS, RN
Production Project Manager: Cynthia Rudy
Design Coordinator: Joan Wendt
Art Director: Jennifer Clements
Manufacturing Coordinator: Kathleen Brown
Marketing Manager: Sarah Schuessler
Prepress Vendor: SPi Global

2nd edition

Library of Congress Cataloging-in-Publication Data
Names: Cox-Davenport, Rebecca A., editor.
  Title: Lippincott fast facts for NCLEX-RN / [edited by] Rebecca A. Cox-Davenport.
  Other titles: Lippincott's fast facts for NCLEX-RN. | Fast facts for NCLEX-RN
  Description: Second edition. | Philadelphia : Wolters Kluwer, [2017] | Preceded by Lippincott's fast facts for NCLEX-RN. c2012. | Includes bibliographical references.
  Identifiers: LCCN 2015049523 | ISBN 9781496325365
  Subjects: | MESH: Nursing Care—methods | Outlines
  Classification: LCC RT55 | NLM WY 18.2 | DDC 610.73076—dc23 LC record available at http://lccn.loc.gov/2015049523

RRS1704

Contributors

Rachel J. Coats, MS, RN, CEN, CNE
Lecturer of Nursing
Lander University
Greenwood, South Carolina

Rebecca A. Cox-Davenport, PhD, RN
Assistant Professor of Nursing
Wilson College
Chambersburg, Pennsylvania

Paula B. Haynes, MS, APRN, FNP-C, CDE, CNE
Assistant Professor
Lander University
Greenwood, South Carolina

Britney B. Kepler, DNP, PMHNP-BC
Assistant Professor
University of Pittsburgh
Pittsburgh, Pennsylvania

Theresa G. Lawson, PhD, APRN, FNP-BC, CNE
Associate Professor of Nursing
Lander University
Greenwood, South Carolina

Karen Montalto, PhD, MSN, RN
Assistant Dean and Director, Office of Nursing Student Success
Rutgers, The State University of New Jersey
Camden, New Jersey

Leslie MacTaggart Myers, DNP, APRN, ANP-BC, CNE
Associate Professor of Nursing/OB-GYN Nurse Practitioner
Lander University
Greenwood, South Carolina

Jodi Orm, RN, MSN, CNE
Assistant Professor of Nursing
Director of Simulation Education
Lake Superior State University
Sault Ste. Marie, Michigan

Patricia Zrelak, PhD, RN, NEA-BC, CNRN, SCRN
Quality and Safety Research Lead
Center for Health Policy and Research
University of California Davis
Davis, California

Contributors and Consultants to the Previous Edition

Vicky H. Becherer, RN, MSN
Julie Calvery Carman, APN, FNP-BC, MS
Marsha L. Conroy, RN, MSN
Maggie Thurmond Dorsey, RN, EdD
Sally E. Erdel, RN, MS, CNE
Margaret Fried, RN, MA
Kathy Henley Haugh, RN, PhD
Corlis Hayden, RN, MSN
Connie S. Heflin, RN, MSN, CNE
Soosannamma Joseph, RN, MS
Carolyn Kingston, RN, MSN
Kathleen Lehmann, RN, BSN, BA, MEd
Marilyn Little, APRN, BS, MSN
Jennifer McWha, RN, MSN
Susan A. Moore, RN, BSN, MS, MSN
Noel C. Piano, RN, MS
Elizabeth R. Pratt, RNC-INP, BSN, MSN
Nan C. Riedé, RN, MSN, CPN, PLNC
Ora V. Robinson, RN, PhD
Mary Frances Schneider, RN, BSN, MS
Lisa A. Seldomridge, RN, PhD
Barbara Selvek, RN, MSN, CCRN
Allison J. Terry, RN, MSN, PhD
Mary L. Terwilliger, RN, MSN
Peggy Thweatt, RN, BSN, MSN
Sandra K. Voll, RNC, MS, WHNP, CNM, FNP
Karen A. Wolf, APRN-BC, FNAP, PhD
Michele Woodbeck, RN, MS
Patricia Zrelak, CNRN, CNAA-BC, PhD

Faculty Reviewers

Nadine M. Aktan, PhD, FNP-BC
Chair and Professor of Nursing
William Paterson University
Wayne, New Jersey

Catherine Bock, RN, MAEd
Faculty, BSN Program
Kwantlen Polytechnic University
Surrey, British Columbia

Joy Borrero, RN, MSN, APRN
Associate Professor of Nursing
Suffolk County Community College
Brentwood, New York

Kerry Lynn Durnford, MN, RN
Nursing Faculty
School of Health and Human Services
Aurora College
Yellowknife, Northwest Territories

Leslie Graham, RN, MN, CNCC, CHSE
Professor, Durham College
Adjunct Professor, University of Ontario, Institute of Technology
RPN to BScN Coordinator
BScN Collaborative Nursing Program
Oshawa, Ontario

Theresa Hoadley, PhD, RN
Professor
Saint Francis Medical Center College of Nursing
Peoria, Illinois

Cathy Hogan, PhD, MPH, RN
Assistant Professor
Maryville University
St. Louis, Missouri

Jessica Jaeger, RN, MSN, CNE
Associate Professor
Ivy Tech Community College
Lafayette, Indiana

Joanne Lavin, RN, EdD, CNS
Adult Psychiatric Mental Health Nursing
Associate Director
CUNY SPS RN-BS Nursing Program
City University of New York
New York, New York

Carol McAuley, MSN, RN, CRRN
Associate Professor of Nursing
Washington State Community College
Marietta, Ohio

Tammie McCoy, PhD, RN
Professor and Chair, Bachelor of Science in Nursing Program
Mississippi University for Women
Columbus, Mississippi

Sandy McNeely, PhD(c), MSN, RN, CNE
Assistant Clinical Professor of Nursing
RN to BSN Track Manager
UH School of Nursing
University of Houston
Houston, Texas

Norma Melanson, BScN, MAEd, MN, PhD
Full Professor
Université de Moncton
Moncton, New Brunswick

Jeanette Murray, RN, BScN, MA
Educator Emerita
Thompson Rivers University
Kamloops, British Columbia

Ronald A. Owens, RN, BN, MN
Faculty
Memorial University of Newfoundland
School of Nursing
St. John's, Newfoundland and Labrador

Diana Paladino, MSN, BSN, RN
Director of the Undergraduate Nursing Program
Carlow University
Pittsburgh, Pennsylvania

Jessica Parrott, DNP, RN, CPNP-PC, CNE
Associate Professor
Norfolk State University
Norfolk, Virginia

Louise J. Rawluk, RN, BScN, MN
College Nursing Professor
Grande Prairie Regional College
Grande Prairie, Alberta

Jacquelyn Reid, MSN, EdD, CNE, APRN
Professor
Indiana University Southeast
New Albany, Indiana

Tracey Siegel, EdD, MSN, RN, CNE
Program Coordinator
Middlesex County College Nursing Program
Edison, New Jersey

Kimberley Staples, RN, MSN
Nursing Instructor
Grande Prairie Regional College
Grande Prairie, Alberta

Nicholas Torres, RN, BSN
Larkin School of Nursing
South Miami, Florida

Teri Bair Wisdorf, MSN, RN
Nursing Faculty
Century College
White Bear Lake, Minnesota

Student/Recent Graduate Reviewers

Rebecca Adams
Springfield Hospital

Todd Chandler
Idaho State University
Pocatello, Idaho

Ashley Falkner
Bradley University
Peoria, Illinois

Caitlin Hale, RN
ICU Staff Nurse
Clark Memorial Hospital
Charlestown, Indiana

Susan Huckleberry, RN
Home Health Nurse
Arkansas State University
Mountain Home, Arkansas

Franklin Quider
Capital Community College
Hartford, Connecticut

Benjamin Snyder, RN
Brookwood Hospital
Birmingham, Alabama

Steve Walters, RN
Orthopedic Nurse
Beebe Healthcare
Lewes, Delaware

Preface

DON'T GUESS. KNOW!

The NCLEX-RN® assesses how a registered nurse applies information to practice. There are no "knowledge-based" questions on the NCLEX-RN®; however, the test taker must possess the *knowledge* necessary to understand and process the best response to a situation. There are many strategies for answering NCLEX-style questions, but unless a test taker *knows* the information related to the question's topic, the person is still forced to guess the answer.

How to Use This Book

Lippincott Fast Facts for NCLEX-RN® is a complete reference designed to help you pass the NCLEX the first time! *Fast Facts* is a quick and easy bulleted review to use when studying for the NCLEX-RN®. With over 5,000 facts, this book covers important aspects of nursing care, organized around the major subject areas tested on the exam: adult health, maternal-neonatal nursing, pediatric nursing, psychiatric nursing, pharmacology, management of care, and client safety. *Fact Facts* uses information specifically chosen for its relevance to the NCLEX. This information will allow you to better prioritize facts about clinical situations on the NCLEX.

Each fact is accurate and up-to-date and has been thoroughly reviewed by nursing experts well versed in the NCLEX-RN® test plan. A small open box precedes each stand-alone fact, serving to keep each point separate and distinct. You may use the box to check off the fact when you feel you've sufficiently learned or mastered the information, or leave it blank to return to later when you need a refresher or further review.

At the end of each chapter, there is a short quiz composed of NCLEX-style questions. These questions were selected specifically because they cover content deemed challenging by *Lippincott PassPoint-RN*, an online adaptive quizzing engine. Use the questions to test your mastery of the information just learned. The information correlating to the question is also highlighted in the chapter by this icon: ⊚. As you study, pay special attention to information highlighted with the icon, because it is considered especially difficult.

Every NCLEX exam is different. Some students pass the NCLEX exam in 75 questions, while others pass by a narrow margin. The information that the test taker knows has a significant impact on test outcomes. Read the bullet points in this book and commit them to memory. Remember, the information listed was selected by nursing experts in their field.

Become a Stronger Test Taker

The appendix contains a guide to help improve your test-taking performance. You will learn to apply strategies to improve the way you approach exam questions and to eliminate bad habits you may have developed. Also in the appendix is a reference covering the types and styles of questions found on the NCLEX and key strategies for how to answer questions correctly. This includes alternate-format type questions (graphic option, chart/exhibit, drag-and-drop, hot spot, fill-in-the-blank, audio, and multiple response/multiple choice) that may appear on the actual exam.

Lippincott Fast Facts for NCLEX-RN® is the perfect tool to have on hand when studying. Use it alone, or quiz other students to review and prepare for the NCLEX. The format is more comprehensive and more portable than flash cards. Use this excellent review to make the most of your study time and increase your chance of success on the NCLEX-RN®!

Acknowledgments

I wish to thank my nursing students. Your insights have helped me to create and refine ways to help you develop into better test-takers. Thank you for always indulging me when I say "Let's try it this way!" I would like to extend another thank you to the *Fast Facts* chapter authors. You were wonderful to work with, and I appreciate your hard work on all of these facts! My last thank you goes to my supportive rock of a husband, Kevin. I appreciate your help and encouragement when I take on a new project. I could not do what I do without you.

About the Author

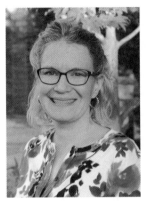

Rebecca A. Cox-Davenport, PhD, RN, earned a PhD in nursing from the University of Nevada, Las Vegas; an MSN in Nursing Education from Waynesburg University; a BSN from the University of Pittsburgh; and a diploma from Lancaster General Hospital School of Nursing. She is an Assistant Professor in Nursing at Wilson College in Chambersburg, Pennsylvania. Dr. C-D cares deeply for her students and their learning. Her research interests include improving student testing, building student communities, and student stress reduction interventions. Dr. C-D has worked in NCLEX preparation for 10 years and runs a tutoring service for students struggling to pass the NCLEX exam. In addition to teaching nursing, Dr. C-D has practiced in the areas of intensive care, emergency care, and hospice nursing.

Contents

1

Adult Care

CARDIOVASCULAR SYSTEM

KEY TERMS

- ☐ **Preload** is the stretching of muscle fibers in the ventricles as the ventricles fill with blood.
- ☐ **Afterload** is the amount of resistance to ejection of blood from the ventricle (during systole).
- ☐ **Cardiac output** is the amount of blood pumped by each ventricle (L/min).
- ☐ **Excitability** is the ability to respond to an electrical impulse.
- ☐ **Conductivity** is the ability of a cell to transmit an electrical impulse to another cardiac cell.
- ☐ **Contractility** is the ability of a cell to contract after receiving a stimulus and is influenced by preload.
- ☐ **Syncope** is a brief loss of consciousness caused by a lack of blood to the brain and can occur abruptly and can last for seconds to minutes.
- ☐ **Aneurysm** is an outpouching of a vessel.

Anatomy and Physiology Review

- ☐ During diastole (relaxation), all heart chambers relax at the same time allowing blood to flow into the ventricles to fill in preparation for contraction.
- ☐ During systole (contraction), the atria contract first, followed by the ventricles, to allow complete filling prior to ejection.
- ☐ The right side of the heart pumps venous (deoxygenated) blood to the lungs.
- ☐ The pulmonary artery is the only artery that carries deoxygenated blood.
- ☐ The left side of the heart pumps oxygenated blood to the body. The apex of the heart is the point of maximal impulse where heart sounds are heard loudest.
- ☐ Because the atria meet little resistance when pumping blood into the ventricles, their walls are relatively thin in comparison to the ventricles.
- ☐ Preload is determined by the volume of blood in the ventricle at the end of diastole.

Heart Valves

☐ Heart valves permit blood flow in one direction; they open and close in response to blood flow.

☐ See Table 1.1 for more information on heart valves.

Cardiac Cycle

☐ Right side (simultaneously occurring with left side):

  ○ Deoxygenated blood flows from the coronary sinus (heart) and the superior and inferior vena cava (body) into the right atrium.

  ○ The right atrium contracts to open the tricuspid valve allowing deoxygenated blood into the right ventricle.

  ○ The right ventricle contracts to open the pulmonic valve allowing deoxygenated blood to pump through the pulmonary arteries to the lungs; O_2 and CO_2 exchange occurs in the lungs.

  ○ Oxygenated blood flows from the lungs into the pulmonary veins.

TABLE 1.1 Heart Valves
Atrioventricular valves   With the closure of the atrioventricular valves, the first (S1) heart sound "lub" is heard loudest at the apical area (left fifth intercostal space at the midclavicular line)

Mitral	■ Also known as the bicuspid or left atrioventricular valve ■ Prevents backflow from the left ventricle into the left atrium ■ Heard best at the left fifth intercostal space at the midclavicular line
Tricuspid	■ Prevents backflow from the right ventricle into the right atrium ■ Heard best at the left fourth intercostal space at the sternal border

Semilunar valves   With the closure of these semilunar valves, the second (S2) heart sound "dub"

Pulmonic	■ Prevents backflow from the pulmonary artery into the right ventricle ■ Heard best at the second intercostal space to the left of the sternum
Aortic	■ Prevents backflow from the aorta into the left ventricle ■ Heard over at the second intercostal space to the right of the sternum

- Left side (simultaneously occurring with right side):
  - ○ Via the pulmonary veins, oxygenated blood is delivered to the left atrium.
  - ○ The left atrium contracts to open the bicuspid (mitral) valve allowing the oxygenated blood into the left ventricle.
  - ○ The left ventricle contracts to open the aortic valve; oxygenated blood is pumped into the aorta and out to the body.

Cardiac Conduction System

- Electrical stimulation causes troponin to expose actin-binding sites, which allows muscle contraction to occur in the heart.
- The firing of the sinoatrial node sets off a chain reaction in cardiac conduction.
- When an impulse leaves the sinoatrial node, it travels through the atria along Bachmann bundle and the internodal pathways on its way to the atrioventricular node.
- After the impulse passes through the atrioventricular node, it travels to the ventricles, first down the bundle of His, then along the bundle branches, and, finally, down the Purkinje fibers.
- The P wave represents atrial depolarization.
- Normal PR interval is 0.12 to 0.20 seconds.
- The QRS wave represents ventricular depolarization.
- Normal QRS interval is 0.06 to 0.12 seconds.

Heart Sounds

- The S_4 heart sound occurs as a result of increased resistance to ventricular filling after atrial contraction related to decreased compliance of the ventricle.
- The S_4 heart sound, also called an atrial gallop, is an adventitious heart sound that you'll hear best over the tricuspid or mitral area when the client lies on the left side.
- The S_3 heart sound, also known as ventricular gallop, is commonly heard in children and may be normal in women during the last trimester of pregnancy; however, it may be a cardinal sign of heart failure in other adults.
- A murmur is a low-pitched, rough, and rasping sound.
- A pericardial friction rub has a scratchy, rubbing quality.
- A dilated aorta causes turbulent blood flow, and a murmur can be also auscultated in heart sounds.
- See Table 1.2 for clinical manifestations of heart valve disorders.

Coronary Arteries

- Originate from the aorta; supply oxygenated blood to the heart.
- The coronary arteries receive blood supply during diastole.

TABLE 1.2	Clinical Manifestations of Heart Valve Disorders	
Atrioventricular Early clinical manifestations are usually mild, but usually progress with aging.		
Mitral	■ Angina ■ Fatigue ■ Dyspnea ■ Cough ■ Syncope ■ Palpitations	
Tricuspid	■ Jugular vein distention ■ Systemic edema	
Semilunar Mild and moderate disease usually does not have any symptoms, but may with exercise.		
Pulmonic	■ Jugular vein distention ■ Weight gain ■ Systemic edema	
Aortic	■ Angina ■ Fatigue ■ Dyspnea ■ Cough ■ Syncope ■ Palpitations	

☐ With a normal heart rate, there is time for myocardial perfusion during diastole.

☐ Increased heart rate = decreased diastolic time = inadequate time for myocardial perfusion = risk for myocardial ischemia.

☐ Obstruction of blood flow to one of these arteries causes acute coronary syndrome, which may result in an acute myocardial infarction (MI).

☐ See Table 1.3 for more information on coronary arteries.

Diagnostic Testing

☐ Stress test measures the heart's response to exertion, either by exercise or medication.

☐ Thallium stress nuclear imaging test that indicates blood flows into the myocardium during exercise and at rest.

☐ Teach the client to be NPO for 4 hours and no caffeine 12 hours prior to stress tests.

TABLE 1.3 Coronary Arteries	
Artery	Location and Function
Left anterior descending artery	■ Extends down the anterior wall ■ Primary source of blood for the anterior wall of the heart
Left main coronary artery	■ Extends from the point of origin to the first major branch ■ Splits into the left anterior descending and circumflex arteries ■ Supplies blood to the left atrium, most of the left ventricle, and most of the interventricular septum
Right coronary artery	■ Travels to the inferior wall ■ Supplies blood to the right side of the heart
Circumflex artery	■ Circles around to the left lateral wall ■ Supplies the lateral wall of the heart
Posterior descending artery	■ Branches from the right coronary artery ■ Supplies blood to the posterior wall of the heart

☐ Multiple-gated acquisition, or MUGA scan, uses a radioactive isotope attached to RBCs to give an accurate measurement of cardiac muscle movement and ejection fraction.

Cardiac Catheterization

☐ Used to visualize coronary arteries, valves, myocardium function, and disease of the aorta as well as interventional procedures to open blocked coronary arteries.

☐ It is most important for the nurse to determine if the client has allergies to iodine or shellfish before cardiac catheterization because it involves the injection of a radiopaque dye.

☐ After the procedure, maintain client on bed rest and monitor vital signs, bleeding at the puncture site, hematoma, distal pulse to the puncture site, nausea, pain, and complications such as MI or stroke.

Electrophysiology Studies (EPS)

☐ EPS stimulate the heart with electricity to help determine the cause of arrhythmias and possibly treat with an ablation.

☐ EPS are usually performed through venous system passing a catheter to the heart.

☐ After the procedure, maintain client on bed rest and monitor vital signs, cardiac monitor, bleeding at the insertion site, and angina.

Transesophageal Echocardiography (TEE)

☐ Ultrasonography is combined with endoscopy to provide a better view of the heart's structures.

☐ Used to evaluate valvular disease or repairs, but it's also used to diagnose thoracic and aortic disorders, endocarditis, congenital heart disease, intracardiac thrombi, and tumors.

☐ After the procedure, maintain client on bed rest due to sedation and keep NPO because the client will not have a gag reflex after the TEE.

Coronary Artery Disease (CAD)

☐ Atherosclerosis, or plaque formation, is the leading cause of CAD.

☐ A myocardial infarction is commonly a result of CAD.

☐ In atherosclerosis, hardened blood vessels cannot dilate properly; therefore, they constrict blood flow and block oxygen transport. As a result, oxygen cannot reach the heart muscle, resulting in angina.

☐ Diabetes mellitus is a risk factor for CAD that can be controlled with diet, exercise, and medication.

☐ Sublingual nitroglycerin is administered to treat acute angina.

☐ Inadequate oxygen supply to the myocardium is responsible for the pain accompanying angina.

☐ Coronary artery bypass surgery and percutaneous transluminal coronary angioplasty are invasive, surgical treatments for CAD.

☐ Clients complaining of angina should be placed on a cardiac ECG monitor immediately.

☐ An electrocardiogram showing ST elevation in leads II and III and a VF suggests occlusion of the right coronary artery.

☐ An electrocardiogram showing ST elevation in leads V_2, V_3, and V_4 suggests an anterior wall MI. An anterior wall MI may result in a decrease in left ventricular function.

☐ Total cholesterol level above 240 mg/dL is considered elevated and is a risk factor for developing CAD.

☐ Total cholesterol level below 200 mg/dL is considered below the nationally accepted level and carries a lesser risk.

☐ A lipid panel tests the amount of total cholesterol, low-density lipoprotein cholesterol, high-density lipoprotein cholesterol, and triglycerides.

Acute Coronary Syndrome (ACS)/Myocardial Infarction (MI)

☐ ACS or MI occurs when part of the heart muscle is not receiving blood flow and begins to die.

☐ In ACS, the blood supply to the heart muscle is suddenly blocked, usually as the result of the rupture of plaque in a diseased artery that forms an obstructive thrombus.

- ☐ MI results from prolonged myocardial ischemia due to reduced blood flow through one of the coronary arteries.
- ☐ ACS and MI are most often caused by atherosclerosis (plaque attracts platelets and causes thrombus formation); thrombus obstructs blood flow.
- ☐ The most common symptom of ACS is angina; others include nausea/indigestion, jaw pain, arm pain, shortness of breath, sweating, anxiety, and pallor.
- ☐ Women often have unusual symptoms including abdominal pain, nausea, palpitations, numbness, and/or referred pain especially to the back.
- ☐ The first priority for a client with chest pain is to obtain a 12-lead ECG within 10 minutes.
- ☐ Obtain a series of blood specimens for cardiac enzymes and biomarkers.
- ☐ Troponin is the best indicator for myocardial injury, measures protein found in myocardial cells, and rises within 2 to 8 hours after myocardial injury.
- ☐ CK-MB is a cardiac-specific isoenzyme released due to damage to cardiac cells and rises 4 to 6 hours after injury.
- ☐ Myoglobin is a heme protein found in cardiac and skeletal muscle that facilitates oxygen transport; less specific rises in 1 to 3 hours after injury; negative results may be used for rule out.
- ☐ Apply supplemental oxygen to assist in oxygenation and prevent further damage to the myocardium.
- ☐ Administer nitroglycerin (vasodilator), morphine (decreases pain and the work of the heart), and aspirin (antithrombus).
- ☐ Unstable angina occurs when there is partial occlusion of a coronary artery; ECG and cardiac enzymes show no evidence of infarction.
- ☐ NSTEMI (non-ST segment elevation myocardial infarction): elevated cardiac biomarkers without ECG evidence of MI.
- ☐ STEMI (ST-segment elevation myocardial infarction): evidence of MI is noted by ST-segment elevation on the ECG; significant damage to the myocardium is present.
- ☐ The treatment for a STEMI is immediate percutaneous coronary intervention (PCI) during the catheterization to open the coronary artery that has been blocked and promote reperfusion of the damaged area.
- ☐ If the catheterization is not immediately unavailable, thrombolytic therapy (tPA) (alteplase/reteplase/tenecteplase) should be initiated.
- ☐ Core measures for MI include aspirin on arrival and prescribed at discharge, an angiotensin-converting enzyme (ACE) inhibitor or

angiotensin II receptor blockers (ARBs) for left ventricular systolic dysfunction, smoking cessation, beta-adrenergic blockers and a statin prescribed at discharge, tPA within 30 minutes of arrival, and PCI within 90 minutes of arrival.

☐ Arrhythmias caused by oxygen deprivation to the myocardium are the most common complication of an MI.

☐ Because the pumping function of the heart is compromised by an MI, heart failure is the second most common complication of MI.

Cardiopulmonary Resuscitation (CPR)

☐ The sequence for CPR is compressions, airway, and breathing (CAB).

☐ Chest compression depth on an adult should be at least 2 inches (5 cm).

☐ All rescuers, trained or not, should deliver high-quality chest compressions by pushing hard to a depth of at least 2 inches (5 cm), at a rate of at least 100 compressions per minute, allowing full chest recoil after each compression and minimizing interruptions in chest compressions.

☐ Trained rescuers should also provide cardiopulmonary resuscitation with a compression to ventilation ratio of 30:2.

☐ Rescuers of adult victims should begin compressions rather than opening the airway and delivering breaths.

Heart Failure (HF)

☐ Cardiac output decreases on one or both sides of the heart causing a backflow of blood into other organs and structures.

☐ Left-sided HF causes primarily pulmonary symptoms, and right-sided HF causes more systemic ones.

☐ Jugular venous pressure is measured with the head of the bed inclined between 30 and 45 degrees. A centimeter ruler is used to obtain the vertical distance between the sternal angle and the point of highest pulsation. Greater than 3 cm is considered elevated or having jugular venous distention (JVD).

☐ Right HF clinical manifestations include JVD, dependent edema, weight gain, nausea, and decreased urine output. Inadequate liver deactivation of aldosterone leads to fluid retention and oliguria.

☐ The most accurate area on the body to assess dependent edema in a bedridden client is the sacral area.

☐ Left HF clinical manifestations include crackles, dyspnea, hypoxia, cough, weight gain, and weakness.

☐ Pharmacology includes diuretics, ACE inhibitors, ARBs, beta-adrenergic blockers, digoxin, aldosterone antagonists, and other vasodilators.

☐ Monitor vital signs, pulse oximetry, daily weights, I&O, edema, jugular veins, skin turgor, and respiratory and cardiovascular assessments.

☐ Teach clients to take medication as prescribed, to report weight gain of 3 pounds (2 kg), to follow a low-sodium diet, and to exercise.

Cardiac Arrhythmias

☐ Causes for arrhythmias include an electrolyte imbalance, cardiac ischemia, HF, cardiomyopathy, genetic influences, drug and alcohol use, and medications.

☐ Bradyarrhythmias decrease the heart rate less than 60 bpm. The low heart rate can cause symptoms of reduced cardiac output.

☐ Tachyarrhythmia's ineffective filling time causes a decrease in cardiac output.

☐ Common atrial arrhythmias include atrial flutter and fibrillation. In atrial flutter, there are flutter waves that are "sawtooth" in appearance. Atrial fibrillation is defined as chaotic, asynchronous, electrical activity in the atrial tissue.

☐ Common ventricular arrhythmias include ventricular fibrillation and ventricular tachycardia and can greatly impact cardiac output.

☐ A junctional rhythm originates from the atrioventricular (AV) node and is not always dangerous. The underlying cause should be treated.

☐ A bundle-branch block has an increased QRS complex duration.

☐ A shortened PR interval indicates a junctional rhythm.

☐ Pathologic Q waves are present with MI.

☐ Ischemic changes are represented on an electrocardiogram by T-wave inversion.

☐ In the presence of a new-onset arrhythmia, assess a client for clinical manifestations of decreased cardiac output including diaphoresis, angina, dizziness, syncope, and pallor.

☐ Monitor vital signs, obtain a 12-lead ECG, establish large-bore IV access, apply oxygen, draw electrolyte levels, and prepare for advanced life support and pacing.

☐ Medications include antiarrhythmics, electrolyte replacement, calcium channel blockers, beta-adrenergic blockers, digoxin, and anticoagulants.

Abdominal Aortic Aneurysm (AAA)

☐ The portion of the aorta distal to the renal arteries is more prone to an aneurysm because the vessel is not surrounded by stable structures, unlike the proximal portion of the aorta.

☐ Risk factors include hypertension, smoking, male gender, and genetic factors like Marfan syndrome.

- ☐ Abdominal pain is the most common symptom but could also have flank pain and a prominent pulsating mass in the abdomen.
- ☐ Rupture is a life-threatening emergency due to hemorrhage leading to hypovolemic shock.
- ☐ CT scan and ultrasound can confirm AAA location and size.
- ☐ Computed tomographic angiography (CTA) will give detailed pictures of the aneurysm.
- ☐ Hypertension should be avoided or controlled in a client with an AAA because it can cause the weakened vessel to rupture.
- ☐ Assess a client for an AAA, inspect for a pulsating mass, and auscultate for a bruit just left of midline in the lower abdomen. Avoid palpation if AAA is suspected.
- ☐ Severe lower abdominal and back pain indicates an aneurysm rupture, secondary to blood loss within the abdominal cavity.
- ☐ Clinical manifestations include severe lower back pain, hypovolemic shock (decreased blood pressure, increased heart rate, anxiety, confusion, and diaphoresis), and decreased hemoglobin and hematocrit counts.
- ☐ An endovascular repair is the treatment for an AAA.
- ☐ Large-bore IV insertion and rapid fluid resuscitation including blood products are the priorities with rupture.

Cardiomyopathy
- ☐ Cardiomyopathy is an abnormality in the heart muscle reducing the heart's ability to pump.
- ☐ Types include dilated, hypertrophic, and restrictive.
- ☐ Causes include exposure to toxins, medications, disease processes from diabetes or hypertension, alcoholism, and genetic influences.
- ☐ Although the cause of pregnancy related cardiomyopathy isn't entirely known, cardiac dilation and heart failure may develop in the mother during the last month of pregnancy or the first few months after birth.
- ☐ Heart failure most commonly occurs in clients with cardiomyopathy because the structure and function of the heart muscle are affected.
- ☐ Clinical manifestations include dyspnea, fatigue, tachycardia, heart murmur, JVD, change in level of consciousness (LOC), hypoxia, and auscultated crackles.
- ☐ The primary goal in the treatment of cardiomyopathy is to improve myocardial filling and cardiac output.
- ☐ The only definitive treatment for cardiomyopathy that can't be controlled medically is a heart transplant because the damage to the heart muscle is irreversible.

- Due to the high incidence of cardiac arrhythmias, a client may have an implantable cardioverter defibrillator (ICD).
- Monitor heart and lung sounds, vital signs, pulse oximetry, I&O, dyspnea, fatigue, and cardiac monitor.
- Teach clients to eat a low-sodium and calorie-restricted diet to prevent excess weight, and to weigh themselves daily, avoid alcohol, and quit smoking.
- Pharmacology goals include decreasing blood pressure and heart rate using ACE inhibitors, ARBs, beta-adrenergic blockers, and digoxin. Diuretics and aldosterone blockers may also be prescribed.

Cardiogenic Shock
- Cardiogenic shock is related to a reduced cardiac output and ineffective pumping of the heart. At least 40% of the heart muscle must be involved for cardiogenic shock to develop.
- Of all clients with an acute MI, 15% suffer cardiogenic shock secondary to the myocardial damage and decreased function.
- Early clinical manifestations are a decrease in cardiac output and cerebral blood flow causing restlessness, agitation, or confusion.
- Other clinical manifestations include diaphoresis, shortness of breath, pallor, tachycardia, decreased blood pressure, and decreased urine output.
- Diagnostic tests include blood pressure, 12-lead ECG, echocardiogram, and cardiac cath.
- Monitor vital signs, perform cardiac monitoring, and obtain arterial blood gases (ABGs), cardiac enzymes, and pulmonary artery pressures.
- Prepare for mechanical ventilation, cardiac catheterization, and possible interventional cardiac surgery.
- The first treatment goal for cardiogenic shock is to increase myocardial oxygen supply to prevent further muscle damage.

Septic Shock
- Septic shock is a bloodstream infection primarily caused by a widespread inflammatory response from bacteria.
- Clients at highest risk for septic shock are the elderly and the immunocompromised and also clients with diabetes, invasive lines, and on long-term antibiotic use.
- Clinical manifestations of septic shock include hypotension, tachycardia, change in LOC, low urine output, hypoxemia, restlessness, and agitation.
- Priority in septic shock is reversing hypoxia with supplemental oxygen or mechanical ventilation and treating hypotension.

- A large-bore IV access is necessary to infuse fluids, crystalloids, and vasopressors. Prepare for mechanical ventilation.
- Treatment with antibiotics will follow obtaining cultures.
- Laboratory tests include serum lactate level (positive is greater than 2 mmol/L), complete blood count (CBC) with differential, pan (every) cultures, and ABG.
- Monitor vital signs, pulse oximetry, I&O, central venous pressure, and LOC.

Hypertension

- Hypertension is usually exhibited by headaches, visual disturbances, and a flushed face.
- An occipital headache is typical of hypertension secondary to continued increased pressure on the cerebral vasculature.
- The brachial artery is most commonly used to measure blood pressure due to its easy accessibility and location.
- The radial and ulnar arteries can be used in extraordinary circumstances to obtain a blood pressure reading, but the measurement may not be as accurate.
- Teach clients to take medications as prescribed, self/home monitor blood pressure, exercise, stop smoking, use the Dietary Approaches to Stop Hypertension (DASH) diet, and avoid over-the-counter medications not prescribed.
- Low-sodium diet includes no more than 1,500 mg/day.
- See Tables 1.4 and 1.5 for facts on the stages and types of hypertension.

TABLE 1.4 Stages of Hypertension	
Prehypertension	Systolic 120–139 mm Hg *or* Diastolic pressure of 80–89 mm Hg represents
Stage 1 mild	Systolic 140–159 mm Hg *or* Diastolic 90–99 mm Hg
Stage 2 moderate	Systolic ≥160–179 mm Hg *or* Diastolic ≥100–109 mm Hg
Stage 3 severe/emergent	Systolic ≥180 mm Hg *or* Diastolic ≥110 mm Hg

TABLE 1.5	Types of Hypertension
Primary hypertension	■ Persistently elevated blood pressure with an unknown cause ■ Accounts for ~90% of hypertension cases ■ Characterized by a progressive, usually asymptomatic blood pressure increase over several years
Secondary hypertension	■ Occurs secondary to a known, correctable cause
Malignant hypertension	■ Rapidly progressive ■ Uncontrollable ■ Causes a rapid onset of complications

Endocarditis

- ☐ The endocardium is the innermost layer of the heart made of endothelial tissue and also lines the valves.
- ☐ Bacterial endocarditis is more common in clients with prosthetic heart valves, cardiac devices, or structural defects and IV drug users; increased risk after indwelling catheters, hemodialysis, prolonged intravenous therapy, and invasive procedures involving mucosal surfaces.
- ☐ Fungal endocarditis is most common in clients taking immunosuppressant medication or corticosteroids.
- ☐ Rheumatic endocarditis is associated with acute rheumatic fever occurring most often in children after an episode of streptococcal pharyngitis (group A beta hemolytic).
- ☐ Organisms invade the clot formation/lesion caused by a deformity or injury of the endocardium. The organism is covered by new clots and concealed from normal defenses.
- ☐ Early clinical manifestations include fever, chills, fatigue, dyspnea, and new-onset heart murmur.
- ☐ Later clinical manifestations include petechiae, Osler nodes under the skin in fingers, and joint pain.
- ☐ Assess for murmur, LOC, heart failure, cardiac monitor, temperature, and I&O.
- ☐ Obtain CBC and blood cultures; administer IV antibiotics or antifungals and cooling measures.
- ☐ Treatment includes IV antibiotics for 2 to 6 weeks with a follow-up echocardiogram to evaluate heart damage.

Myocarditis

- ☐ The myocardium is the thick middle layer of the heart responsible for pumping action and forms most of the heart wall; made of striated muscle fibers that cause the heart to contract.

- ☐ Myocarditis results from infection (most commonly viral), immune reaction, or toxins.
- ☐ Clinical manifestations include dyspnea, angina, fatigue, joint pain, fever, and arthralgia.
- ☐ Diagnostic tests include CBC with differential, blood cultures, 12-lead ECG, and echocardiogram.
- ☐ Monitor cardiovascular assessment to focus on signs and symptoms of heart failure.
- ☐ Minimize myocardial oxygen consumption by encouraging bed rest, assist with ADLs, and give supplemental oxygen to increase delivery to heart muscle if indicated.

Pericarditis
- ☐ The pericardium is composed of an outer fibrous layer and an inner double layer. Between the inner double layers is the pericardial space. The fluid in this space lubricates the surface of the heart, reducing friction.
- ☐ This pericardial sac may become inflamed following various disorders such as a viral illness or trauma and may also occur after MI.
- ☐ Pericarditis is often asymptomatic. Most common symptom is chest pain that worsens with deep breathing or movement. A friction rub is commonly heard at the left lower sternal border.
- ☐ Treatment of choice is NSAIDs to reduce inflammation and pain.

Cardiac Tamponade
- ☐ Cardiac tamponade occurs when fluid collects around the heart reducing pericardial space and impairing cardiac filling.
- ☐ Associated with decreased cardiac output, which in turn reduces blood pressure.
- ☐ Clinical manifestations include shortness of breath, sharp chest pain, hypotension, signs of shock, decreased LOC, absent peripheral pulses, pulsus paradoxus, and a narrow pulse pressure.
- ☐ Diagnostic tests include 12-lead ECG, echocardiogram, and chest X-ray.
- ☐ Monitor vital signs, cardiac monitor, heart sounds, urine output, and LOC.
- ☐ Apply high-flow oxygen, large-bore IV access for IV fluids, and vasopressors.
- ☐ Treatment for cardiac tamponade is a pericardiocentesis or a pericardial window to remove the fluid, as well as the cause of the fluid accumulation must be treated.

Varicose Veins
- ☐ Primary varicose veins have a gradual onset and progressively worsen. Secondary varicose veins are caused by injury to the vein wall.

- ☐ Leg fatigue and pressure are classic signs of varicose veins, related to valve weakness, increasing blood volume, and edema.
- ☐ Sharp pain and cool feet are clinical manifestations of alteration in arterial blood flow not venous issue.
- ☐ Edema and blue pigmented veins are signs and clinical manifestations of varicose veins.
- ☐ Teach clients to exercise, wear compression stockings, and elevate their legs when seated.
- ☐ Assess for skin ulcers and superficial venous thrombus.
- ☐ Ligation and stripping of the vein can rid the vein of varicosity, but it won't prevent other varicose veins from forming.
- ☐ Sitting and bed rest are contraindicated in the postoperative management of a client who has undergone ligation and stripping because both promote decreased blood return to the heart and venous stasis.

Pulmonary Edema

- ☐ Caused by increased pulmonary pressures due to fluid volume overload, decreased left-sided cardiac output, or pulmonary injury, allows fluid to accumulate in the interstitial and alveolar spaces.
- ☐ Pulmonary edema is a life-threatening complication of heart failure.
- ☐ Pulmonary edema can develop in minutes, secondary to a sudden fluid shift from the pulmonary vasculature into the interstitium and alveoli of the lung.
- ☐ Production of pink, frothy sputum is a classic sign of acute pulmonary edema.
- ☐ Early clinical manifestations include sudden onset of dyspnea, coughing, and restlessness.
- ☐ Late clinical manifestations include low blood pressure, tachycardia, diffuse crackles, and a cough producing pink and frothy sputum.
- ☐ Diagnostic tests include chest X-ray, ECG, echocardiogram, ABG, blood cultures, and cardiac markers.
- ☐ Apply supplemental oxygen, cardiac monitor, position in high Fowlers, and have suction equipment available.
- ☐ Monitor vital signs, lung sounds, oxygenation, cardiac rhythm, I&O, and daily weight.
- ☐ Medications ordered include morphine, diuretics, nitrates, and antihypertensives.
- ☐ Teach clients to quit smoking, follow a low-sodium diet, take antihypertensive medication, and exercise.

Anticoagulation Studies

☐ Activated partial thromboplastin time (APTT), partial thromboplastin time (PTT), prothrombin time (PT), bleeding time, and activated clotting time are tests that measure clotting time.

☐ Increased international normalized ratio (INR) values may indicate disseminated intravascular coagulation, cirrhosis, hepatitis, vitamin K deficiency, salicylate intoxication, or uncontrolled oral anticoagulation with warfarin.

RESPIRATORY SYSTEM

Anatomy and Physiology Review

☐ The upper airway (nose, paranasal sinuses, pharynx, tonsils, adenoids, larynx, and upper trachea) warms and filters inhaled air.

☐ The lower airway (lower trachea and lungs) contains the bronchioles and alveoli needed for gas exchange.

☐ The body requires oxygen to use carbohydrates, fats, and proteins for energy; carbon dioxide is produced as a result of this oxidation.

☐ Carbon dioxide and oxygen exchange occur by diffusion in the alveoli.

☐ Blood must perfuse, or flow around each alveolus, for the exchange of carbon dioxide and oxygen to occur across the alveolar-capillary membrane.

☐ The diaphragm and the external intercostal muscles are the primary muscles used in breathing.

☐ The diaphragm and the external intercostal muscles contract when the client inhales and relax when the client exhales.

☐ A ruptured diaphragm leads to hyperresonance on percussion, hypotension, dyspnea, dysphagia, and shifting of heart and bowel sounds in the lower to middle chest.

☐ See Table 1.6 for a list of abnormal breath sounds.

TABLE 1.6	Abnormal Breath Sounds
Sound	**Characteristics**
Crackles	■ Short explosive or popping sounds ■ Caused by fluid in the airway, atelectasis, and interstitial fibrosis
Rhonchi	■ Low-pitched sounds with a snoring quality ■ Suggests secretions in the large airways
Wheezes	■ High-pitched, whistling sounds ■ Results from narrowed airways, as in asthma, COPD, or bronchitis

Geriatric Considerations
- [ ] Reduction in vital capacity and ciliary action are normal physiologic changes in the older adult.
- [ ] Other normal physiologic changes in the older adult include decreased elastic recoil of the lungs, fewer functional capillaries in the alveoli, and an increase in residual volume.

Sputum Testing
- [ ] When possible, sputum samples should be in the morning before the client has had anything by mouth.
- [ ] If a sputum specimen will be collected by expectoration, the client should be instructed to take several deep abdominal breaths; when ready to cough, the client should take one more deep abdominal breath, bend forward, and cough into the provided sterile container.
- [ ] A client should be instructed to drink plenty of fluids the night before a sputum test.
- [ ] Coughing can be induced with a nebulizer treatment or suctioning.

Oxygen (O_2) Delivery
- [ ] Hemoglobin carries oxygen to all tissues in the body.
- [ ] Pulse oximetry (SpO_2) measures the oxygen saturation of hemoglobin.
- [ ] SpO_2 levels less than 90% indicate inadequate oxygenation to the tissues.
- [ ] Supplemental O_2 is considered to be a medication; its effects should be closely monitored.
- [ ] A nasal cannula is used to deliver 1 to 6 L of oxygen per minute and delivers oxygen concentration of 20% to 40%.
- [ ] A simple mask is used to deliver 6 to 8 L/min and oxygen concentration of 40% to 60%.
- [ ] A nonrebreather mask is used in emergent client conditions to deliver 12 to 15 L/min with oxygen concentration of 80% to 100%.
- [ ] A Venturi mask is used to deliver 4 to 8 L/min, oxygen concentration of 24%, 26%, 28%, 30%, 35%, or 40%, and delivers precise oxygen concentrations, which is used most commonly in clients with chronic obstructive pulmonary disease (COPD).
- [ ] Oxygen toxicity causes direct pulmonary trauma, reduces the amount of alveolar surface area available for gaseous exchange, and can result in increased carbon dioxide levels and decreased oxygen uptake.
- [ ] The administration of too much oxygen can decrease the respiratory drive and cause high $PaCO_2$ in the client with COPD.

Bronchoscopy
- [ ] A rigid or flexible scope passed down the bronchus to visualize structures, biopsy, and collect sputum samples.

- ☐ Client will be NPO for 6 to 12 hours before the procedure.
- ☐ After the procedure, monitor client's vital signs, pulse oximetry, lung sounds, and cardiac monitoring due to possible complications such as pneumothorax and arrhythmias.
- ☐ Keep the client NPO until the gag reflex returns.

Endotracheal (ET) Intubation

- ☐ Indications: severe respiratory distress, airway obstruction, airway management, and respiratory failure.
- ☐ To care for a client who has been intubated: secure the ET tube and note measurement at the lip, visualize symmetry of the chest, listen to bilateral breath sounds, and verify placement with capnography and X-ray.
- ☐ Provide humidity, perform suction only as needed, and reposition client to prevent atelectasis and pressure ulcers.
- ☐ Prevent ventilator-associated pneumonia (VAP) by performing oral hygiene and keeping the head of bed at 30 to 45 degrees.
- ☐ A prone position (lying on the abdomen) improves oxygenation in a client with acute respiratory distress syndrome who's receiving mechanical ventilation because it recruits new alveoli in the posterior region of the lung.

Positive End-Expiratory Pressure (PEEP)

- ☐ PEEP improves oxygenation by delivering positive pressure to the lung at the end of expiration, helps open collapsed alveoli, and helps them stay open so gas exchange can occur in these newly opened alveoli.
- ☐ Usually PEEP is set from +5 to +10 cm H_2O.
- ☐ Avoid high levels of PEEP to prevent barotrauma and pneumothorax.
- ☐ PEEP can reduce cardiac output by increasing intrathoracic pressure and reducing the amount of blood delivered to the left side of the heart.

Continuous Positive Airway Pressure (CPAP)

- ☐ Commonly used by clients who have sleep apnea.
- ☐ CPAP makes it easier to breathe by providing pressurized oxygen continuously through both inspiration and expiration; the client has less resistance to overcome in taking in a next breath.
- ☐ Oxygen can be provided through a CPAP mask to improve oxygenation in hypoxic clients.

Bilevel Positive Airway Pressure (BiPAP)

- ☐ Commonly used to treat clients in fluid overload due to heart failure.
- ☐ BiPAP delivers both continuous positive airway pressure (CPAP) and expiratory positive airway pressure (similar to PEEP).

☐ BiPAP provides the differing pressures throughout the respiratory cycle, attempting to optimize a client's oxygenation and ventilation.

☐ Inspiratory and expiratory pressures are set separately to optimize the client's ventilatory status in BiPAP.

☐ The fraction of inspired oxygen is adjusted to optimize oxygenation in BiPAP.

Thoracentesis

☐ Thoracentesis is used to remove excess pleural fluid and restore proper lung inflation.

☐ Causes include pleural effusion, cancer, pneumonia, heart failure, and trauma.

☐ During the procedure, keep the client still, obtain baseline vital signs, monitor continuous pulse oximetry, administer sedation if needed, provide support, and record the amount of fluid extracted.

☐ Position client sitting on the side of the bed arms on bedside table.

☐ After the procedure, monitor vital signs, pulse oximetry, lung sounds, and respiratory effort. Position the client with their unaffected lung down for 30 to 60 minutes.

Chest Tubes

☐ To prevent complications after thoracic surgery or trauma, chest tubes are placed to remove air, fluid, and blood from the pleural cavity.

☐ The chest drainage unit should be kept below the level of the client's chest.

☐ Monitor respiratory rate, work of breathing, breath sounds, and pulse oximetry frequently.

☐ Assess the insertion site for subcutaneous emphysema, drainage, and tube security. Keep all tubing free of kinks and occlusions. Take steps to prevent fluid-filled dependent loops, which can impede drainage.

☐ Fluctuations, referred to as tidaling, in the fluid level of the water-seal chamber are expected with respiratory effort. The water level will increase and decrease with inspiration and expiration.

☐ If there is no tidaling, assess for tubing obstruction or displacement.

☐ If continuous bubbling in the water-seal chamber occurs, the system should be examined for an air leak; examine the system from the insertion site to the drainage unit.

☐ If the chest tube becomes disconnected, place the open end in a bottle of sterile water to prevent excess air from entering the pleural space.

☐ Never clamp a chest tube, except momentarily, when changing the system, while assessing for location of air leak or with a doctor's order to test a client's tolerance of chest tube removal.

☐ Administer ordered analgesia.

Suctioning

- ☐ Performed to remove secretions and/or induce cough to prevent airway obstruction.
- ☐ Client should be well oxygenated prior to suctioning.
- ☐ Sterile gloves should be worn and suction catheter lubricated when performing suctioning.
- ☐ Advance the catheter without suction during inspiration; apply suction for only 15 seconds at a time while withdrawing the catheter.
- ☐ Suction pressure should be no more than 120 mm Hg.
- ☐ Assess for improvement in breath sounds, increased SpO_2, and the character of removed secretions.

Arterial Blood Gas (ABG)

- ☐ Before obtaining an arterial blood sample from a client's radial artery, the Allen test is performed to assess circulation.
- ☐ Normal arterial blood gas values include a pH of 7.35 to 7.45.
- ☐ Normal $PaCO_2$ or PCO_2 (partial pressure of CO_2 in arterial blood) is 35 to 45 mm Hg.
- ☐ Normal PaO_2 or PO_2 (partial pressure of O_2 in arterial blood) values are 80 to 100 mm Hg.
- ☐ Normal HCO_3^- (bicarbonate) levels are 22 to 26 mEq/L.

ABG Analysis

- ☐ Is the pH below 7.35 (acidotic) or above 7.45 (alkalotic).
- ☐ Is the PCO_2 below 35 mm Hg (alkalotic) or above 45 mm Hg (acidotic).
- ☐ Is the HCO_3^- below 22 mEq/L (acidotic) or above 26 mEq/L (alkalotic).
- ☐ Match the PCO_2 or the HCO_3^- with the pH.
- ☐ If the PCO_2 and the pH are both acidotic or both alkalotic, the disturbance is a respiratory issue.
- ☐ If the HCO_3^- and the pH are both acidotic or both alkalotic, the disturbance is metabolic.
- ☐ If the pH is normal, you must determine whether the PCO_2 or HCO_3^- is most likely causing the disturbance.
- ☐ If the HCO_3^- or PCO_2 value moves in the opposite direction of the pH, there is compensation.
- ☐ A PaO_2 below 80 is evidence of hypoxemia.
- ☐ Respiratory acidosis: acidotic (low) pH and acidotic (high) PCO_2 and normal HCO_3^-.
  - ○ Partly compensated: HCO_3^- is high.
  - ○ Caused by increased CO_2 due to hypoventilation; treat by increasing ventilation.

- Respiratory alkalosis: alkalotic (high) pH and alkalotic (low) PCO_2 and normal HCO_3^-.
  - Partly compensated: HCO_3^- is low.
  - Caused by hyperventilation; treat the causes (anxiety, infection, stimulants).
- Metabolic acidosis: acidotic (low) pH and acidotic (low) HCO_3^- and normal PCO_2.
  - Partly compensated: PCO_2 is low.
- Metabolic alkalosis: alkalotic (high) pH and alkalotic (high) HCO_3^- and normal PCO_2.
  - Partly compensated: PCO_2 is high.
  - Fully compensated = normal pH.

Tuberculosis (TB)

- Infectious disease caused by *Mycobacterium tuberculosis* primarily affecting the lungs.
- Droplet particles spread via airborne transmission and cause an inflammatory reaction.
- Risk factors: those who are immunocompromised (human immunodeficiency virus [HIV], cancer), substance abuse, homeless, poverty, comorbidities, or immigrants.
- Classic clinical manifestations are fever, night sweats, cough, fatigue, and weight loss; hemoptysis may be present.
- Once a client has tested positive via a skin test, blood test, or sputum culture, a chest X-ray will be performed to assess for lung lesions.
- Tuberculin skin test (Mantoux method): intradermal injection of 0.1 mL purified protein derivative (PPD) is administered into the inner aspect of the midforearm, creating a wheal.
- The result is read 48 to 72 hours after placement. A reaction with induration of 5 mm or greater in immunosuppressed (HIV) and 10 mm or greater in those with normal immunity is considered positive.
- Treated with anti-TB agents for 6 to 12 months; TB drug resistance is an increasing concern.
- Most common medications are isoniazid, rifampin, pyrazinamide, and ethambutol.
- The client should be on droplet/AFB precautions (negative pressure room), and particulate respirators (N95) should be implemented to prevent transmission.
- Promote airway clearance by encouraging increased fluid intake.
- Educate about transmission prevention (hygiene, covering nose/mouth) and importance of adherence to the medication regimen (multiple medication regimen).

- □ It is mandatory that all cases of TB be reported to the health department.
- □ Some people carry dormant tuberculosis that may develop into active disease.
- □ The tubercle bacilli may remain latent for years and then activate when the client's resistance is lowered, as when a client is being treated for cancer.
- □ The sputum culture for *M. tuberculosis* is the only method of confirming the diagnosis and cure of tuberculosis.

Pneumonia

- □ Inflammation of the lungs caused by microorganisms that enter the pulmonary circulation.
- □ Community-acquired pneumonia occurs within the community setting or within the first two days of hospitalization commonly caused by *Streptococcus pneumonia*.
- □ Health care–associated pneumonia occurs in a client who is not hospitalized but has close contact with health care such as hemodialysis, chemotherapy, or nursing home residence.
- □ Hospital-acquired pneumonia develops greater than 48 hours after admission to the hospital.
- □ Ventilator associated is hospital acquired with the presence of an endotracheal tube.
- □ Aspiration pneumonia occurs with the entry of substances, such as gastric contents, into the airway that cause inflammatory changes and lead to bacterial growth.
- □ Risk factors include clients with immobility, decreased LOC, increased age, cardiac and lung disease, weakened immune system, and alcoholism.
- □ Clinical manifestations include fever, chills, cough, chest pain, and varying degrees of respiratory distress such as tachypnea, dyspnea, and orthopnea.
- □ Elderly clients with pneumonia may first appear with only an altered mental status and dehydration due to a diminished immune response.
- □ Obtain a chest X-ray, sputum culture, and blood specimens including two sets of blood cultures, CBC with differential, and possibly ABG.
- □ Critical treatment includes broad-spectrum antibiotic therapy and fever control and may need oxygen therapy, fluid replacement, nebulizer treatment, and/or inhaler (bronchodilator).
- □ Hydration, oxygen therapy, deep breathing exercises, coughing, position changes, and ambulation are particularly important for the geriatric client to prevent mortality.
- □ Potential complications include sepsis, respiratory failure, and pleural effusion.

- ☐ Monitor vital signs to include oxygen saturation, secretions, cough, dyspnea, altered mental status, and hemodynamic status.
- ☐ Assist with the removal of secretions; promote rest, fluid intake, and nutrition.
- ☐ The pneumococcal vaccine is recommended for children younger than 5, clients 65 and older, immunocompromised clients, and those who are at high risk for pneumonia such as chronic heart and lung disease.
- ☐ Teach clients about the use of antibiotics, signs of deterioration (difficulty breathing, worsening cough, increasing fever), smoking cessation, and importance of activity and deep breathing exercises including incentive spirometry.

Severe Acute Respiratory Syndrome (SARS)

- ☐ Viral respiratory illness spread by respiratory droplets and contact with contaminated surfaces.
- ☐ Clinical manifestations are fever, coughing, and difficulty breathing; others include body aches, diarrhea, and headache; client often develops pneumonia.
- ☐ No treatment; provide supportive care.
- ☐ Use infection control strategies to include contact and airborne isolation, personal protective equipment (PPE), and hand hygiene.

Asthma

- ☐ Airway inflammation characterized by edema, bronchoconstriction, hyperreactivity, and airway changes.
- ☐ Asthma is classified as mild intermittent, mild persistent, moderate persistent, and severe persistent based on frequency and severity of symptoms and lung function.
- ☐ Clinical manifestations are cough, wheezing, and difficulty breathing and also chest tightness and prolonged expiration.
- ☐ The client with asthma should use a peak flow meter to measure the highest volume of airflow with forced expiration. A result in the green zone means asthma is well controlled, yellow zone means asthma is getting worse, and red zone means take immediate action.
- ☐ Acute symptoms should be treated with a short-acting beta-2 agonists (albuterol) inhaler or nebulizer.
- ☐ Other medications include steroids (inhaled, PO, parenteral), long-acting beta agonists (salmeterol), mast cell stabilizers (cromolyn), and leukotriene modifiers (montelukast).
- ☐ Status asthmaticus is an asthma exacerbation that may lead to complete airway obstruction due to severe bronchospasm and mucus.
- ☐ Prepare for possible intubation and mechanical ventilation.

- ☐ Initial treatment for status asthmaticus is a bronchodilator and systemic corticosteroids (methylprednisolone sodium succinate) and also IV fluids and oxygen; magnesium sulfate (smooth muscle relaxer) may be administered to induce bronchodilation.
- ☐ Elevate head of bed or assist to a tripod position, encourage abdominal and pursed-lip breathing, and promote increased fluid intake.
- ☐ Monitor vital signs, lung sounds, and continuous pulse oximetry.
- ☐ Assist the client to identify factors that may have caused the exacerbation (flowers, smoke, perfume, cleaning agents, food, pets, etc.).

Atelectasis

- ☐ Atelectasis develops when there's interference with the normal negative pressure that promotes alveolar expansion due to hypoventilation or obstruction.
- ☐ Risk factors include obesity, lung disease, immobility, and smoking.
- ☐ Clinical manifestations include auscultating crackles, low-grade fever, and decreased lung sounds especially at the lung bases.
- ☐ Atelectasis is the most common respiratory disorder to occur in the first 24 to 48 hours after surgery and increases the client's risk for pneumonia.
- ☐ Medicate clients for pain, ambulate, teach to splint incision, encourage increased fluid intake, encourage client to cough and deep breathe, and use incentive spirometer.
- ☐ To use the incentive spirometer, place the client in a high or semi-Fowler position, observe a return demonstration to assess the client's technique, and assist the client to create goals.
- ☐ The incentive spirometer should be used every 1 to 2 hours while the client is awake.
- ☐ Monitor lung sounds, LOC, vital signs, pulse oximetry, and presence of oversedation.

Chronic Obstructive Pulmonary Disease (COPD)

- ☐ Progressive respiratory conditions that cause obstruction of airflow that includes chronic bronchitis and emphysema.
- ☐ Chronic bronchitis is inflammation of the bronchi that causes a productive cough.
- ☐ Emphysema is irreversible destruction of the alveoli causing impaired gas exchange.
- ☐ Most often caused by tobacco smoke and also dust, chemicals, pollution, genetics including alpha-1-antitrypsin deficiency, and age.
- ☐ The chronic bronchitis "blue bloater" client is usually overweight and cyanotic. Most often comfortable at rest and worsens with

activity. Auscultation of the lungs reveals rhonchi and wheezing. Hypersecretion of mucus causes plugging. More common in winter.

- [ ] The emphysema "pink puffer" client is typically thin and uncomfortable at rest, with evident use of accessory muscles. Auscultation of the lungs reveals clear sounds. Chest radiograph demonstrates hyperinflation (barrel-shaped chest).
- [ ] Client tends to maintain a forward-leaning position to increase airflow.
- [ ] Thick green or yellow sputum is indicative of infection associated with acute bronchitis.
- [ ] Decrease client dyspnea by assisting with deep breathing exercises, chest physiotherapy, and suctioning.
- [ ] Treated with bronchodilators and corticosteroids; may need oxygen therapy.
- [ ] A client with emphysema should receive only 1 to 3 L/min of oxygen, if needed. Increasing oxygen doses may cause the client to lose the hypoxic drive.
- [ ] Clients with COPD often retain CO_2 (hypercapnia) as a result of decreased respiratory drive with the administration of too much oxygen (more than 3 L/min).
- [ ] Smoking cessation counseling and materials should be provided.
- [ ] Teach clients to avoid respiratory irritants, to exercise regularly, and the importance of vaccination for flu and pneumonia.

Lung Cancer

- [ ] Most commonly caused by cigarette smoke; other environmental agents less common.
- [ ] Clinical manifestations: a new or changing cough, dyspnea, hemoptysis, and chest pain.
- [ ] Diagnosed with bronchoscopy, biopsy, and needle aspiration.
- [ ] Surgery is the best treatment option if the tumor is localized. Chemotherapy is used in addition to surgery. Radiation therapy is indicated when surgery is not an option.
- [ ] Pneumonectomy is the removal of an entire lung; lobectomy is the removal of a single lobe.
- [ ] Clients should be positioned with "good lung down" after a pneumonectomy.
- [ ] Nursing care should focus on pain relief and prevention of complications.
- [ ] Decrease dyspnea by assisting with deep breathing exercises, chest physiotherapy, and suctioning. A bronchodilator and oxygen therapy may be indicated.

- Provide support to the client and family in regard to prognosis, treatment options, quality of life, and end-of-life options.
- Adenocarcinoma is a slow-growing cancer, rarely metastasizes, and has the best prognosis of all lung cancer types.
- Assess lung sounds, presence of dyspnea, pulse oximetry, and changes in LOC, and apply oxygen as necessary.

Pulmonary Embolism (PE)

- Obstruction of pulmonary vasculature most commonly due to a venous thrombus embolism (VTE) most often comes from the deep veins in the leg (DVT).
- Clinical manifestations include dyspnea, chest pain, anxiety, panic, tachycardia, and tachypnea.
- Sudden reduction in adequate oxygenation may cause feelings of apprehension or a sense of "impending doom."
- A PE is often an emergent condition as it can lead to rapid deterioration and death due to region of lung tissue unavailable for perfusion.
- Emergent management includes applying supplemental oxygen and IV access (preferably two sites); managing hypotension with IV fluids and possible vasopressor therapy; and obtaining 12-lead ECG, ABG, and blood specimens (CBC, serum electrolytes, and coagulation studies to include D-dimer).
- D-dimer is indicated for possible thrombotic disorders, but a positive result requires further testing; a CT scan is warranted when a PE is suspected.
- A stable PE is treated with anticoagulation therapy (heparin for at least 5 days then warfarin for at least 3 to 6 months).
- An unstable PE is treated with tPA (Activase) or a surgical embolectomy.
- Due to the risk in most cases, surgical removal is only performed if tPA is contraindicated.
- An inferior vena cava filter (umbrella filter) may be inserted to prevent another VTE/PE. The filter allows blood to pass while catching or breaking up large emboli.
- Monitor coagulation (PT/INR & PTT), vital signs, pulse oximetry, and pain level.
- Preventing a DVT is the best way to prevent a VTE/PE (leg exercises, ambulation, compression stockings, and leg elevation). Educate clients not to cross legs or wear tight clothing.

Ventilation-Perfusion Mismatch

- An adequate ventilation-perfusion (V/Q) ratio is necessary for gas exchange.
- Mismatch may occur due to altered ventilation or altered perfusion.

- ☐ A mismatch that shows impaired perfusion with normal ventilation indicates a state in which the alveoli do not have adequate blood supply, such as pulmonary embolism or cardiogenic shock.
- ☐ A mismatch that shows impaired ventilation but normal perfusion indicates a pathologic state in the bronchial tree, such as pneumonia or atelectasis.
- ☐ Inadequate ventilation and perfusion are seen with asthma, pneumonia, pneumothorax, and severe respiratory distress.

Acute Respiratory Failure

- ☐ Failure of the lungs to adequately oxygenate or ventilate and characterized by decreased PaO_2 (hypoxemia), increased $PaCO_2$ (hypercapnia), and pH less than 7.35.
- ☐ Caused by impaired central nervous system, neuromuscular dysfunction, musculoskeletal dysfunction, pulmonary dysfunction, pneumonia, heart failure, COPD, and pulmonary embolus.
- ☐ Early clinical manifestations include change in LOC, restlessness, dyspnea, air hunger, and tachycardia.
- ☐ Late clinical manifestations include cyanosis, diaphoresis, and respiratory arrest.
- ☐ Other assessment findings include accessory muscle use, diminished breath sounds, inability to speak full sentences, and forward-leaning position with hands on knees.
- ☐ Monitor respiratory status including level of responsiveness, arterial blood gas, and vital signs with pulse oximetry.
- ☐ Be prepared to assist with intubation and manage mechanical ventilation; transfer to ICU.
- ☐ For the intubated client, prevent complications with frequent respiratory assessment, a turning schedule, mouth care, skin care, and range of motion.

Tension Pneumothorax

- ☐ Tension pneumothorax is an accumulation of atmospheric air in the thoracic cavity.
- ☐ Clinical manifestations include severe respiratory distress, hypotension, eventual tracheal shift, paradoxical chest wall movement on the injured side, and diminished breath sounds over the affected area.
- ☐ Spontaneous pneumothorax occurs when the client's lung collapses, causing an acute decrease in the amount of functional lung used in oxygenation.
- ☐ The only way to re-expand the lung in spontaneous pneumothorax is to place a chest tube in the pleural cavity so the air in the pleural space can be removed.

- ☐ Diagnostic tests include chest X-ray, chest CT, and ABG.
- ☐ Monitor vital signs, pulse oximetry, respiratory rate and effort, and lung sounds.
- ☐ Priority is to maintain oxygenation and breathing. Apply oxygen, assist with placement of chest tube, and insert large-bore IV catheter. Prepare for possible mechanical ventilation.

Hemothorax

- ☐ A massive hemothorax produces signs of shock (such as tachycardia and hypotension) and dullness on percussion on the injured side.
- ☐ Clinical manifestations include tachypnea, decreased breath sounds on the injured side, respiratory distress, and, possibly, mediastinal shift.
- ☐ Diagnostic tests include chest X-ray, chest CT, MRI, hemoglobin and hematocrit, and coagulation studies.
- ☐ The placement of a chest tube will drain the blood from the space and re-expand the lung.
- ☐ Monitor vital signs, pulse oximetry, signs of shock, respiratory assessment, and lung sounds.
- ☐ Prepare for fluid volume replacement, blood transfusion, and possible intubation.

Cystic Fibrosis (CF)

- ☐ Autosomal recessive disease caused by gene mutations that lead to thick secretions in the lungs and other areas of the body.
- ☐ Clinical manifestations include cough, production of thick secretions, wheezing/rhonchi, and hyperinflated lungs.
- ☐ Clients with CF are at risk for chronic respiratory infections; treat with antibiotics and maintain airway clearance with chest physiotherapy, deep breathing, and coughing.
- ☐ Encourage adequate fluid intake and nutrition.
- ☐ Clients with cystic fibrosis may receive chest percussion with a high-frequency chest wall oscillation vest.

NEUROSENSORY SYSTEM

KEY TERMS

- ☐ **Homonymous hemianopia** is a type of visual field blindness involving either the two right or the two left halves of the visual fields of both eyes due to damage to the optic nerves.
- ☐ **Astereognosis** is the inability to identify common objects through touch alone.

- **Ataxia** is the inability to coordinate muscle movements.
- **Oculogyric crisis** is a fixed position of the eyeballs that can last for minutes or hours and is related to the administration of antipsychotic medications.
- **Nystagmus** refers to jerking movements of the eye.
- **Diplopia** means double vision.
- **Exophthalmos** refers to bulging eyeballs, as seen in Graves disease.
- **Accommodation** refers to convergence and constriction of the pupil while following a near object.
- **Cornea** is the nonvascular, transparent fibrous coat where the iris can be seen.
- **Fovea** is the point of central vision.
- **Sclera** is the fibrous tissue that forms the outer protective covering over the eyeball.
- **Quadriplegia** occurs as a result of cervical spine injuries.
- **Aphasia** refers to difficulty expressing or understanding spoken words.
- **Receptive aphasia** is the inability to understand words or word meaning.
- **Dysarthria** is garbled speech.
- **Hemiparesis** describes weakness of one side of the body.
- **Contusion** is a bruise on the brain's surface.
- **Lucid interval** is described as a brief period of unconsciousness followed by alertness after several hours; the client again loses consciousness.
- **Amnesia** is an interval in which the client is alert but can't recall recent events.
- **Enucleation** refers to surgical removal of the entire eye.

Brain

- The basic functional unit of the brain is the neuron, which forms into bodies called ganglia.
- Coordination and balance are functions of the cerebellum.
- The midbrain, pons, medulla oblongata, and reticular formation regulate vital functions.
- The brain stem contains the medulla and the vital cardiac, vasomotor, and respiratory centers.
- Nursing care of a client with damage to the hippocampus, amygdala, and fornix should focus on frequent monitoring of vital signs.
- Problems initiating movement are associated with the basal ganglia and memory problems with the hippocampus.

TABLE 1.7	Lobes of the Brain
Lobes	Function
Parietal	■ Regulates sensory function including the ability to sense hot or cold objects ■ Important for a person's ability to sense body's position in space
Frontal	■ Manages concentration, memory, abstract thought, and motor function ■ Responsible for majority of affect, personality, judgment, and inhibition
Occipital	■ Primarily responsible for vision function ■ Responsible for some memory
Temporal	■ Regulates memory of sound ■ Assists with interpreting language and music

Basal Ganglia

☐ Motor movement is regulated by the basal ganglia.

☐ The basal ganglia consist of the caudate nucleus, putamen, and globus pallidus.

☐ See Table 1.7 for facts covering lobes of the brain.

Cerebrospinal Fluid (CSF)

☐ White blood cells or pus in CSF indicates infection.

☐ Blood may be found in CSF with trauma or subarachnoid hemorrhage.

☐ Increased glucose concentration in CSF is a nonspecific finding indicating infection or subarachnoid hemorrhage.

☐ Clear liquid from the nose (rhinorrhea) or ear (otorrhea) can be determined to be CSF or mucus by the presence of glucose.

☐ See Table 1.8 for facts covering cranial nerves.

Spinal Cord

☐ The spinal cord is the connection between the brain and the periphery of the body.

☐ The bones of the vertebral column protect the spinal cord and typically consist of 7 cervical, 12 thoracic, and 5 lumbar vertebrae in addition to the sacrum.

☐ Vertebrae are separated by intervertebral disks.

☐ Motor pathways from the brain to the spinal cord are formed by upper motor neurons.

☐ Lower motor neurons receive impulses from the spinal cord and run to the myoneural junction at the muscle.

TABLE 1.8 Cranial Nerves	
Cranial Nerve	What it Controls
Olfactory (I)	■ Controls smell
Optic nerve (II)	■ Visual fields and visual acuity
Oculomotor nerve (III)	■ Controls pupillary constriction and accommodation; controls eye movement
Trochlear nerve (IV)	■ Coordinates eye movement
Trigeminal nerve (V)	■ Innervates the muscles of chewing and facial sensation
Abducens (VI)	■ Controls eye movement
Facial (VII)	■ Controls expression in forehead, eye, and mouth; taste; salivation; tearing
Acoustic (VIII)	■ Controls hearing and balance
Glossopharyngeal (IX)	■ Controls swallowing, salivating, and taste
Vagus (X)	■ Controls swallowing, gag reflex; talking; sensations of the throat, larynx, and abdominal viscera; activities of thoracic and abdominal viscera such as heart rate and peristalsis
Spinal accessory (XI)	■ Controls shoulder movement and head rotation
Hypoglossal (XII)	■ Controls tongue movement

Peripheral Nervous System

☐ The peripheral nervous system includes cranial nerves, spinal nerves, and the autonomic nervous system.

☐ The autonomic nervous system regulates functions of the internal organs and is divided into the sympathetic nervous system and the parasympathetic nervous system. (See Table 1.9 for more facts related to autonomic nervous system activity.)

The Babinski Reflex

☐ To test for the Babinski reflex, use a tongue blade to slowly stroke the lateral side of the underside of the foot.

☐ Start at the heel and move toward the great toe.

TABLE 1.9 Autonomic Nervous System Activity

Structure	Parasympathetic Effect	Sympathetic Effect
Heart rate and contractility	Decreased	Increased
Blood pressure	Decreased	Increased
Bronchioles	Baseline	Dilated
Peristalsis	Increased	Decreased
Bladder sphincter	Relaxed	Contracted
Liver glycogen to glucose	No change	Increased
Adrenal hormone production	No change	Secretion of epinephrine and norepinephrine

☐ The normal Babinski reflex response in an adult is plantar flexion of the toes.
☐ Upward movement of the great toe and fanning of the little toes, called the Babinski reflex, are abnormal.

Testing Cranial Nerves
☐ Cranial nerves III, IV, and VI function: ask client to follow the cardinal fields of gaze and assess eye movements.
☐ Cranial nerve V motor function: ask client to clench jaw.
☐ Cranial nerve V facial sensation with touch: facial pain could indicate trigeminal neuralgia.
☐ Cranial nerve VII motor function: ask the client to frown, smile, and raise his eyebrow.
☐ Cranial nerve IX function: test sensation of the gag reflex by placing an applicator against the pharynx and assessing swallowing ability.
☐ Cranial nerve X function: the same test evaluates the motor of the gag reflex.
☐ Cranial nerve XI function: ask the client to shrug shoulders and turn head from side to side.
☐ Cranial nerve XII function: ask client to move tongue out and side to side.

Lumbar Puncture
☐ A lumbar puncture is the removal of CSF that results in pressures lower in the lumbar area than in the brain and put the client at risk for herniation of the brain.

- Lumbar puncture is contraindicated with increased intracranial pressure.
- A lumbar puncture is performed if brain imaging is negative or inconclusive in the presence of symptoms that suggest subarachnoid hemorrhage or for suspected meningitis.
- Blood in the CSF is diagnostic for subarachnoid hemorrhage.
- Position client on side with knees and chin to chest.
- Common side effects are client reports of headache. Have client lie flat, encourage increased fluid intake, and give analgesia.
- Assess for CSF leakage from the puncture site.

Diagnostic Testing
- Radiopaque dyes, used in myelography and cardiac catheterization, are usually iodine based and may cause a reaction in those clients who are allergic.
- Allergy to shellfish may be a contraindication to tests using iodine-based dyes.
- The percentage of functional brain tissue is determined by a series of tests including electroencephalography (EEG), cerebral angiography, nuclear scan and MRI.

Plasmapheresis
- In plasmapheresis, antibodies are removed from the client's plasma.
- In some clients with nervous system disease processes, plasmapheresis diminishes symptoms.

Stroke
- A brain attack or cerebrovascular accident (CVA) is a loss of functioning resulting from disruption of blood supply to a part of the brain.
- Strokes are divided into two major types: ischemic and hemorrhagic.
- Uncontrolled hypertension is the major cause of hemorrhagic stroke.
- Increased intracranial pressure is a concern following a hemorrhagic stroke.
- Both diabetes and heart disease increase the probability of stroke by hastening atherosclerosis.
- Asynchronous atrial contraction that occurs with atrial fibrillation predisposes to mural thrombi, which may embolize, leading to a thromboembolic stroke.
- Clinical manifestations include rapid onset of headache, changes in LOC, speech, vision, and motor function.
- A brain stem infarction leads to vital sign changes such as bradypnea.
- Diagnostic tests include CT scan, angiography, lumbar puncture, and MRI.

- A client with an ischemic stroke in evolution may be prescribed with tissue plasminogen activator, a thrombolytic agent, as treatment.
- Clients may also be treated with anticoagulants like heparin and antiplatelets aspirin.
- Assess frequently for increased intracranial pressure, neuro checks, rate and depth of breathing, and changes in vital signs.
- Because of a potential loss of the gag reflex and potential altered LOC in a client with stroke in evolution, tracheal suction should be available at all times.
- Speech therapists will evaluate the client's ability to swallow after the gag reflex returns and make recommendations about diet and fluid consistency.
- Care should be taken to position the client to prevent contractures and spasticity.
- Deep vein thrombosis (DVT) may develop in clients with a stroke but is more likely to occur in the lower extremities related to immobility.
- Low-dose heparin therapy and sequential compression boots will help prevent DVT. Clients may experience receptive aphasia, expressive aphasia, or global aphasia.

Hemiplegia or Hemiparesis

- Hemiplegia is paralysis, and hemiparesis is weakness on one side of the body.
- A loss of muscle contraction decreases venous return and may cause swelling of the affected extremity.
- Contralateral hemiplegia and numbness or tingling in the face or arm may occur, depending on the level of brain stem injury.
- Teach client to protect affected extremity from injury and neglect.
- Due to the weight of the flaccid extremity, the shoulder of a client with a stroke may disarticulate.
- A sling will support the flaccid extremity of a client with a stroke.

Transient Ischemic Attack (TIA)

- A TIA is a brief episode of neurologic dysfunction caused by localized cerebral ischemia that is not permanent.
- Symptoms of a TIA result from a transient lack of oxygen to the brain and usually resolve within 24 hours; the average time to resolution is less than 1 hour.
- Assess neuro checks and vital signs frequently.
- Teach clients the signs and symptoms of stroke and risk factor to prevent stroke.

Expressive (Broca) Aphasia

☐ Expressive (Broca) aphasia results from damage to Broca area, located in the frontal lobe of the brain's dominant hemisphere.

☐ Typically, the client with expressive aphasia has difficulty expressing speech. Speech will also be slow, nonfluent, and labored.

☐ Comprehension of written and verbal communication is intact in the client with expressive aphasia.

☐ Answer the call bell in person and place a notice on the call bell system to make other personnel aware.

☐ Provide other forms of communication with the client including pad and pencil or picture system.

Receptive (Wernicke) Aphasia

☐ With receptive (Wernicke) aphasia, which results from injury to Wernicke area, the client can't comprehend written or verbal communication.

☐ With receptive Wernicke aphasia, the client's speech is normal but he conveys information poorly.

☐ The Wernicke area is located in the temporal lobe of the dominant hemisphere.

Global Aphasia

☐ Global aphasia results from extensive damage to both Broca and Wernicke areas.

☐ Global aphasia is a combination of receptive and expressive aphasia.

☐ Clients with global aphasia have difficulty in both understanding and producing communication.

Dysphagia

☐ An intact gag reflex shows a properly functioning cranial nerve IX (glossopharyngeal).

☐ Speech may be normal while the gag reflex is absent.

☐ A nurse should not offer food or fluids without assessing for an intact gag reflex.

☐ Thickened liquids are easiest to form into a bolus and swallow.

☐ A mechanical soft diet may be too hard to chew and too dry to swallow when dysphagia is present.

☐ Thickened liquids would be least likely to lead to aspiration in a client who has a neurologic condition resulting in dysphagia.

☐ Nutrition may be delivered by a feeding tube when dysphagia exists.

Diabetes Insipidus

☐ Diabetes insipidus is a deficiency of antidiuretic hormone (ADH) from the posterior pituitary gland.

- [ ] Clinical manifestations include excessive thirst and the large volumes of dilute urine.
- [ ] Diabetes insipidus may occur with increased intracranial pressure, brain tumors, and head trauma.
- [ ] Diabetes insipidus produces low urine specific gravity, increased serum osmolarity, and dehydration.
- [ ] Prevent dehydration by replacing lost volume with IV fluid or oral fluid intake.

Hypophysectomy

- [ ] A client who had a transsphenoidal hypophysectomy, or removal of the pituitary gland.
- [ ] After a hypophysectomy, the body cannot synthesize ADH and may experience diabetes insipidus.
- [ ] Monitor for frequent swallowing after brain surgery, which may indicate CSF or blood leaking from the sinuses into the oropharynx.

Mannitol

- [ ] Mannitol promotes osmotic diuresis by increasing the pressure gradient, drawing fluid from intracellular to intravascular spaces.
- [ ] Mannitol may be ordered for a client with a subdural hematoma, to decrease intracranial pressure.
- [ ] Mannitol can reduce intraocular pressure, prevent acute tubular necrosis, and draw water into the vascular system to increase blood pressure.

$PaCO_2$

- [ ] Lowering $PaCO_2$ through hyperventilation in some clients may lower the increased intracranial pressure caused by dilated cerebral vessels.
- [ ] Oxygenation is evaluated through PaO_2 and oxygen saturation.

Increased Intracranial Pressure (ICP)

- [ ] Normal intracranial pressure is between 5 and 15 mm Hg.
- [ ] Increased ICP causes decreased cerebral perfusion, promotes further swelling, and may force the brain to shift.
- [ ] The earliest clinical manifestation of increasing ICP is a change in LOC.
- [ ] Cushing's response is a late clinical manifestation marked by widened pulse pressure and decreasing heart rate.
- [ ] Fixed and dilated pupils are symptoms of increased ICP or cranial nerve damage.
- [ ] Profuse or projectile vomiting is a symptom of increased ICP and should be reported immediately.

- [ ] The nurse should always reassess the client's airway, breathing, and circulation when the intracranial pressure is elevated.
- [ ] Any sudden change in condition such as confusion or increased drowsiness is significant.
- [ ] The head of the bed should be elevated between 15 and 30 degrees to facilitate venous drainage.
- [ ] External stimulation, such as visitors, should be limited because it may increase ICP.
- [ ] Straining when having a bowel movement, sneezing, coughing, and suctioning may lead to increased ICP and should be avoided when potential increased ICP exists.
- [ ] In the client with increasing ICP, the nurse should first attempt repositioning the client to avoid neck flexion, which increases venous return and lowers ICP.
- [ ] Prevent nausea and subsequent vomiting, which could increase ICP, as will avoiding bending or placing the head in a dependent position.
- [ ] Prevent the Valsalva maneuver, which could lead to bradycardia and reflex tachycardia.
- [ ] Loop diuretics and osmotic diuretics are often used to promote a negative fluid balance, and corticosteroids may be used to prevent cerebral edema.
- [ ] Avoiding temperature elevation is important in order to avoid increases in cerebral metabolism that may cause cerebral edema that would cause increased ICP.

Laminectomy
- [ ] Surgical removal of the lamina creating space in the vertebral canal.
- [ ] Progressive neurologic deficits including worsening muscle weakness, paresthesia, and loss of bowel and bladder control, and symptoms of spinal cord compression.
- [ ] Lower back pain, pain radiating across the buttocks, and positive Kernig sign usually occur in clients with herniated nucleus pulposus without spinal cord compression.
- [ ] In most cases after laminectomy, clients are able to ambulate on the first postoperative day.
- [ ] Frequent repositioning using a logroll technique, use of a specialized brace for the lower back when out of bed, and a firm mattress will help minimize complications.
- [ ] Swelling or pressure on the peripheral nerves controlling micturition, anesthesia, or use of an indwelling urinary catheter may lead to urine retention with frequent overflow of small amounts of urine after lumbar laminectomy.

- Frequent voiding of small amounts of urine after a lumbar laminectomy may indicate urine retention.
- Teach clients to strengthen the abdominal muscles and erector spinal muscles after laminectomy to prevent lower back pain.
- Teach client to not lift more than 10 pounds (4.5 kg) for several weeks after laminectomy surgery is contraindicated.

Skull Fracture
- Clear fluid draining from the ear or nose of a client may mean a CSF leak, which is common in basilar skull fractures.
- Blood or fluid draining from the ear may indicate a basilar skull fracture.
- Nothing is inserted into the ears or nose of a client with a skull fracture because of the risk of infection.

Hematoma
- An epidural hematoma occurs when blood collects between the skull and dura mater.
- A subdural hematoma is when venous blood collects between the dura mater and arachnoid mater.
- In a subarachnoid hemorrhage, arterial blood collects between the pia mater and arachnoid membrane.
- The extent of intracranial bleeding and location of the injury are determined by computed tomography or magnetic resonance imaging.
- Monitor for changes in LOC, and headache may indicate expanding lesions such as subdural hematoma.
- Management of these may include supportive care, control of ICP, or surgical intervention.

Spinal Cord Injury
- All clients with a head injury are treated as if a cervical spine injury is present until X-rays confirm their absence. Injuries at levels between C1 and C4 lead to tetraplegia (formerly known as quadriplegia) with total loss of respiratory function.
- A client with a spinal cord injury at levels from C5 to C6 has tetraplegia with gross arm movement and diaphragmatic breathing.
- Paraplegia with intercostal muscle function loss occurs with injuries at levels between T1 and L2.
- Injuries below L2 cause paraplegia and loss of bowel and bladder control.
- If the client has a suspected cervical spine injury, the jaw-thrust maneuver should be used to open the airway rather than head-tilt/chin-lift, which could worsen a cervical spine injury.

- ☐ If the tongue or relaxed throat muscles are obstructing the airway, a nasopharyngeal or oropharyngeal airway can be inserted.
- ☐ The head-tilt/chin-lift maneuver wouldn't be used until cervical spine injury is ruled out.
- ☐ After a spinal cord injury, ascending cord edema may cause a higher level of injury.
- ☐ The diaphragm is innervated at the level of C4, so assessment of adequate oxygenation and ventilation is necessary.
- ☐ Other assessment parameters for the client with C5 fracture also include bladder distention, neurologic deficit, and the client's feelings about the injury.
- ☐ The bladder treatment program for a client in rehabilitation for spinal cord injury should begin early and should include intermittent catheterization every 2 to 4 hours.
- ☐ Indwelling catheters may predispose the client with a spinal cord injury to infection and are removed as soon as possible.
- ☐ Credé maneuver is applied after voiding to enhance bladder emptying.
- ☐ It isn't necessary to measure the urine of a paraplegic client with intermittent catheterization.
- ☐ It is important to maintain high PaO_2 because hypoxemia can worsen the neurologic deficit in the spinal cord.
- ☐ Initially, a client with a cervical spine injury at the level of C5 may need mechanical ventilation due to cord edema, which may resolve in time.
- ☐ Clients with tetraplegia have paralysis or weakness of the diaphragm, abdominal muscles, or intercostal muscles.
- ☐ In clients with tetraplegia, maintenance of airway and breathing takes top priority.
- ☐ Clients with spinal cord injuries are at risk for neurogenic shock because of the loss of autonomic nervous system function below the level of the injury.
- ☐ DVT is a common complication in clients with spinal cord injuries. This may lead to VTE resulting in pulmonary embolism.
- ☐ Measures should be taken to prevent the development of skin breakdown related to immobility.
- ☐ Monitor for signs of autonomic dysreflexia.

Autonomic Dysreflexia

- ☐ Autonomic dysreflexia refers to uninhibited sympathetic outflow in clients with spinal cord injuries.
- ☐ Clinical manifestations include pounding headache, nasal congestion, anxiety, flushing of the skin, piloerection, elevated blood pressure, bradycardia, and profuse sweating.

□ Autonomic dysreflexia can occur in clients with spinal cord lesions above T6.

□ Typically caused by a noxious stimuli such as a full bladder, fecal impaction, pain, or stimulation of the skin such as a pressure ulcer.

□ Putting the client in high Fowler position will decrease cerebral blood flow, decreasing hypertension during an episode of autonomic dysreflexia.

□ Assess client for a fecal impaction. If a fecal impaction is present, a topical anesthetic agent should be inserted prior to removing the impaction.

□ Examine the skin for any areas of irritation or pressure.

□ The bladder should be assessed immediately for urinary retention.

□ Elevating the client's legs, putting the client flat in bed, or putting the bed in Trendelenburg position increases cerebral blood flow and will worsen hypertension in autonomic dysreflexia.

Neurogenic Shock

□ Clinical manifestations are due to loss of adrenergic stimulation below the level of the lesion.

□ Spinal or neurogenic shock is characterized by hypotension, bradycardia, dry skin, flaccid paralysis, and the absence of reflexes below the level of injury.

□ Spasticity and the return of reflexes are signs of resolving shock.

□ Monitor client airway, cardiac output, tissue perfusion, and body temperature.

□ Be prepared to mechanically ventilate the client.

Cervical Collars

□ Most soft collars do not limit cervical motion but act as a reminder against excessive motion.

□ More rigid devices such as the Philadelphia collar provide reasonable immobilization of the midcervical segments for flexion and extension, but not for lateral flexion.

□ Clients on cervical precautions should be strictly logrolled, maintained on strict bed rest in a flat position, and should have frequent neuro checks.

□ Teach the client to assess skin under the cervical collar for breakdown or irritation.

Halo Vest

□ The purpose of the halo vest is to immobilize the neck.

□ The wrench must be attached at all times to remove the halo vest in case the client needs cardiopulmonary resuscitation.

- [ ] The halo vest is designed to improve mobility; the client may use a wheelchair.
- [ ] The Minerva vest will provide significant immobilization, including lateral flexion.
- [ ] Hydrogen peroxide, especially when applied full strength to halo vest pin sites, can disrupt the healing process and normal flora.
- [ ] Range-of-motion exercises to the neck are prohibited in the client with a halo vest but should be performed to other areas.
- [ ] Assess for signs and symptoms of infection at pin site, loosening of the pins at the insertion site, or loosening of the immobilization constructs.
- [ ] Client will need assistance to loosen straps on vest to wash under the vest, one side at a time with the client lying flat.
- [ ] Client may wear a cotton T-shirt under the vest to prevent irritation.
- [ ] Teach client to care for skin and prevent skin breakdown.

Unconscious Client
- [ ] Will not have the ability to expectorate. Airway management takes priority in an unconscious client.
- [ ] Airway, breathing, and circulation are the priorities over other client needs.

Alzheimer Disease
- [ ] Cognitive impairment that greatly impacts memory, behavior, judgment, and language.
- [ ] Clinical manifestations include impaired short-term memory, disorientation, and confusion. Later symptoms include loss of long-term memory and loss of speech.
- [ ] When communicating with a client with advancing Alzheimer disease, listening and deciphering word substitutions are the most helpful, because the client may have difficulty expressing thoughts.
- [ ] Sentences should be repeated as often as needed with advancing Alzheimer disease clients.
- [ ] In questioning the client with advancing Alzheimer disease, yes-or-no and multiple-choice questions are very helpful.
- [ ] Sentences should be short and literal for clients with advancing Alzheimer disease, following the subject-verb-object format.
- [ ] Protect the client from injury including aspiration risk.

Guillain-Barré Syndrome
- [ ] An autoimmune disease that typically follows a viral or bacterial infection.

- [ ] Clinical manifestations include ascending paralysis, loss of reflexes, and possible failure of the muscles of respiration.
- [ ] Frequently assess cardiac and respiratory status, and have suction available.
- [ ] Assess for DVT and place client on venous thromboembolism precautions.
- [ ] Respiratory support through mechanical ventilation may be necessary until the symptoms improve.
- [ ] Plasmapheresis may be used to reduce the circulating antibody levels.

Myasthenia Gravis

- [ ] An autoimmune disorder that results in the destruction of acetylcholine receptors.
- [ ] Ptosis and diplopia are common early signs of myasthenia gravis.
- [ ] Dysphagia, dysphonia, generalized weakness, and respiratory distress occur later.
- [ ] Symptoms are typically milder in the morning and may be exacerbated by stress or lack of rest.
- [ ] Stress, including pregnancy, may precipitate crisis in myasthenia gravis.
- [ ] Diagnostic tests include electromyography (EMG) and a cholinesterase inhibitor test (Tensilon challenge test).
- [ ] Treated with anticholinesterase or cholinergic drugs such as pyridostigmine bromide.
- [ ] Plasmapheresis is used in myasthenia gravis to separate and remove circulating acetylcholine receptor antibodies from the blood in clients who are refractory to the usual therapies or in crisis.
- [ ] In a myasthenia gravis crisis, assess respiratory status and give respiratory support like suction, chest physical therapy, and postural drainage.

Parkinson Disease

- [ ] Caused by the inability of the substantia nigra in the basal ganglia region to produce sufficient dopamine.
- [ ] Parkinson disease has a gradual onset and is characterized by the slowing of voluntary muscle movement (bradykinesia), muscular rigidity, postural instability, and resting tremor.
- [ ] Diminished distal sensation doesn't occur.
- [ ] The nurse should recognize that a client whose face is expressionless and masking and whose speech is soft and monotone is showing common symptoms of Parkinson disease.
- [ ] Early clinical manifestations include coarse resting tremors of the fingers and thumb such as pill rolling movements of the hand.

☐ Akinesia and aspiration are late signs of Parkinson disease.

☐ Dementia occurs in up to 75% of clients with Parkinson disease.

☐ Antiparkinsonian medications are prescribed to act on neurotransmitter pathways including dopamine and cholinergic activity.

☐ Levodopa is the primary medication prescribed and works by converting to dopamine in the basal ganglia.

☐ The eating problems associated with Parkinson disease include dysphagia, risk of choking, drooling, aspiration, and constipation.

☐ Clients with Parkinson disease are at a high risk for falls related to changes in their posture and gait pattern.

☐ A semisolid diet with thickened liquids may be better tolerated once dysphagia progresses.

Multiple Sclerosis (MS)

☐ A chronic autoimmune disease that is more common in women than in men caused by loss of the myelin sheath (demyelination).

☐ Characterized by multiple areas of demyelination and scarring (sclerosis) of the underlying nerve fibers characterized by patterns of relapses and remissions.

☐ There is no known cure for MS, although treatment can help promote remissions and prevent exacerbations.

☐ Early clinical manifestations include fatigue, slurred speech, patchy blindness (scotoma), and double vision (diplopia).

☐ Exacerbated by exposure to stress, fatigue, and heat.

☐ Elevated gamma globulin fraction in CSF without an elevated level in the blood occurs in MS.

☐ Disease-modifying therapies reduce the frequency of relapses and include immunosuppressant medications or immunomodulators.

☐ Many medications may be prescribed for symptom management such as analgesics for pain and baclofen for spasticity.

☐ The nurse should be mindful to assist the client with improving coping mechanisms and optimizing day-to-day functioning.

Seizures

☐ The priority during and after a seizure is to maintain a patent airway.

☐ Timing the seizure activity and noting the origin of motor dysfunction are important nursing interventions but are not the first priority.

☐ Nothing should be placed in the client's mouth during a seizure because teeth may be dislodged or the tongue pushed back, further obstructing the airway.

- [ ] An aura (such as a certain smell or a vision such as flashing lights) occurs in some clients as a warning before a seizure.
- [ ] Atonic seizure, or drop attack, refers to an abrupt loss of muscle tone.
- [ ] Postictal experience occurs after a seizure, during which the client may be confused, somnolent, and fatigued.
- [ ] Surgical excision of an epileptic focus is considered when seizures are not controlled with anticonvulsant medication therapies.
- [ ] Incontinence may occur during or after a seizure.
- [ ] Status epilepticus (acute prolonged seizure activity not responsive to usual therapies) occurs with the abrupt cessation of anticonvulsant drugs, fever, infections, or alcohol intake.
- [ ] Treat status epilepticus with benzodiazepines such as diazepam.
- [ ] Medication classes include Iminostilbenes (carbamazepine), GABA analogs (gabapentin), Valproic acid, Barbiturates (phenobarbital), Benzodiazepines (diazepam), and Hydantoins (phenytoin).
- [ ] Teach clients to take seizure medications at the same time each day, to not discontinue abruptly, and to have blood levels check frequently.

Mild Traumatic Brain Injury (Concussion)
- [ ] Concussion may be associated with a brief loss of consciousness, physical and cognitive problems, and loss of memory about the events immediately before and after the injury.
- [ ] A slight headache may last for several days after concussion; severe or worsening headaches should be reported.
- [ ] Neurologic symptoms usually resolve within 72 hours of injury.
- [ ] Orientation and LOC are assessed frequently for 24 hours after a head injury.

Cauda Equina Syndrome
- [ ] Occurs when there is compression on the nerve roots and affects areas below the level of the compressed nerve roots.
- [ ] Cauda equina syndrome is an emergency that requires surgical intervention.
- [ ] If not treated, cauda equina syndrome may lead to permanent loss of bladder and bowel control and paralysis of the legs.
- [ ] Nursing care includes inserting a urinary drainage device, frequency of vital sign measurements, and administering anti-inflammatory medication.

Back Pain
- [ ] Symptoms of back pain and neurologic deficits may be symptoms of metastasis in a client with breast or lung cancer.

- ☐ The provider should be notified if the client with cancer is experiencing back pain and neurologic deficits.
- ☐ A client with intervertebral disk prolapse, showing new symptoms of loss of bladder control and paralysis of both legs, requires the health care provider to be notified immediately.

Ménière Disease

- ☐ Ménière disease is caused by an abnormal fluid balance in the inner ear.
- ☐ Clinical manifestations include tinnitus, dizziness, and vertigo.
- ☐ The client is at risk for injury and should be protected from falling.
- ☐ Ménière disease may cause hearing loss, causing impaired social interaction.
- ☐ Teach client that a low-sodium diet may reduce symptoms.
- ☐ Treated with antihistamines, antiemetics, or diuretics.
- ☐ Diazepam may be prescribed to control acute episodes of severe vertigo.

Eye Drops

- ☐ Eye medications can have systemic absorption. Press the inner corner of the eye nearest the nose to prevent absorption.
- ☐ Teach client to keep eyes closed for 1 minute to enhance absorption.
- ☐ Driving may be contraindicated after instillation of atropine eye drops due to blurred vision.
- ☐ Corneal damage may occur with the prolonged use of topical anesthetics.

Cataracts

- ☐ Prolonged use of ophthalmic steroidal anti-inflammatory agents is a risk factor for cataracts.
- ☐ Pain should not be present after cataract surgery.
- ☐ Pain after cataract surgery may be an indication of hyphema (blood in the anterior chamber) or infection.
- ☐ Blurred vision, glare, and itching may be present after cataract surgery.
- ☐ Maintaining nothing-by-mouth status for at least 8 hours before surgical procedures to the eye prevents vomiting and aspiration.
- ☐ Using makeup, bending, straining, lifting, vomiting, and sleeping on the affected side may increase intraocular pressure and put strain on the sutures after cataract surgery.
- ☐ Teach clients to report flashes of light and floating shapes and also signs and symptoms of infection such as purulent drainage, edema, and erythema of the sclera and conjunctiva.

Glaucoma

☐ Glaucoma is a group of conditions characterized by damage to the optic nerve and increased intraocular pressure.

☐ Normal intraocular pressure is 10 to 21 mm Hg.

☐ Without lifelong treatment, glaucoma may progress to irreversible blindness.

☐ Clients with glaucoma may be asymptomatic.

☐ Clinical manifestations include complaints of halos around lights, peripheral vision loss or blind spots, reddened sclera, firm globe, decreased accommodation, halos around lights, and occasional eye pain.

☐ Treatment for glaucoma won't restore visual damage, but will slow disease progression.

☐ Medications include prostaglandin agonists (latanoprost), carbonic anhydrase inhibitors (brinzolamide), alpha agonists (brimonidine tartrate), beta-adrenergic blockers (timolol), and cholinergic agonists (pilocarpine).

☐ The client is at risk of injury from stumbling over peripheral objects that are not visible.

☐ Adverse effects of medications to treat open-angle glaucoma are common.

☐ Angle-closure glaucoma is an ocular emergency with acute pain, rapidly progressing visual impairment, conjunctival redness, and pupil changes.

☐ Family members of clients with open-angle glaucoma should be screened for open-angle glaucoma every 2 years.

Retinal Detachment

☐ A retinal detachment is usually associated with retinal holes created by vitreous traction.

☐ Clinical manifestations include abrupt flashing lights, floaters, loss of peripheral vision, and a sudden shadow or curtain in the vision.

☐ If any part of the retina is lifted or pulled from its normal position, it is considered detached and will cause some vision loss.

☐ Surgical repair (scleral buckling) is necessary.

☐ Postoperatively, client will need an eye patch. Teach the client to avoid eye strain including reading and activities that require fine detail.

☐ Clients with an oil or gas bubble placed in the eye will need to be kept at the prescribed position.

☐ Teach client not to do activities that will increase intraocular pressure such as bending at the waist, lift objects, blowing the nose, Valsalva maneuver, and sexual intercourse.

Enucleation

- ☐ Enucleation of the eye refers to surgical removal of the entire eye.
- ☐ The client needs instructions about the eye socket and ocular prosthesis.
- ☐ There are no activity restrictions following enucleation surgery.
- ☐ Clients typically have a large ocular pressure dressing in place for 1 week, and then, an ophthalmic antibiotic ointment is applied in the socket.
- ☐ Clients experience a loss of depth perception after enucleation.

Assessment of the Eye

- ☐ When using a Snellen chart, describing a client's visual acuity as 20/40 indicates that the client can see at 20 feet what the person with normal vision sees at 40 feet.
- ☐ Alterations in near vision may be due to loss of accommodation caused by the aging process (presbyopia) or farsightedness.
- ☐ A tonometer is a device used in glaucoma screening to record intraocular pressure.
- ☐ An ophthalmoscope examines the interior of the eye, especially the retina.
- ☐ A slit lamp evaluates structures in the anterior chamber of the eye.
- ☐ Loss of accommodation is a normal response to aging due to a loss of lens elasticity.

Ocular Foreign Bodies

- ☐ One or both eyes may be patched to prevent pain with extraocular movement or accommodation when the client has a foreign body in the eye.
- ☐ Chemicals or small foreign bodies in the eye may be irrigated with normal saline solution.
- ☐ Assessment of visual acuity is not the priority in an emergency, although it may be done after treatment.
- ☐ Protruding objects in the eye should not be removed by the nurse because the vitreous body may rupture.

Hearing Loss

- ☐ Hearing loss in an elderly client typically involves high-frequency sounds first.
- ☐ Lowering the pitch of your voice and facing the client are essential to enable the client with hearing loss to use other means of understanding, such as lip reading, affect, and gestures.
- ☐ Alternative means of communication such as writing may also be used to assess the client while waiting for the family to bring the hearing aid from home.

Stapedectomy

☐ Vertigo is the most frequent complication of stapedectomy.

☐ After stapedectomy, the client should move slowly to avoid triggering or worsening vertigo and should ask for assistance with ambulation.

☐ Ringing in the ears (tinnitus) rarely follows stapedectomy and should be reported to the health care provider.

☐ Hearing typically decreases after stapedectomy because of ear packing and tissue swelling, but commonly returns over the next 2 to 6 weeks.

☐ Excessive drainage and pain should be reported to the provider.

☐ The client should avoid getting water in the ear and avoid nose blowing for 2 weeks after surgery.

Ear Irrigation

☐ Irrigation of the ear canal is contraindicated if the tympanic membrane is perforated.

☐ Irrigation solution entering the inner ear may cause dizziness, nausea, vomiting, and infection; warming the irrigation solution may prevent this.

☐ Ear pain, hearing loss, and otitis externa are not contraindications to irrigation of the ear canal.

Eardrops

☐ The eardrops may be warmed to prevent pain or dizziness, but this action is not essential.

☐ The client should be placed in a lateral position to prevent the eardrops from draining out of the ear for 5 minutes.

☐ An ear wick may be used to allow medications to enter the ear canal if the ear canal is excessively swollen.

INTEGUMENTARY SYSTEM

KEY TERMS

☐ **Petechiae** are small macular lesions 1 to 3 mm in diameter.

☐ **Ecchymosis** is a purple-to-brown bruise and macular or papular and varied in size.

☐ **Purpura** is a purple macular lesion larger than 1 cm.

☐ **Paronychia** is a bacterial infection of the nail fold.

☐ **Erosion** refers to loss of part or the entire skin surface, usually from infection or pressure.

☐ **Splinter hemorrhages** are reddish brown narrow streaks under the nails that run in the same direction as nail growth and are caused by minor trauma but can also occur in clients with bacterial endocarditis.

Functions of the Integumentary System

☐ The skin, hair, and nails make up the integumentary system, which serves as protection for the body's inner organs.

☐ The integumentary system helps regulate body temperature through the sweat glands.

☐ The integumentary system contains three types of glands: sebaceous, eccrine, and apocrine.

☐ Sebaceous, or oil, glands lubricate the hair and the epidermis and are stimulated by sex hormones.

☐ The skin provides the first line of defense against microorganisms. (See Table 1.10 for facts covering layers of the skin.)

Lesion Configurations

☐ Dermatomal lesions form a line or an arch that follows a dermatome.

☐ An annular lesion is circular or ring shaped.

☐ A diffuse rash usually has widely distributed scattered lesions.

☐ Confluent lesions are touching or adjacent to each other.

☐ Linear rashes are lesions arranged in a line.

☐ See Table 1.11 for more types of skin lesions.

Burns

☐ The destruction of skin that causes loss of intracellular fluid and electrolytes. Characterized by the extent (area) and depth of the burn; however, most burns are a combination of thicknesses.

☐ During the first 48 hours after a burn, capillary permeability increases, allowing fluids to shift from the plasma to the interstitial spaces.

☐ In early burn care, the client's greatest need is fluid resuscitation because of large-volume fluid loss through the damaged skin.

TABLE 1.10 Layers of the Skin

Skin layer	Purpose
Epidermis	■ Outer layer of the skin ■ Acts as a protective barrier against the environment
Dermis	■ Middle layer of the skin ■ Contains nerves and blood vessels ■ Origin of hair, nails, sebaceous glands, eccrine sweat glands, and apocrine sweat glands
Hypodermis	■ Third layer of the skin ■ Also known as subcutaneous tissue ■ Provides heat, insulation, and shock absorption ■ Acts as a nutritional reservoir

TABLE 1.11	Types of Skin Lesions
Lesion	**Description**
Pustule	■ A small, pus-filled lesion (called a follicular pustule if it contains a hair)
Cyst	■ A closed sac in or under the skin that contains fluid or semisolid material
Papule	■ A solid, raised lesion that is <1 cm in diameter
Vesicle	■ A small, fluid-filled blister that is <0.5 cm in diameter
Bulla	■ A large, fluid-filled blister that is 0.5 cm or more in diameter
Ulcer	■ A craterlike lesion of the skin that usually extends at least into the dermis
Macule	■ A flat nonpalpable area of color change on the skin <1 cm with a well-circumscribed border
Wheal	■ A raised, reddish area with irregular borders that varies in size and shape
Nodule	■ A raised lesion detectable by touch that's usually 0.5–2 cm in diameter and extends deeper into the dermis
Fissure	■ A linear crack-like lesion of the skin that may extend into the dermis

☐ Burn shock can occur, with fluid volume deficit and hyponatremia.

☐ Escharotomy is a surgical incision used to relieve pressure from edema and is needed with circumferential burns that prevent chest expansion or cause circulatory compromise.

☐ A burn injury causes a hypermetabolic state resulting in protein and lipid catabolism that affects wound healing.

☐ Potassium also leaks from the cells into the plasma after a burn, causing hyperkalemia.

☐ To maintain asepsis of a blistered area, the nurse should cover it with a clean dry dressing.

☐ Removing the raised skin of a blistered area would cause further skin damage.

☐ Pulmonary complications from inhalation injuries should be considered in certain clients.

TABLE 1.12 Burn Classifications

Classification	Description
Superficial partial-thickness burn	▪ Involves the epidermal layer and possibly a portion of the dermis ▪ Reddened, blanches with pressure, dry, minimal to no edema
Deep partial-thickness burn	▪ Involves the epidermal and dermal layers ▪ Blistered with mottled red base, broken epidermis with weeping surface, edema
Full-thickness burn	▪ Involves epidermal, dermal, subcutaneous layers; may involve nerve endings, muscle, and bone ▪ Dry, charred, or leathery; edema

Rule of Nines

☐ A common method for estimating the extent of burns in adults is the rule of nines.

☐ According to the rule of nines, the posterior trunk, anterior trunk, and legs are each 18% of the total body surface.

☐ The head, neck, and arms are each 9% of total body surface according to the rule of nines.

☐ The perineum is 1% of total body surface according to the rule of nines.

☐ See Table 1.12 for burn classifications.

Types of Rashes

☐ A bull's-eye rash located primarily at the site of the bite is a classic sign of Lyme disease.

☐ Diffuse pruritic wheals are associated with an allergic reaction.

☐ Pityriasis rosea starts with a "herald patch" and then erupts in a Christmas tree pattern on the trunk.

Herpes Zoster

☐ The varicella-zoster virus causes herpes zoster, also referred to as shingles.

☐ Clinical manifestations include unilaterally clustered vesicles along peripheral sensory nerves usually on the trunk or face that produce burning, stinging, stabbing, or aching pain.

☐ The infection can be stopped if antiviral medications are administered within 24 hours of the vesicular lesions appearing.

☐ The papulovesicular lesions of disseminated varicella (chickenpox) are distributed over the trunk, face, and scalp and do not follow a dermatome.

☐ In disseminated varicella, the virus is present in the vesicular fluid and the respiratory secretions. Clients should be placed on standard plus airborne and contact precautions until lesions are dry and crusted.

☐ Clients with localized herpes zoster (shingles) should not be able to spread the virus to others as long as they have had a previous varicella infection. Clients should be placed on contact precautions until lesions are dry and crusted.

Dermatitis

☐ Contact dermatitis is an inflammatory disorder that results from contact with an irritant.

☐ Atopic dermatitis is a hereditary disorder associated with a family history of asthma, allergic rhinitis, or atopic dermatitis.

☐ Seborrheic dermatitis is a chronic inflammatory dermatitis.

Pressure Ulcers

☐ Pressure (or decubitus) ulcers are localized areas of skin breakdown that occur as a result of prolonged pressure. (See Table 1.13 for stages of pressure ulcers.)

☐ Risk factors include clients on complete bed rest, low serum albumin, incontinence, and decreased sensation.

☐ In pressure ulcers, necrotic tissue develops because the vascular supply to the area is diminished.

☐ When moving a client, lift, rather than slide, the client to avoid shearing forces that pull the skin.

☐ A client in bed for prolonged periods should be repositioned every 1 to 2 hours.

Skin Infections

☐ Candidiasis is a fungal infection of the skin or mucous membranes and is commonly found in the oral, vaginal, and intestinal mucosal tissue, but also occurs in abdominal skin folds, beneath the breasts, and in the gluteal cleft.

☐ Tinea is a fungal infection of the skin that affects the head, body, groin, feet, and nails. (See Table 1.14 for types of tinea infections.)

☐ Molluscum contagiosum is a viral skin infection with small, umbilicated (depressed), papular lesions.

Psoriasis

☐ Psoriasis is a chronic skin condition characterized by red plaques with silver scales that will bleed if removed.

TABLE 1.13	Pressure Ulcer Staging
Stage	**Description**
Unstageable	■ Involves full-thickness tissue loss, with the base of the ulcer covered by slough and/or eschar
Stage I	■ Intact skin with nonblanchable redness of a localized area ■ Usually found over a bony prominence ■ May be painful, firmer or softer, and warmer or cooler than the surrounding tissue
Stage II	■ Partial-thickness loss of dermis presenting as a shallow open ulcer with a red wound bed without slough
Stage III	■ Full-thickness skin loss ■ Bone, muscle, and tendon are NOT exposed. ■ Slough may be present but does not obscure the depth of tissue loss. ■ May include tunneling or undermining
Stage IV	■ Involves full-thickness skin loss, with exposed muscle, bone, and tendon ■ May be accompanied by eschar, slough, undermining, and tunneling
Suspected deep tissue injury	■ Involves maroon or purple intact skin or a blood-filled blister ■ May be painful; mushy, firm, or boggy; and warmer or cooler than other tissue before discoloration occurs

TABLE 1.14	Tinea Infections
Name	**Location**
Tinea capitis	■ Fungal infection of the scalp ■ Characterized by hair loss in the area of infection
Tinea corporis	■ Commonly called "ringworm" ■ Fungal infection of the body ■ Characterized by round, red, scaly lesions that may itch ■ Lesions have slightly raised, red borders consisting of scales.
Tinea cruris	■ Commonly called "jock itch" ■ Fungal infections of the inner thigh and inguinal creases
Tinea pedis	■ Commonly called "athlete's foot" ■ Superficial fungal infection of the feet ■ Causes itching, burning, and a foul odor

- □ Clients with psoriasis also have thick, discolored nails with splintered hemorrhages that easily separate from the nail bed.
- □ The nails also show "ice pick" pits and ridges of the nail bed.
- □ Treatment includes topical and systemic corticosteroids, UV light therapy, topical retinoids, topical calcitriol (vitamin D), biologic therapy (secukinumab), and immunosuppressant therapy (methotrexate).
- □ Assess for signs and symptoms of depression.
- □ Teach client to manage risk factors by smoking cessation, eating a balanced diet, exercise, stress management, and elimination of alcohol from diet.

Scabies

- □ Scabies are mites that burrow under the skin, generally between the webbing of the fingers and toes, near the wrists, and skin folds such as the groin, buttocks, and abdomen.
- □ Clinical manifestations include small, red, pruritic dots between the fingers and toes with itching typically increasing at night.
- □ Clients are prescribed a topical scabicide medication to apply to the skin, which is left on for 12 to 24 hours and then washed off.
- □ Teach clients to wash clothing and launder bed linens in hot water and dry on the hot cycle in the dryer.
- □ Household members and people in close contact should be treated for scabies as well.

Wounds

- □ The correct way to culture a wound is to roll the swab from the center of the wound outward.
- □ Irrigating the wound washes away drainage, debris, and many of the microorganisms colonizing or infecting the wound.
- □ Wound incision and drainage and wound culturing are done when infection is present or suspected.
- □ Wounds should be cleaned from the least contaminated area to the most contaminated area (e.g., from the center outward).
- □ For healing to occur, necrotic (dead) tissue must be removed from the wound. This is done by debridement.
- □ See Table 1.15 for the phases of wound healing.

Cryosurgery

- □ Cryosurgery leaves a wound resembling a burn, with swelling, blistering, and tenderness.
- □ Oozing and pain after cryosurgery suggest an infection.

TABLE 1.15	**Phases of Wound Healing**
Phases	**Criteria**
Inflammatory	■ First phase of wound healing ■ Immediately follows the injury and lasts 4–6 d ■ Involves control of bleeding and the release of chemicals needed for healing
Proliferative	■ Lasts from the 4th to the 21st day after injury ■ Granulation tissue appears (scabs form). ■ Wound edges start to pull together.
Contraction	■ May begin around the 7th day after injury ■ Involves a significant decrease in the wound surface
Remodeling	■ May lead to scar flattening and correction of any deformities that occurred during the third phase

Vitamin and Mineral Sources

☐ Proper diet and nutrition is important for proper wound healing.

☐ The vitamins and minerals found in food sources and supplements are also important to wound healing. (See Tables 1.16 and 1.17 for food sources of minerals and vitamins.)

TABLE 1.16	**Food Sources of Minerals**
Minerals	**Source**
Calcium	■ Milk and dairy products (ice cream, cottage cheese, yogurt) ■ Dark green, leafy vegetables (best nondairy sources)
Iron	■ Red meat, pork, fish, shellfish, poultry, lentils, beans and soy foods, some flours are fortified.
Magnesium	■ Whole grains, nuts, seeds, green leafy vegetables, potatoes, beans, avocados, bananas, milk, and chocolate
Phosphorus	■ Dairy foods, meat, and fish
Potassium	■ Broccoli, potatoes with skins, green leafy vegetables, citrus fruits, bananas, dried fruits, and legumes
Tyramine	■ Wine, cheese, preserved fruits, meats, and vegetables
Zinc	■ Red meat, poultry, oysters and other seafood, nuts, dried beans, milk and other dairy products, whole grains, and fortified breakfast cereals

TABLE 1.17	Food Sources of Vitamins
Vitamins	**Source**
Vitamin A	▪ Milk, eggs, fortified cereal, dark orange or green vegetables, orange-colored fruits
Thiamin B$_1$	▪ Fortified breads, cereals and pasta, lean meats, dried beans, soy foods, peas, whole grains
Riboflavin B$_2$	▪ Meat, eggs, legumes, nuts, dairy, green leafy vegetables, fortified cereals
Niacin B$_3$	▪ Red meat, poultry, fish, legumes, fortified hot and cold cereals
Vitamin B$_6$	▪ Potatoes, bananas, beans, seeds, nuts, red meat, poultry, fish, eggs, spinach, and fortified cereals
Folate B$_9$	▪ Liver, dried beans, other legumes, green leafy vegetables, orange juice, fortified bread, rice, and cereals
Vitamin B$_{12}$	▪ Fish, red meat, poultry, milk, cheese, eggs, and fortified breakfast cereal
Vitamin C	▪ Citrus fruits, tomatoes, broccoli, and spinach
Vitamin D	▪ Sunlight needed to manufacture, egg yolks, oily fish (tuna, sardines), fortified milk and orange juice
Vitamin E	▪ Vegetable oils, nuts, green leafy vegetables
Vitamin K	▪ Green leafy vegetables, brussel sprouts, and broccoli (naturally synthesized by GI tract bacteria)

MUSCULOSKELETAL SYSTEM

KEY TERMS

☐ **Arthrodesis** is the surgical fusion of a joint.

☐ **Fasciotomy** is a surgical incision through the skin and subcutaneous tissue into the fascia to relieve pressure and restore neurovascular circulation.

☐ **Nodule** is a small lump or collection of tissue or bone visible on X-ray or palpable to the touch of the skin or bone such as Heberden nodules found in osteoarthritis.

☐ **Open reduction** is the surgical incision into a fracture site so that the bones can be realigned.

□ **Paresthesia** is described as numbness or tingling, often the result of electrolyte, neuromuscular, or vascular changes.

Types of Musculoskeletal Pain

□ Bone pain is often described as dull, deep, and "boring" or aching in nature.

□ Muscular pain is often described as soreness and aching or cramping.

□ Bone fracture pain is sharp and piercing and relieved by immobilization.

□ Joint pain is often felt with arthritic changes and increases with movement.

Osteomyelitis

□ Osteomyelitis is an infection of the bone resulting in inflammation, necrosis, and formation of new bone.

□ Bone infections are difficult to treat because bone has poor blood circulation.

□ The client with diabetes mellitus who has a foot ulcer or any wound in the extremities is at high risk for acute or chronic osteomyelitis. Most common organism is *Staphylococcus aureus.*

□ Early X-ray findings show soft tissue edema, and bone scans are used for the detection of tumors, osteomyelitis, arthritis, and unexplained bone pain.

□ If not treated promptly, an abscess can form.

□ Acute clinical manifestations are localized pain, edema, erythema, and fever greater than 101°F (38.3°C).

□ Chronic clinical manifestations are skin ulceration, localized pain, and drainage.

□ Treatment includes antibiotic therapy for 3 to 6 weeks and surgery if no response to antibiotics.

□ Care is focused on relieving pain, improving mobility, and controlling infection.

□ Teach client to call practitioner if pain increases or they can no longer bear weight on the extremity.

Osteoporosis

□ Chronic metabolic disorder with bone loss leads to fracture.

□ Screen with bone mineral density testing (T-score).

□ A T-score lower than −2.5 or below is positive; Medicare reimburses for screening every 2 years in those 65 and older.

□ Risk factors for primary osteoporosis include being postmenopausal, thin build, chronic low calcium and vitamin D intake, and prolonged immobility.

- ☐ Causes of secondary osteoporosis are due to the effects of another medical condition or the medical treatment of that condition: diabetes mellitus, hyperthyroidism, hyperparathyroidism, Cushing syndrome, rheumatoid arthritis, bone cancer, chronic corticosteroid use, heparin, anticonvulsants, cytotoxic agents, immunosuppressants, loop diuretics, smoking, more than 3 alcoholic drinks per day, and aluminum-based antacids.
- ☐ Teach clients to engage in weight-bearing activity and daily intake of 1,200 mg of calcium to maintain adult bone mass.
- ☐ Vitamin D is also needed for the absorption of calcium.
- ☐ Medications include bisphosphonates (alendronate), and calcitonin slows bone loss.

Gout

- ☐ Caused by hyperuricemia, affected by diet, medication, overproduction, and inadequate kidney excretion.
- ☐ Acute arthritis is the most common early clinical manifestation of gout.
- ☐ Other clinical manifestations include recurrent attacks, severe joint inflammation, tophi (crystalline deposits accumulating in joint tissue), nephropathy, uric acid, and urinary stones.
- ☐ Acute attacks are managed with colchicine, indomethacin, and possibly a corticosteroid.
- ☐ Allopurinol or probenecid may be instituted to excrete uric acid after the acute attack is over.
- ☐ Drugs to lower uric acid level should not be started during an attack as it may make it worse.
- ☐ Encourage clients to decrease consumption of purine-rich foods like meats, seafood, organ meats, and alcohol.
- ☐ During acute attacks, pain management with NSAIDs or COX-2 inhibitors (celecoxib) is the priority.
- ☐ Teach client to manage and prevent gout attacks to prevent persistently painful joints.
- ☐ Teach clients to increase intake of fluids to promote the excretion of uric acid, avoid fasting, and also avoid overeating.

Rheumatoid Arthritis

- ☐ Rheumatoid arthritis is a systemic inflammatory joint disease.
- ☐ Clinical manifestations include symmetrical swelling of the joints of both hands, morning stiffness lasting longer than 30 minutes, and fever.
- ☐ Laboratory results reveal an elevated sedimentation rate, positive antinuclear antibodies, and increased C-reactive protein.

- Laboratory results may also reveal a decreased erythrocyte count and hematocrit.
- Treatment includes COX-2 inhibitor NSAIDs (celecoxib), DMARDs (methotrexate), biologics (etanercept given subcut), and steroids (prednisone).
- It is essential to assess for pain, mobility, and joint damage.
- Teach clients about the effects of bone marrow suppression from medication therapy and nonpharmacologic pain management (heat, cold, and massage).

Osteoarthritis

- Osteoarthritis occurs with degeneration and loss of articular cartilage in synovial joints.
- As osteoarthritis progresses, the cartilage covering the ends of bones is destroyed and bones rub against each other causing a "grating" type of pain.
- Osteoarthritis is the most common form of arthritis and can be debilitating.
- Elderly are most commonly affected.
- Primary osteoarthritis may be caused by the overuse of joints, aging, or obesity.
- Secondary arthritis can be caused by congenital abnormalities and diabetes mellitus.
- Clinical manifestations include joint pain after exercise usually relieved by rest, asymmetrical flexion, and deviation deformities.
- Teach the client to stay hydrated, use heat to ease stiff joints, and utilize range-of-motion exercises to prevent contractures.
- Treatment includes NSAIDs and joint interventions including cortisone injections and joint replacement.
- Primary prevention of injury from osteoarthritis includes warming up before exercise and avoiding repetitive tasks. Encourage client to lose weight, and use assistive devices as needed to take stress off joints.
- Teach the client to manage pain and avoid overexertion.

Herniated Nucleus Pulposus

- Gel like inner material of the outer wall of intervertebral disc pushes through a tear in the disc causing pressure on the nerve root.
- Often referred to as "herniated disc."
- The most common areas of herniation are L4–L5 and L5–S1. Clinical manifestations include chronic back pain, pain traveling the length of a nerve to the leg, numbness, weakness, tingling, and loss of reflexes.

□ Diagnostic tests include myelography, magnetic resonance imaging (MRI), and computed tomography (CT) scan.

□ Conservative treatment may include bed rest, pain medication, heat and cold therapy, and physiotherapy.

□ Aggressive treatment may include surgery such as a bone fusion or endoscopic spinal surgery.

□ Teach client to utilize heat and cold therapy and the use of good body mechanics to prevent strain on the back that may result in increased pressure on nerve roots.

Preventing Spinal Injuries

□ Proper body mechanics involves bending at the knees, carrying objects close to the body, and avoid twisting movements and carrying heavy objects.

□ Pelvic tilt exercises are recommended to strengthen back muscles.

□ Increasing fiber and fluid intake helps soften stool, thereby preventing straining, which increases intraspinal pressure.

□ Place items within reach of the client, use a professional alert system in the home, and install bars in bathrooms to prevent falls.

□ Application of cold decreases swelling and numbs nerves and may be used for back pain, sprains, muscle spasms, and arthritic joints.

Compartment Syndrome

□ A medical emergency in which tissue pressure increases in a confined body space restricting arterial blood flow.

□ The earliest clinical manifestation is paresthesia progressing to severe pain and paralysis.

□ Compartment syndrome may lead to the death of tissues within 2 to 4 hours.

□ Treatment of compartment syndrome includes fasciotomy and possibly a thrombectomy and embolectomy.

□ Priority assessment of neurovascular status includes the 6 Ps—**P**ain, **P**allor, **P**aralysis, **P**aresthesia, **P**ulselessness, and **P**olar (cold).

□ Teach the client especially with casts and crushing injury to report increased pain and numbness.

□ Postfasciotomy care focuses on the prevention of infection and restoration of circulation to the limb.

Fractures

□ Clinical manifestations include redness, warmth, numbness or loss of sensation, and a new sharp pain related to movement.

□ Classic fractures that occur with trauma are those of the humerus and clavicle.

- ☐ A transverse fracture commonly occurs with such bone diseases as osteomalacia and Paget disease.
- ☐ Linear, longitudinal, and oblique fractures generally occur with trauma.
- ☐ Spiral fractures are commonly seen in the upper extremities and are related to physical abuse.
- ☐ Initial treatment of obvious and suspected fractures includes providing support above and below the injury by immobilizing and splinting the limb.
- ☐ Any attempt to realign or rest the fracture at the stem may cause further injury and complications.
- ☐ The fractured body part should be elevated only after immobilization to reduce swelling.
- ☐ Apply ice intermittently for the first 24 to 72 hours to reduce swelling.
- ☐ To maintain proper alignment, a screw, plate, nail, or wire may be inserted to prevent the bones from separating.
- ☐ Monitor neurovascular status for compartment syndrome symptoms, lung sounds, respiratory effort, and vital signs.
- ☐ Serous drainage around the pin insertion site is a normal finding.
- ☐ Pain management is generally focused on the utilization of NSAIDs.

Casting

- ☐ Immobilization of a fracture with a cast to promote healing is a common intervention.
- ☐ Assessment involves checking neurovascular status routinely (the 6 Ps) due to edema in a confined space of the cast.
- ☐ As a fiberglass cast dries, a client may report sensations of heat from the cast.
- ☐ Plaster casts could take 24 hours to dry (48 hours for weight bearing). Rest cast on a pillow to prevent denting into the skin.
- ☐ Fiberglass casts dry in 30 minutes (weight bearing 1 hour).
- ☐ The casted extremity should be elevated above heart level for the first 24 to 48 hours.
- ☐ Assess for foul odor and drainage from under the cast; fever, malaise, and elevated white blood cell count may indicate infection.
- ☐ Immediate intervention is necessary with signs and symptoms of compartment syndrome.
- ☐ If pulses aren't palpable, verify the assessment with Doppler ultrasonography.

- ☐ If pulses can't be found with Doppler ultrasonography, immediately notify the health care provider.
- ☐ To prevent foot drop in a leg with a cast, the foot should be supported with 90 degrees of flexion.
- ☐ A client with a hip spica cast should avoid gas-forming foods to prevent abdominal distention.
- ☐ Client teaching includes monitoring for infection, ROM exercises, cast care, and mobility assistance including crutch walking.
- ☐ After cast removal, the dry, peeling skin will heal in a few days with normal cleaning.
- ☐ Teach the client that a plaster cast becomes weaken if allowed to become wet.

Skeletal Traction
- ☐ Traction is the application of a pulling force for alignment or reduction of a fracture or to treat severe muscle spasms.
- ☐ Weights should be hanging freely and not resting on the floor.
- ☐ Realignment, weight reduction, or removal of traction is typically not performed by the nurse, and an order is necessary for changes.
- ☐ Assessment of mobility and circulation is essential in each shift.
- ☐ Intervention is necessary if there are signs of decreased circulation (6 Ps).
- ☐ Assessment for signs of infection such as erythema and swelling is essential in each shift.
- ☐ Severe muscle spasms may indicate improper alignment, and the health care provider should be notified.
- ☐ Opioid and nonopioid pain management may be used as well as muscle relaxants while the client is in traction.
- ☐ Teach the client that good nutrition high in fiber and hydration are essential to prevent constipation.

Fat Emboli
- ☐ A serious complication of long-bone fractures is the development of fat emboli, in which the fat molecules enter the venous circulation and travel to the lung, obstructing pulmonary circulation.
- ☐ Clinical manifestations of fat emboli include tachypnea, tachycardia, shortness of breath, and a petechial rash on the chest and neck.
- ☐ Fat emboli cause blood vessel injury and acute respiratory distress syndrome.
- ☐ Bed rest, oxygen, hydration, and possible steroid therapy may be utilized for treatment.
- ☐ Teach the client to alert with any fat emboli symptoms.

Total Hip Arthroplasty

- ☐ Most frequently performed on clients over 60 years old.
- ☐ Positioning is one of the most important interventions to prevent contractures, loss of alignment, and promote healing.
- ☐ Before surgery, never place client on the affected side; only turn clients from the unaffected side to back while in bed.
- ☐ After surgery, keep legs and hips abducted to maintain the prosthesis in the acetabulum.
- ☐ After surgery, the client's activity is usually ordered as limited weight bearing.
- ☐ The hip shouldn't be flexed more than 90 degrees after a hip replacement.
- ☐ The client is allowed to move with restrictions for approximately 2 to 3 months after a hip replacement.
- ☐ Progressive weight bearing reduces the complications of immobility after a hip replacement.
- ☐ Anticoagulants (heparin or enoxaparin) and pneumatic compression boots are used to prevent DVT after hip surgery.
- ☐ Frequently assess lung sounds, pulse oximetry, and the affected limb for presence of edema and neurovascular status.
- ☐ Encourage cough and deep breathing exercises and incentive spirometer.
- ☐ Teach the client that after discharge, they will need assistance to put on shoes and should not cross legs or flex the hip more than 90 degrees.

Crutch Walking

- ☐ To avoid damage to the brachial plexus nerves in the axilla, the palms of the hands should bear the client's weight on crutches.
- ☐ Two fingers should fit between the axilla and the top of the crutch.
- ☐ Touchdown weight bearing involves no weight on the extremity, but the client may touch the floor with the affected extremity.
- ☐ Partial weight bearing allows for 30% to 50% weight bearing on the affected extremity.
- ☐ Partial weight bearing pattern is the advancement of the crutches with the "bad leg" to absorb most of the weight.
- ☐ Full weight bearing allows for full weight to be put on the affected extremity.
- ☐ Nonweight bearing is no weight on the extremity.
- ☐ Teach clients to pace activity and to slowly build strength while beginning to use crutches.

- On stairs, advance the "good leg" first and move the crutches with the affected extremity to go up. To go down, advance the affected extremity first, "bad leg," with the crutches.

Dislocated Hip
- The leg is usually adducted and shortened with a dislocated hip.
- If a hip is dislocated, the surgeon realigns under moderate sedation.
- Immobilization is necessary with an abduction splint.
- Healing takes about 6 weeks.
- A dislocated hip will create problems with walking, and pain is often due to a pinched nerve in the joint.

Carpal Tunnel Syndrome
- Acute wrist flexion places pressure on the inflamed median nerve, causing the pain and numbness of carpal tunnel syndrome (Phalen sign).
- Tapping gently over the median nerve tests for Tinel sign is another sign of carpal tunnel syndrome.
- Interventions include assessment adapting the client's environment to be ergonomically appropriate.
- The use of specially designed wrist rest devices and geometrically designed computer keyboards may be necessary.
- The client's chair height should allow good body alignment.
- The client should take regular breaks away from activities that cause repetitive stress.
- Teach the client to stretch fingers and wrists and stay relaxed.
- Surgical intervention involves cutting the transverse carpal ligament, releasing pressure on the median nerve.

Amputation
- Most amputations are related to complications resulting from peripheral vascular disease (PVD).
- Diabetes mellitus is often an underlying cause of PVD.
- Monitor for common post-op complications including hemorrhage, infection, contractures, DVT, and phantom limb pain.
- Assessment of pain and pain management is necessary. Residual limb pain is common after limb amputation and may be more severe with traumatic injury.
- If the limb was severed traumatically, peripheral circulation should be adequate.
- Teach clients to prevent contractures especially in proximal joints to amputation.
- With leg amputations, encourage client to lay supine and prone to prevent hip contractures from sitting in wheelchair or prolonged stump elevation on a pillow.

☐ Teach client to promote wound healing, and enhance ROM of the residual and nonaffected limbs.

☐ Long-term teaching includes stump shaping and the use of prosthetic devices for mobility.

Torn Meniscus

☐ The medial and lateral menisci are two large C-shaped cartilages on the top of the tibia.

☐ A torn meniscus happens when twisting or flexing of the knee joint occurs.

☐ Clinical manifestations include increased pain and edema.

☐ Treatment may include physical therapy or surgery.

☐ Straight-leg raising and quadriceps setting exercises help maintain the strength of the affected extremity in a client with a torn meniscus.

☐ Weight bearing may begin as soon as the day of surgery in a client with a torn meniscus.

☐ Mild to moderate pain is normal after arthroscopic knee surgery and can be relieved by oral narcotic analgesics or NSAIDs.

☐ To minimize swelling after arthroscopic knee surgery, the client should ice and elevate the extremity for at least 24 hours after surgery.

☐ Swelling and coolness of the joint and limb may indicate complications from tourniquet use during arthroscopic knee surgery.

GASTROINTESTINAL SYSTEM

Abdominal Ultrasound

☐ Images the liver, gallbladder, spleen, pancreas, and kidneys.

☐ Can show an enlarged gallbladder, presence of gallstones, thickening of gallbladder wall, or distention of the gallbladder lumen.

☐ Can also diagnose appendicitis, abdominal abscess, pancreatitis, and renal calculi.

☐ Client is usually NPO before the procedure.

Endoscopy

☐ A flexible fiberoptic endoscope is used to visualize the structures of the GI tract.

☐ Procedures such as sclerotherapy to stop bleeding, dilation to a stricture, or biopsy of tissue can be performed with endoscopy.

☐ Prior to endoscopy, clients should avoid NSAIDs or anticoagulants several days before the tests.

☐ The day before, clients should avoid anything PO containing dark colors such as red, orange, blue, and purple dyes.

- For an esophagogastroduodenoscopy (EGD), a client is NPO for at least 6 hours prior except for most medications.
- After an EGD, clients are NPO until their gag reflex returns.
- For a colonoscopy, the client is on clear liquids the day before the procedure and will complete a bowel prep prescription the evening before and/or morning of the procedure.
- The client will be NPO except ice chip and sips of water for 6 hours before colonoscopy.
- After either endoscopy, monitor the sedated client's vital signs, pulse oximetry, and depth of respirations. Monitor for bowel perforation symptoms including abdominal pain, rigid abdominal muscles, and hypotension. The client is at high risk for injury due to sedation.

Barium Tests

- A barium swallow (upper GI) view structures such as the esophagus, stomach, and the duodenum.
- A barium enema visualizes the structure of the descending colon and rectum.
- Contraindicated if the client has a perforation in the bowel, has a bowel obstruction, or is severely constipated.
- Client is usually NPO before the procedure.
- Teach the clients that barium causes constipation, and encourage the client to drink fluids, eat fiber, and monitor their BM and flatus until the barium passes.

Appendicitis

- An infection of the appendix caused by bowel wall swelling, kinking of the appendix, and external occlusion of the bowel by adhesions.
- Clinical manifestations include moderate to severe right lower quadrant pain (McBurney point), anorexia, nausea, low-grade fever, and elevated WBC count. The pain with appendicitis begins in the epigastrium or periumbilical region, then shifts to the right lower quadrant, and becomes steady.
- Lying flat or sitting may increase the amount of pain experienced. Client usually presents lying still with the legs drawn up toward the chest.
- Assess for peritonitis symptoms including firm, tender, and rigid abdomen. Also an increase in pain, fever, and heart rate.
- Enemas are contraindicated in any acute abdominal condition of unknown origin (such as suspected appendicitis) and after recent colon or rectal surgery.
- Treatment includes removal of the infected appendix and antibiotic therapy.

Gastritis

- Gastritis is an inflammation of the gastric mucosa that may be acute, often resulting from exposure to local irritants.
- Gastritis may be chronic, associated with autoimmune infections or atrophic disorders of the stomach.
- Reducing the amount of stress, eating a balanced diet, and exercise are important in the recovery phase.
- A gastric resection may be performed when serious erosion has occurred.
- *Helicobacter pylori* infection can lead to chronic atrophic gastritis.
- Chronic gastritis can occur at any age but is more common in older adults and may be caused by conditions that allow reflux of bile acids into the stomach.
- With gastritis, the stomach lining becomes thin and atrophic, decreasing stomach acid secretion.
- Medications include H2 receptor antagonists (famotidine), proton pump inhibitors (pantoprazole), and antacids (magnesium hydroxide).
- With *H. pylori* infection, antibiotic therapy is necessary.
- Teach the client to eat bland foods, reduce stress, exercise, and eliminate caffeine, alcohol, and nicotine.
- Clients with chronic gastritis may need vitamin B_{12} (cyanocobalamin) injections.

Gastroesophageal Reflux Disease (GERD)

- Associated with the backward flow of stomach contents into the esophagus most often by an excessive relaxation of the lower esophageal sphincter (LES).
- Diagnosed through esophageal pH monitoring or an EGD.
- Clinical manifestations include indigestion, epigastric pain, and eructation.
- Client may also exhibit coughing, hoarseness or wheezing at night, and painful swallowing.
- Treatment includes avoidance of fatty foods, caffeine, carbonation, chocolate, smoking, alcohol, and acidic foods like citrus fruits.
- To further prevent reflux, the client should eat smaller meals, remain upright for 2 to 3 hours after eating, and avoid eating for 2 to 3 hours before bedtime.
- Medications include antacids, histamine receptor antagonists (H2 blockers), prokinetic drugs (metoclopramide), and proton pump inhibitors (omeprazole).
- Contact the health care provider with chest or abdominal pain, bloody emesis or dark stools, dysphagia, shortness of breath, or nausea and vomiting.

Hiatal Hernia

☐ Hiatal hernia is the protrusion of the stomach through a weakening in the esophageal hiatus of the diaphragm.

☐ Obesity may cause increased abdominal pressure that pushes the lower portion of the stomach into the thorax.

☐ An upper GI series is used to diagnose hiatal hernia.

☐ Clinical manifestations, diet therapy, and medications are similar to GERD.

☐ Client should be counseled to lose weight and stop smoking.

☐ The surgical repair procedure for hiatal hernia is the laparoscopic Nissen fundoplication.

☐ In the post-op period, assess for bleeding, position head of the bed at 30 degrees, and encourage splinting with cough and deep breathing exercises.

Peptic Ulcer Disease

☐ A break in the integrity of the gastric mucosa allows stomach acid to come in contact with the epithelium of the stomach causing epithelial inflammation and necrosis.

☐ Risk factors include stress (including burns and trauma), increased intracranial pressure, *H. pylori* bacteria, alcohol, nicotine, and medications like NSAIDs, bisphosphonates, and corticosteroids.

☐ Clinical manifestations include dyspepsia, nausea, vomiting, hematemesis, melena, and abdominal pain.

☐ Gastric ulcers have greater epigastric pain that is aggravated within 30 to 60 minutes of eating and hematemesis.

☐ Duodenal ulcers have pain below the epigastrium, and pain begins 90 minutes after eating, pain at night, and melena.

☐ Assess for symptoms of perforation into the peritoneal cavity, hemoglobin and hematocrit levels, and vital signs.

☐ Diagnose with an EGD (with biopsy). The client may also have a bleeding scan if GI bleed is suspected.

☐ Treatment for gastric ulcers includes antibiotic therapy, mucosal barrier fortifiers (sucralfate), proton pump inhibitors (omeprazole), H2 blockers (ranitidine), and prostaglandin analogs (misoprostol).

☐ Monitor for symptoms of gastric or bowel perforation causing peritonitis.

Peritonitis

☐ Peritonitis is an inflammation of the peritoneal cavity and infection of the peritoneum.

☐ Peritonitis is commonly caused by a perforated ulcer or appendix rupture.

- ☐ Also caused by rupture of the gall bladder due to cholelithiasis and rupture of the intestines due to an incarcerated hernia or obstruction.
- ☐ Clinical manifestations include abdominal pain, rigid abdominal muscles, Turner sign (bluish discoloration of the left flank area), fever, and progressive abdominal distention.
- ☐ Client will instinctively lie still with knees flexed to reduce abdominal pain.
- ☐ Treatment involves IV antibiotics, IV fluids to maintain hydration and to replace electrolytes, pain management, and surgery to remove cause.
- ☐ Peritonitis can advance to septic shock and circulatory failure; management of fluid and electrolyte balance is the priority focus.
- ☐ Assess vital signs, pulse oximetry, nasogastric tube drainage, pain, and symptoms of shock.

Diverticulosis

- ☐ Outpouching or herniation of the bowel wall is diverticulum.
- ☐ Undigested food can block a diverticulum, decreasing blood supply to the area and predisposing the area to bacterial invasion causing diverticulitis.
- ☐ Clients at increased risk for diverticulosis are elderly clients and clients with low-fiber diets.
- ☐ Often, there are no symptoms; however, clinical manifestations include constipation and intermittent lower abdominal pain.
- ☐ A barium enema will cause diverticula to fill with barium and be easily seen on an X-ray.
- ☐ Diverticulitis clinical manifestations include anorexia, fever, and LLQ abdominal pain.
- ☐ Observe older clients carefully for sudden changes in mental status that would indicate infection.
- ☐ Diverticulitis is treated with antibiotics, IV fluids, analgesia, and anticholinergic medications.
- ☐ Assess vital signs, blood in stools, and the abdomen for distention and pain with palpation. Teach the client to rest, and avoid laxatives, enemas and straining.
- ☐ During acute diverticulitis, provide a low-fiber diet as the bowel heals. Then, encourage a high-fiber diet.
- ☐ Teach the client to stay well hydrated by drinking eight 8-oz glasses of water per day and gradually increase fiber in the diet to improve intestinal motility to prevent future episodes.
- ☐ Clients should start with a small amount of fiber and gradually increase the amount as tolerated to a maximum of 25 to 30 g of fiber daily.

Crohn Disease

- ☐ A recurrent GI tract inflammation with remissions and exacerbations commonly involves any segment of bowel from the mouth to the anus and affects the entire thickness of the bowel.
- ☐ The inflammation of the bowel is exacerbated with an acute infection resulting in an abscess.
- ☐ Clinical manifestations include abdominal pain, low-grade fever, diarrhea, steatorrhea, and rectal bleeding.
- ☐ Colonoscopy is the definitive test to diagnose Crohn disease.
- ☐ Laboratory tests reveal low hematocrit and hemoglobin due to chronic bleeding, and an increased WBC, ESR, and C-reactive protein is consistent with inflammatory disease.
- ☐ Teach the client to document stools and monitor changes in bowel habits.
- ☐ Medications include antibiotics, corticosteroid therapy, analgesics, antidiarrheal therapy, aminosalicylate therapy, and immunosuppressant therapy.
- ☐ Clients many also need iron, vitamin B_{12}, and calcium with vitamin D nutritional supplements.
- ☐ Bowel rest (NPO) may decrease acute inflammation followed by a low-residue and low-fat diet.
- ☐ Surgical management including bowel resection, strictureplasty, fistula closure, and draining abscess.
- ☐ Teach client stress management including exercise and smoking cessation.

Ulcerative Colitis

- ☐ Ulcerative colitis can affect the entire length of the large intestine through the layers of mucosa and submucosa.
- ☐ Colon becomes edematous, and ulcers occur along the lining of the colon.
- ☐ Clinical manifestations include colicky abdominal pain, blood and mucus in the stool, diarrhea, fever, dehydration, and weight loss.
- ☐ High-residue food, such as grains and nuts, should be avoided.
- ☐ A colonoscopy with biopsy can be performed to determine the state of the colon's mucosal layers, presence of ulcerations, and level of cytologic involvement.
- ☐ Client should be kept NPO and may need to be placed on TPN for nutrition.
- ☐ Clients with ulcerative colitis should follow a low-residue, high-protein diet.

- Clients should avoid caffeine, dairy, high-fiber foods, carbonated foods, and alcohol.
- Bowel perforation, obstruction, hemorrhage, cancer, and toxic megacolon are common complications of ulcerative colitis that may require surgery.
- A temporary or permanent ileostomy could be placed to manage inflammation.

Dehydration
- Dehydration can occur with GI disorders due to excessive diarrhea, nausea, and vomiting.
- Clinical manifestations include poor skin turgor, dry mucous membranes, lethargy, concentrated urine, decreased blood pressure, and increased heart rate (shock).
- Dehydration is a cause of acute kidney injury (AKI) and occurs rapidly in older adults.
- Fluid resuscitation is necessary using isotonic crystalloid solution such as 0.9% normal saline or lactated Ringer's solution.
- Assess hourly urine output, lung sounds, and cardiac status including cardiac monitor and vital signs.

Intrinsic Factor
- Stomach acid secretion is the source of intrinsic factor. A decrease in intrinsic factor causes a reduction in the absorption of vitamin B_{12}.
- Pernicious anemia is a low hemoglobin and red blood cell count due to inadequate amount of vitamin B_{12} to manufacture red blood.
- Clients at risk for pernicious anemia include clients with a gastrectomy, gastric bypass, and gastritis.
- Client may require lifelong vitamin B_{12} (cyanocobalamin) injections.

Colon Cancer
- Surface blood vessels of polyps and cancers are fragile and often bleed with the passage of stools.
- Screening tests for clients over the age of 50 include a colonoscopy recommended every 10 years, and annual occult blood test should be performed.
- Clinical manifestations include anorexia, changes in bowel elimination, fatigue, rectal bleeding, anemia, abdominal distention, and weight loss.
- Complete or partial intestinal obstruction may occur.
- Risk factors include familial history; personal history of breast, ovarian, and endometrial cancer; Crohn disease; and intestinal

polyps. Therapy for colon cancer can involve radiation, chemotherapy, and surgical bowel resection.

☐ Client and family teaching for ostomy care is essential to be able to manage ostomy before discharge.

☐ Ostomy should start functioning within 2 to 3 days after surgery.

☐ Monitor fluid and electrolyte status, vital signs, wound drainage, and incision site.

☐ To reduce risk of colon cancer, fats should account for no more than 25% of total daily calories and the diet should include 25 to 30 g of fiber per day.

Ostomy Care

☐ Assess client's readiness to learn, available support, resources, hobbies and activities, and physical limitations.

☐ The stoma should be pink and moist, and skin around the stoma should be intact and without redness.

☐ Teaching involves skin barrier use to protect skin around ostomy.

☐ The ostomy pouch should be emptied when one-third to one-half full.

☐ Consistency of the stool depends on ostomy placement along the colon tract.

☐ The wafer attached to the skin should be changed every 3 to 7 days.

☐ Teach client to avoid gas-producing foods such as carrots, cabbage, onions, and cauliflower.

Gastric Cancer

☐ The client with suspected gastric cancer may report a feeling of fullness in the stomach, but usually not enough to cause the client to seek immediate medical care.

☐ Other clinical manifestations include anorexia and weight loss.

☐ Diagnosed with an EGD with biopsy.

☐ Clients with peptic ulcer disease have a higher incidence of gastric cancer.

☐ After gastric resection, a client may require total parenteral nutrition or jejunal tube (J-tube) feedings to maintain adequate nutritional status and promotes healing.

☐ Teach post-op clients about how to prevent dumping syndrome.

Dumping Syndrome

☐ Dumping syndrome is a problem that occurs postprandial after gastric surgery.

☐ Group of vasomotor symptoms that occur after eating as food rapidly dumps into the small intestine including vertigo, tachycardia, syncope, sweating, pallor, and palpitations.

- To reduce the occurrences of the dumping syndrome after gastric resection, clients should be told to lie down for 30 minutes after eating, eat small meals, and drink fluids at least 30 minutes after meals.
- Teach client to avoid simple sugars and eat high-protein, and moderate-fat foods also reduce dumping syndrome.
- Medications include antidiabetic alpha-glucosidase inhibitor (acarbose) to decrease carbohydrate absorption and octreotide 30 minutes before meals to slow intestinal transit time.

Hemorrhoids
- Distended anal veins caused by portal hypertension and other conditions associated with persistently high intra-abdominal pressure.
- Clinical manifestations include rectal bleeding, pain, itch, and visualization of thrombosed veins.
- Teach clients to have diets high in fiber and fluids to promote regular bowel movements.
- Sitz baths four times per day and topical anesthetics such as lidocaine can be used for pain and 1% to 2.5% hydrocortisone cream to relieve itch.
- Clients should wear loose clothing, avoid straining and bending, and avoid standing on their feet for long periods.
- Surgery may be necessary for severe hemorrhoid pain and bleeding that is recurrent.

Pancreatitis
- Inflammation of the pancreas occurs due to an increase in enzyme levels within the pancreas.
- Blockage of the pancreatic ducts to the GI tract causes pancreatic enzymes to autodigest the pancreatic tissue causing inflammation. Pancreatic enzymes are released into the blood, resulting in an elevation of amylase and lipase levels.
- Etiology includes alcohol abuse, pancreatic duct blockage, trauma, manipulation of the pancreas during gastric surgery, drug abuse, and cigarette smoking.
- Severity depends on extent of inflammation and tissue damage and can progress to necrotizing hemorrhagic pancreatitis.
- Abdominal CT scan is used to diagnose pancreatitis.
- Clinical manifestations include acute severe midepigastric abdominal pain made worse by lying flat supine, Cullen sign (bluish area around the umbilicus), and Grey Turner sign (bluish discoloration of the flanks).

- ☐ Impairment of pancreatic beta cells causes the client to become hyperglycemic.
- ☐ Complications include peritonitis, hemorrhage, kidney failure, pleural effusions, atelectasis, pneumonia, and diabetes.
- ☐ Lab tests reveal increased serum amylase, lipase, trypsin, elastase, glucose, bilirubin levels, and WBC count.
- ☐ Keep client NPO during the acute phase. Client may need an NG tube placed to suction.
- ☐ Monitor for symptoms of fluid and electrolyte imbalance especially hypocalcemia.
- ☐ Medications include opioid analgesia, antibiotics, H2 antagonist (famotidine), and proton pump inhibitors (pantoprazole) to control stomach acid secretion. Insulin may also be needed.
- ☐ Position client in a side-lying position with knees flexed, and perform frequent oral care.
- ☐ Teach the client to abstain from alcohol and smoking.
- ☐ Teach client to monitor for symptoms of diabetes, clay-colored stools, dark urine, and jaundice.
- ☐ Once taking PO, the diet should be low in fat and high in calories, carbohydrates, and protein.

Cirrhosis

- ☐ Normal tissue of the liver is replaced with fibrotic tissue due to hepatic inflammation and necrosis.
- ☐ Common causes include alcohol abuse, medications, chemicals, and viral hepatitis.
- ☐ Clinical manifestations include jaundice, dry skin, pruritus, petechiae, ascites, spider angiomas, asterixis, and mental status changes.
- ☐ Laboratory results reveal increased liver enzymes (aspartate aminotransferase [AST], alanine aminotransferase [ALT], and lactate dehydrogenase [LDH]), bilirubin, ammonia, and PT/INR. Decreases are seen in serum protein and albumin.
- ☐ High ammonia levels cause hepatic encephalopathy; combined with increased bleeding time, safety is a primary concern.
- ☐ Complications include portal hypertension leading to esophageal varices, splenomegaly, and ascites.
- ☐ Assess respiratory status, fluid and electrolyte levels, vital signs, bleeding, LOC, and infection symptoms.
- ☐ Teach client to eat a low-sodium, high-protein, and high-carbohydrate diet. Change diet to moderate protein diet if client develops encephalopathy.

- Avoid polypharmacy due to reduction of liver's ability to metabolize medications.
- Lactulose and antibiotics are used to reduce serum ammonia levels.
- Varices can be a significant source of rapid GI bleeding.
- Vasopressin causes constriction of blood vessels to control bleeding, and a Sengstaken-Blakemore tube may be used to provide pressure on blood vessels of the esophagus.

Viral Hepatitis

- Contagious liver infection with multiple strains of the hepatitis virus.
- About 15% of clients develop chronic hepatitis B and are at high risk for cirrhosis and liver cancer.
- HAV vaccine recommended for adults 18 and older; second dose 1 month after first, third 6 to 12 months later; HBV vaccine recommended in childhood with the same schedule.
- Bed rest during the acute phase of hepatitis and nutritious diet with frequent small feedings.
- IV fluids with glucose if the client is experiencing an aversion to food.
- Recovery generally is at home.
- Teach client to complete follow-up blood work, abstain from alcohol, and transmission precautions to prevent the spread of virus.
- Promote rest, a diet high in carbohydrates and calories and moderate in protein, and avoid unnecessary medications.
- Interferon and antiviral treatments are used for HBV and HCV.
- Nonviral hepatitis caused by chemicals with toxic effects on the liver (such as carbon tetrachloride, phosphorus, or chloroform).
- Nonviral hepatitis also caused by medications acetaminophen, methyldopa, isoniazid, and some antibiotics and antimetabolites.
- See Table 1.18 for more on the types of viral hepatitis and routes of transmission.

Cholecystitis

- Acute or chronic inflammation of the gallbladder.
- Clinical manifestations include pain, tenderness in the upper right abdomen, pain radiating to right shoulder, nausea, vomiting, and diarrhea.
- Urine may also be dark and stools light (clay) color due to the excretion of bile pigments in the urine.
- Gallstones (cholelithiasis) can lodge in the bile ducts preventing outflow of digestive enzymes.

TABLE 1.18	Viral Hepatitis and Routes of Transmission	
Hepatitis	Transmission Route	Clinical Manifestations
A (HAV)	Fecal-oral route due to poor hand hygiene practices and poor sanitation	■ Mild GI illness that is self-limiting
B (HBV)	Parentally, through intimate contact	■ Anorexia, nausea and vomiting, fatigue, jaundice, dark urine, light stools, and fever ■ Usually self-limiting (body will clear virus)
C (HCV)	Transfusion of blood and blood products; sharing needles and unintentional needle sticks	■ Usually asymptomatic but usually leads to chronic infection
D (HDV)	Parentally through intimate contact in clients with HBV	■ Needs HBV for infection, usually leads to chronic infection
E (HEV)	Fecal-oral route due to poor hand hygiene practices and poor sanitation	■ Mild GI illness that is self-limiting

☐ Risk factors for cholelithiasis include obesity, female sex, diet high in fat, frequent changes in weight and rapid weight loss, estrogen medications, diabetes, and Mexican and Native American descent.

☐ Gallbladder ultrasound is the diagnostic procedure of choice.

☐ Murphy sign, elicited when the client reacts to pain and stops breathing in response to palpation in the area of the gallbladder, is a common finding in clients with cholecystitis.

☐ Monitored complications such as perforation, fever, abscess, fistula, and sepsis.

☐ Surgery is usually done after the acute infection has subsided in acute cholecystitis.

☐ Laparoscopic cholecystectomy is the standard of treatment. However, some clients may require an open abdominal incision.

☐ Post-op client should ambulate frequently, cough and deep breathe with splinting, and monitor lung sounds, bowel sounds, and bowel movements and/or flatus.

- ☐ Conservative therapy for chronic cholecystitis includes weight reduction, increasing physical activity and following a low-fat diet.
- ☐ Medications postcholecystectomy may include anticholinergic and antispasmodic drugs.
- ☐ Laser pulse technology may be used to fragment stones in the gallbladder or common bile duct.
- ☐ Diarrhea can continue after surgery, but usually resolves.
- ☐ Teach the client to adhere to low-fat, high-carbohydrate and high-protein diet after surgery.

Liver Biopsy

- ☐ Having the client lie on their right side with the bed flat will splint the liver biopsy site and minimize bleeding.
- ☐ Monitor vital signs and for hemorrhage symptoms.

Irritable Bowel Syndrome (IBS)

- ☐ A noninflammatory chronic disorder of the large bowel affecting mostly women.
- ☐ Clinical manifestations include abdominal pain, diarrhea, constipation (could be both), and mucus in stools.
- ☐ Although the cause is unknown, exacerbations are related to diet, stress, anxiety, and hormones.
- ☐ Teach the client to eat at least 30 g of fiber per day, to drink plenty of fluids, and to keep a food diary to better understand which foods cause problems.
- ☐ Medications for the diarrhea form of IBS include antidiarrheal (loperamide), anticholinergics (dicyclomine), SSRI's antidepressants (fluoxetine), and bulk-forming agents (psyllium).
- ☐ Medications for constipation form of IBS include the chloride channel activator lubiprostone and bulk-forming laxatives.
- ☐ Teach clients stress management and to contact practitioner with blood in stools.

GENITOURINARY SYSTEM

KEY TERMS

- ☐ **Anuria** is decreased urine output of less than 50 mL in 24 hours.
- ☐ **Azotemia** is a buildup of nitrogenous waste in the blood with impaired renal function.
- ☐ **Diuresis** is increased urine volume.
- ☐ **Dysuria** is painful urination.

- ☐ **Hematuria** is the presence of red blood cells in the urine.
- ☐ **Nocturia** is nighttime urination.
- ☐ **Nephrosclerosis** refers to hardening of the renal arteries.

Kidneys

- ☐ The cortex of the kidney makes up the outer layer and contains the glomeruli, the proximal tubules of the nephron, and the distal tubules of the nephron.
- ☐ The medulla of the kidney makes up the inner layer and contains the loops of Henle and the collecting tubules.
- ☐ The renal pelvis of the kidney collects urine from the calyces.
- ☐ The nephron of the kidney makes up the functional unit and contains Bowman capsule, the glomerulus, and the renal tubule, which consists of the proximal convoluted tubule and collecting segments.
- ☐ By removing water from the body in the form of urine, the kidneys also help regulate blood pressure.
- ☐ The kidney sensing a decreased blood pressure activates the renin-angiotensin system.
- ☐ The ureter, which transports urine from the kidney to the bladder, is a tubule that extends from the renal pelvis to the bladder floor.
- ☐ The urethra, extending from the bladder to the urinary meatus, transports urine from the bladder to the exterior of the body.
- ☐ Decreased cardiac output causes a decrease in renal perfusion, which leads to a lower glomerular filtration rate (GFR).
- ☐ The kidneys are responsible for excreting potassium.

Cystoscopy

- ☐ During a cystoscopy, a cytoscope is used to directly visualize the bladder by distending the bladder with fluid.
- ☐ Teach the client to void frequently after cystoscopy, and output should be measured.
- ☐ A small amount of blood in the urine may occur during the first 24 hours after cystoscopy.
- ☐ Monitor for bladder perforation symptoms such as increased abdominal pain and hematuria.

Urinary Diagnostics

- ☐ Urinalysis involves an examination of urine for color, appearance, pH, urine specific gravity, protein, glucose, ketones, red blood cells, white blood cells, and casts.
- ☐ Renal angiography provides a radiographic examination of the renal arterial supply by injecting dye into the vascular system.
- ☐ A renal scan involves injecting a radioisotope to allow visual imaging of blood flow distribution to the kidneys.

- ☐ Iodine allergy may manifest with dyspnea, flushing, and pruritus during injection of a contrast medium.
- ☐ Bladder biopsies should not be done when an active urinary tract infection is present because sepsis may result.

Cystitis

- ☐ Inflammation of the bladder due to infection or other factors such as radiation therapy.
- ☐ Obtain a clean-catch urine specimen for urinalysis and culture.
- ☐ A urinalysis reveals WBCs, RBCs, leukocyte esterase, and nitrates.
- ☐ Clinical manifestations include dysuria, frequency, urgency, and nocturia.
- ☐ The older adult may only show acute confusion and worsening incontinence symptoms.
- ☐ Treated with antibiotics for suspected bacterial infection, bladder analgesics (phenazopyridine), and anticholinergic/antispasmodic medications (hyoscyamine).
- ☐ Teach clients to void often, wear cotton underwear, drink increased fluids, void after intercourse, and avoid tub baths.

Pyelonephritis

- ☐ An infection of one or both kidneys and is usually a complication of an ascending bladder infection (UTI).
- ☐ Clinical manifestations include UTI symptoms, flank pain, costovertebral area (CVA) tenderness, fever, nausea, vomiting, and malaise.
- ☐ In addition to urinalysis and urine and blood cultures, the client may also have a renal CT and ultrasound to assess for abscess and renal structure.
- ☐ Treated with IV or oral antibiotics and increased fluid intake (PO or IV).
- ☐ Monitor for urosepsis symptoms including hypotension, tachycardia, and decreased LOC.
- ☐ Chronic pyelonephritis can be a long-term condition requiring antibiotic treatment for several weeks or months as well as close monitoring to prevent permanent damage to the kidneys.
- ☐ Hypertension is associated with chronic pyelonephritis.
- ☐ Maintenance of blood pressure is important to prevent kidney damage.

Renal Calculi

- ☐ Clinical manifestations include nausea, vomiting, diaphoresis, pallor, and severe back and flank pain.
- ☐ Teach the client to increase fluid intake of 3 to 4 quarts (3 to 4 L)/ day to flush the urinary tract and prevent further calculi formation.

- □ Ambulation is encouraged to help pass the calculi through gravity.
- □ Renal calculi are commonly composed of calcium. However, if made of uric acid, the client should avoid high-purine foods such as organ meats.
- □ Teach client to strain all urine to identify renal calculi that have passed through the urine.
- □ Large stones may need lithotripsy to break into smaller fragments.
- □ Manage client's pain with opioid pain medication and anticholinergic/antispasmodic medication (oxybutynin chloride) to reduce spasm.

Nephrotic Syndrome
- □ The glomeruli are damaged, and the kidneys are excessively permeable to plasma protein.
- □ Clinical manifestations include frothy urine (proteinuria) and hypoalbuminemia, which leads to a decreased oncotic pressure, resulting in anasarca (massive generalized edema).
- □ Other clinical manifestations include weight gain, high serum lipids, and hypertension.
- □ Treatment includes steroids, diuretics, ACE inhibitors, and anticoagulation.
- □ Provide low-sodium, low-fat, and high-protein diet and fluids if GFR is normal.
- □ Monitor for kidney failure and intravascular dehydration.

Ileal Conduit
- □ A client who has undergone a radical cystectomy may have an ileal conduit for the treatment of bladder cancer.
- □ The stoma should be red and moist, indicating adequate blood flow; a dusky or cyanotic stoma indicates insufficient blood supply and is an emergency needing prompt intervention.
- □ Report a urine output of less than 30 mL/h or no urine output for more than 15 minutes from an ileal conduit.

Acute Kidney Injury (AKI)
- □ A rapid reduction in the kidney's ability to filter or regulate fluids and waste in the body.
- □ Causes include hypovolemia, hypotension, reduced cardiac output, heart failure, kidney obstruction, nephrotoxins, and infection.
- □ Clinical manifestations include increased blood urea nitrogen (BUN) and creatinine levels, oliguria, dry mucous membranes, drowsiness, headache, muscle twitching, seizures, and metabolic acidosis.

- Some clients could experience polyuria due to damage of the glomerulus and loss of protein.
- Lack of filtration builds up fluid and metabolic waste. Hyperkalemia is the most life-threatening of the fluid and electrolyte changes and is characterized by tall peaked T waves on electrocardiogram.
- Sodium polystyrene sulfonate is administered PO or enema to decrease potassium levels.
- Monitor vital signs, pulse oximetry, pulmonary function, infection symptoms, and skin breakdown (skin is dry and subject to breakdown due to edema).
- Diuretics (furosemide) to increase urine and waste output.
- Calcium carbonate is prescribed to increase calcium and decrease phosphorous.
- Fluid challenges are used to increase mean arterial pressure (MAP) greater than 65 mm Hg to keep kidneys perfused.
- Calcium channel blockers can protect kidney tissue from further damage from nephrotoxins.
- Protein needs will depend on renal function and balancing fluid intake and loss.
- Diet should be low in potassium, sodium, and phosphorus.
- Renal replacement therapy (RRT) (dialysis) may be instituted if fluid volume overload and azotemia become symptomatic (uremia).

Chronic Kidney Disease (CKD)

- Umbrella term that describes chronic and progressive kidney damage leading to end-stage renal disease.
- Risk factors include diabetes, cardiovascular disease, hypertension, chronic pyelonephritis, and exposure to nephrotoxic agents.
- Clinical manifestations are found in every body system due to the buildup of uremic waste and fluid and electrolyte shifts.
- Important changes include lethargy, coma, pulmonary edema, cardiac rhythm alterations, cardiomyopathy, and muscle weakness and cramping.
- Laboratory results reveal an elevated serum creatinine, anemia, metabolic acidosis, and abnormalities in potassium, calcium, and phosphorus levels.
- There are five stages of CKD based on a GFR—an estimate of kidney function.
- A GFR less than 60 mL/min/1.73 m^2 is considered moderate CKD, and the client is watched more closely for deterioration of kidney function.

☐ In stage 4, there is a severe decrease in GFR (15 to 29 mL/min/1.73 m^2) and treating complications becomes necessary.

☐ Nephrosclerosis is due to prolonged hypertension and diabetes.

☐ Treatment of nephrosclerosis is aggressive antihypertensive therapy with ACE inhibitors.

☐ Other medications include calcium channel blockers, alpha-adrenergic and beta-adrenergic blockers, erythropoietin-stimulating agents, phosphate binders, and vasodilators.

☐ Monitor I&O, daily weights (a 1-kg weight gain is 1,000 mL retained fluid), serum electrolyte levels, lung sounds, and cardiac status including peripheral edema.

☐ Teach the client to restrict fluids and phosphorus, potassium, and sodium intake.

Renal Transplant

☐ Treatment of choice for end-stage kidney disease.

☐ Clinical manifestations of acute rejection of a transplanted kidney include pain at the graft site and decreased urine output.

☐ Hyperacute rejection can occur within 24 hours, but is rare due to tissue typing.

☐ Acute rejection occurs within 3 to 14 days.

☐ Chronic rejection is a slow process that occurs after months to years after transplant.

☐ Renal graft rejection will show evidence of deteriorating renal function (elevated protein, BUN, and creatinine levels), elevated WBCs, and flu-like symptoms.

☐ A client who has received a renal transplant may be started on immunosuppressive drug (cyclosporine) therapy to prevent graft rejection.

☐ Fever, a flushed feeling, or lethargy suggests infection, which is the major complication to watch for in clients on cyclosporine therapy.

Uremia

☐ Symptomatic buildup of nitrogen-based waste (end products of protein metabolism) in the blood.

☐ Affects every system in the body and if untreated leads to coma, seizures, and death.

☐ Cardiac arrest may occur from severe electrolyte abnormalities.

☐ Immediate RRT is necessary to filter waste from blood.

Renal Replacement Therapy (RRT/Dialysis)

☐ RRT is used to extract building waste products, fluid, and electrolytes.

- Types include intermittent RRT (IRRT/hemodialysis), continuous renal replacement therapy (CRRT), and peritoneal dialysis (PD).
- IRRT can cause rapid shifts in fluid and electrolyte levels and is performed usually three times per week.
- A dialysis catheter can be used, or a more permanent arteriovenous fistula is created in the arm.
- No blood pressures or invasive procedures should be done to the arm with a fistula.
- Assess the fistula daily: palpate for a thrill and auscultate for a bruit.
- CRRT is done to clients who are too unstable to undergo hemodialysis.
- PD is an option for clients unwilling or unable to utilize IRRT.
- In PD, a long-term catheter is inserted into the abdomen, and daily exchanges of 2 to 3 L of sterile dialysate fluid are performed.
- Postexchange fluid is clear and colorless or straw colored.
- An acute complication of PD is peritonitis.
- First sign of peritonitis is cloudy dialysate drainage fluid. Abdominal pain and rebound tenderness occurs later.
- Assess all RRT clients for anemia due to low erythropoietin levels.
- Teach the client to decrease protein and restrict fluid and sodium, potassium, and phosphorous intake.

Prostatitis
- Inflammation of the prostate gland due to an acute bacterial infection or chronic inflammatory response due to many causes.
- Symptoms include urinary tract infection symptoms (fever, dysuria, frequency, hesitancy, nocturia), difficulty urinating, pain in genitals, and painful ejaculation.
- Treated with antibiotics, alpha-adrenergic blockers (doxazosin), and NSIADs for inflammation and pain.
- Teaching the client to do warm sitz baths promotes comfort.
- Ejaculation can aid in the treatment of prostatitis by decreasing the retention of prostatic fluid.

Benign Prostatic Hypertrophy (BPH)
- Noncancerous enlargement of the prostate.
- Clinical manifestations in urine retention, frequency, dribbling, and difficulty starting the urine stream.
- Clients who cannot void require immediate catheterization.
- Pharmacologic treatment includes alpha-adrenergic blockers (doxazosin), and antiandrogen agents (finasteride; do not handle

the tablet directly) may also be used but can take up to 6 months for full effect.

□ Minimally invasive surgery or transurethral prostatectomy may be used if surgery is necessary.

□ A client with a transurethral resection of the prostate (TURP) will require continuous bladder irrigation post-op.

□ Monitor for hemorrhage, pain, bladder spasms, and strict I&O.

□ The nurse subtracts the amount of infused bladder irrigation from the total volume in the drainage bag to determine urine output.

□ Continuous bladder irrigation shouldn't be stopped as long as the catheter is draining because clots will form.

Biopsy of the Prostate

□ Difficulty urinating suggests urethral obstruction after biopsy of the prostate.

□ Mild pain is expected for 1 to 3 days after biopsy of the prostate.

□ Semen may be discolored for up to a month after biopsy of the prostate.

□ Temperature higher than 101°F (38.3°C) after a biopsy of the prostate should be reported because it suggests infection.

□ After a transrectal prostatic biopsy, blood in the stool is expected for a number of days.

Vasectomy

□ After vasectomy, the client remains fertile for several weeks until sperm stored distal to the severed vas is evacuated.

□ Teach clients to apply ice packs intermittently to ease pain and swelling.

□ The client will have to limit strenuous activities for about 1 week.

□ A vasectomy can be reversed, but the success rate is low.

Testicular Cancer

□ Starting at the age of 18, monthly testicular self-examination is recommended for the detection of testicular cancer.

□ Teach the client to use both hands to palpate.

□ The normal testicle is smooth and uniform in consistency.

□ Alpha-fetoprotein and beta HCG are tumor markers for testicular cancer.

□ A persistent elevation of alpha-fetoprotein after orchiectomy indicates tumor metastasis.

□ Early testicular cancer is curable with surgical intervention. Treatment can also involve radiation and chemotherapy (cisplatin, bleomycin, and etoposide).

□ Encourage the client to perform sperm banking prior to treatment.

□ Encourage counseling due to prolonged treatment at a young age.

Pelvic Inflammatory Disease (PID)

- ☐ Caused by an ascending infection into a woman's pelvic cavity from the lower genital tract.
- ☐ Causes scarring of fallopian tubes, infertility, and recurrent pelvic pain.
- ☐ Often caused by untreated sexually transmitted infections (STI) such as chlamydia or gonorrhea.
- ☐ Symptoms include pelvic pain, lower abdominal pain, pain with movement or lying supine, fever, and STI symptoms.
- ☐ Treated with broad-spectrum antibiotics and analgesia.
- ☐ Teach the client about transmission of STIs. All sexual partners must be notified and treated.

Breast Cancer

- ☐ Women at higher risk for breast cancer include having the BRCA 1 or BRCA 2 gene mutation, having a first-degree relative with breast cancer or BRCA 1 or BRCA 2 gene mutations, and radiation to the chest between 10 and 30 years old.
- ☐ Monthly self-breast exam (SBE) is an option for women starting at age 20.
- ☐ SBE requires palpation of all breast tissue, including the area up to the clavicle, down to the ribs, and into the axilla.
- ☐ Health care provider performs clinical breast exams every 3 years for women age 20 to 30 and annually after age 40.
- ☐ Mammogram screening can begin annually as early as 40 years old, but timing may vary depending on a woman's level of risk.
- ☐ Women at high risk for breast cancer should have a mammogram and a breast MRI annually and usually earlier than age 40.
- ☐ Lumpectomy, mastectomy, radiation, and chemotherapy in various combinations are treatment options for breast cancer.
- ☐ In a modified radical mastectomy, lymph nodes are often removed, and lymph drainage to the affected arm may cause lymphedema.
- ☐ Clients at risk for lymphedema should be taught to avoid anything that constricts the affected arm including blood draws and blood pressure monitoring.
- ☐ Elevation after surgery will assist with decreasing edema.
- ☐ Once lymphedema develops, it is usually chronic.
- ☐ Radiation therapy is used to decrease the risk of a local recurrence.
- ☐ Cyclophosphamide, methotrexate and docetaxel, doxorubicin, epirubicin, and aclitaxel are common chemotherapies.
- ☐ Teach clients about side effects of chemotherapy including bone marrow suppression, hair loss, and immunosuppression.

Brachytherapy (Intracavitary) Radiation

☐ Radioactive material (wires, seeds) is placed directly into a body structure such as uterus.

☐ Clients receiving brachytherapy are placed on strict bed rest, with the head of the bed elevated no more than 15 degrees to avoid displacing the radiation source.

☐ It's important to empty the bowel before treatment with intracavitary radiation because pressure changes in the pelvis associated with bowel movements can alter the position of the applicator and the radiation source.

☐ Limit visitors to 30 minutes and advise to stay 6 feet (1.8 m) away from the client.

☐ Perform only necessary nursing activities to decrease exposure time and do not loiter in the client's room.

☐ Do not touch radiation source with bare hands if dislodged. Use protective gloves and 12-inch (30-cm) forceps to move radiation source to protective container.

☐ Linen and trash should be kept inside the client's room until cleared by the radiation safety personnel.

☐ After cervical radiation, some vaginal bleeding occurs for 1 to 3 months.

☐ It's recommended that fluid intake be increased in a client receiving a radiation implant for the treatment of bladder cancer.

Radiation Care

☐ Skin and tissues can become irritated, become darker in color, and form blister from radiation therapy.

☐ Teach clients to wear loose clothing, use mild soaps, and apply only suggested skin care products over treatment area.

☐ Clients should not apply any skin products to treatment site for at least 2 hours before treatment.

☐ Fatigue is common after radiation. Encourage client to balance necessary activity with periods of rest.

☐ Assess for dehydration, orthostatic blood pressures, daily weight, and urine characteristics in clients reporting nausea, vomiting, and diarrhea after radiation.

☐ Encourage clients to eat frequent small meals and snacks instead of big meals.

Toxic Shock Syndrome

☐ Caused by *S. aureus* bacteria.

☐ Toxic shock syndrome occurs most commonly in menstruating women using tampons.

TABLE 1.19	Vaginal Infections	
Infection	Clinical Manifestations	Treatment
Candidiasis	■ Thick and white discharge that resembles cottage cheese in appearance	■ Antifungal medications (fluconazole PO or miconazole topically)
Bacterial vaginosis (BV)	■ Thin and grayish white discharge, with a marked fishy odor	■ Antibiotic therapy PO or topically (metronidazole)

☐ Tampons, particularly when left in place for more than 8 hours (such as overnight), are believed to provide a good environment for growth of the bacteria, which then enter the bloodstream through breaks in the vaginal mucosa.

☐ Clinical manifestations include hypotension, tachycardia, confusion, muscle aches, malaise, nausea, vomiting, and diarrhea.

☐ Treatment usually involves removing infected item and giving antibiotics like nafcillin or cephalosporin.

☐ Intravenous fluids administered to treat shock.

☐ Monitor vital signs, pulse oximetry, cardiac monitor, and urine output.

☐ See Tables 1.19 and 1.20 for types of vaginal infections and STI.

Dilatation and Curettage (D&C)

☐ Tissue is scraped and removed by suction from the uterus for therapeutic or diagnostic reasons.

☐ Can be performed under general anesthesia but often preformed with light anesthesia and numbing of the cervix.

☐ Teach the client to void prior to the procedure.

☐ Mild analgesics needed after procedure for pain.

☐ Strenuous work and sexual intercourse avoided for 2 weeks postprocedure.

☐ Tampons and tub baths should be avoided for 1 week after a dilatation and curettage procedure.

Endometriosis

☐ Chronic disease affecting women of reproductive age.

☐ Thought to occur due to retrograde menstruation.

☐ Symptoms include pelvic discomfort and pain, possible infertility, and rectal or sacrococcygeal pain.

TABLE 1.20 Sexually Transmitted Infections

Infection	Clinical Manifestations	Transmission	Treatment
Human papillomavirus (genital warts)	■ External genital warts ■ Most common STI	■ Skin-to-skin contact	■ Recurrent, lifelong infection ■ Podofilox topical gel to remove surface lesions
Herpes simplex virus 2 (genital herpes)	■ Painful itchy genital blisters ■ Dysuria	■ Skin-to-skin contact	■ Recurrent, lifelong infection ■ Stress and emotions can influence outbreak timings. ■ Treated with antivirals (acyclovir)
Chlamydia	■ Often no symptoms until progresses to PID or genital inflammation in males ■ May have watery mucus discharge and dysuria	■ Infected vaginal secretions ■ Semen	■ Antibiotics ■ Partner must be treated.
Gonorrhea	■ Often no symptoms until progresses to PID or genital inflammation in males ■ May have yellow-green discharge, pharyngitis, and dysuria	■ Infected vaginal secretions ■ Semen	■ Antibiotics ■ Partner must be treated

Syphilis	■ First stage is a painless chancre sore on genitals. ■ In secondary syphilis, a maculopapular, nonpruritic rash appears on the palms of the hands and soles of the feet.	■ Infected vaginal secretions ■ Semen	■ Antibiotics ■ Partner must be treated.
Trichomonas	■ Greenish gray, watery, and frothy or purulent discharge	■ Infected vaginal secretions ■ Semen	■ Antibiotics (metronidazole) ■ Partner must be treated.
Human immunodeficiency virus	■ Often no symptoms, but may have initial flu-like symptoms	■ Blood ■ Breast milk ■ Infected vaginal secretions ■ Semen	■ A combination of antiretroviral therapies

☐ NSAIDs and oral contraceptives may be utilized.

☐ Surgical intervention may be necessary.

☐ Client teaching is necessary related to psychological consequences.

ENDOCRINE SYSTEM

☐ See Table 1.21 for facts covering glands and their actions.

☐ See Table 1.22 for facts covering pancreatic enzymes and their actions.

☐ See Table 1.23 for facts covering hormones and their function.

Hypothalamus

☐ The hypothalamus controls temperature, respiration, blood pressure, thirst, hunger, and water balance.

☐ The hypothalamus also produces hypothalamic-stimulating hormones, which affect the inhibition and release of pituitary hormones.

Hyperthyroidism

☐ The thyroid gland secretes high levels of T_3 and T_4 thyroid hormone.

☐ Clinical manifestations include nervousness, palpitations, tremor, irritability, bulging eyes, heat intolerance, light sensitivity, weight loss, and fatigue.

☐ Lab test reveals elevated T_3, T_4, radioactive iodine uptake, and a low thyroid-stimulating hormone (TSH) level.

TABLE 1.21 Glands and their Actions	
Gland	**Action**
Hypothalamus	■ Secretes corticotropin-releasing factor, which stimulates the anterior pituitary to secrete corticotropin
Pancreas	■ Secretes enzymes into the duodenum through the pancreatic duct ■ Exocrine function digestive enzymes amylase, lipase, and trypsin ■ Endocrine function, the islets of Langerhans insulin, glucagon, and somatostatin
Parathyroid	■ Secretes parathyroid hormone, depending on the levels of calcium and phosphorus in the blood
Pituitary	■ Secretes vasopressin and oxytocin ■ Controls the rate of thyroid hormone released by secretion of thyroid-stimulating hormone
Thyroid	■ Secretes thyroid hormone ■ Secretes calcitonin

TABLE 1.22   Pancreatic Enzymes and Their Actions

Pancreatic enzyme	Action
Amylase	■ Breaks down starches into smaller carbohydrate molecules
Glucagon	■ Increases blood glucose levels by promoting hepatic gluconeogenesis.
Insulin	■ Moves glucose from the blood into the cells of the body so that the cells can use the glucose as an energy source ■ Changes excess glucose into glycogen and stores it in the liver
Lipase	■ Breaks down fats into fatty acids and glycerol
Trypsin	■ Breaks down proteins

TABLE 1.23   Hormones and Their Functions

Hormone	Function
Corticotrophin	■ Stimulates secretion of hormones from the adrenal cortex
Epinephrine	■ Regulates instantaneous stress reaction ■ Increases metabolism, blood glucose levels, and cardiac output
Follicle-stimulating hormone (FSH)	■ Stimulates graafian follicle growth and estrogen secretion in women and sperm maturation in men
Glucocorticoids (cortisol, cortisone, and corticosterone)	■ Mediates the stress response ■ Promotes sodium and water retention and potassium secretion ■ Suppresses corticotropin secretion
Growth hormone	■ Insulin antagonist that stimulates the growth of cells, bones, muscle, and soft tissue
Insulin	■ Regulates fat, protein, and carbohydrate metabolism and lowers blood glucose levels by promoting glucose transport into cells

(Continued)

TABLE 1.23 Hormones and Their Function (Continued)	
Hormone	**Function**
Luteinizing hormone (LH)	■ Induces ovulation and the development of the corpus luteum in women ■ Stimulates testosterone secretion in men
Mineralocorticoids (aldosterone and deoxycorticosterone)	■ Promotes sodium and water retention ■ Promotes potassium secretion
Norepinephrine	■ Regulates generalized vasoconstriction
Oxytocin	■ Stimulates uterine contractions during labor ■ Stimulates milk secretion in lactating women
Parathyroid hormone (parathormone)	■ Regulates calcium and phosphorus levels ■ Promotes the resorption of calcium from bones
Sex hormones (androgens, estrogens, and progesterone)	■ Develops and maintains secondary sex characteristics ■ Develops and maintains libido
Thyroid-stimulating hormone (TSH)	■ Regulates the secretory activity of the thyroid gland
Thyroxine (T_4) Triiodothyronine (T_3)	■ Thyroid hormones that affect growth and development as well as metabolic rate
Vasopressin (antidiuretic hormone, ADH)	■ Prevents water loss, vasoconstriction

☐ Graves' disease is a type of hyperthyroidism caused by autoimmune disorder.

☐ Clients need a calm, restful environment in which to relax and get adequate rest.

☐ Thyrotoxicosis (thyroid storm) is a form of severe hyperthyroidism that can be precipitated by thyroid surgery, stress, injury, or infection.

☐ Clinical manifestations of thyroid storm are hyperthermia, tachycardia, chest pain, delirium, and palpitations.

☐ A high-calorie, high-protein diet is appropriate for clients with hyperthyroidism.

- [ ] Treatment with irradiation, involving administration of iodine 131 (^{131}I), destroys the thyroid gland.
- [ ] Surgery includes subtotal and total thyroidectomy.
- [ ] Pre-op client should be euthyroid by using antithyroid medication methimazole, sodium or potassium iodine solutions with dexamethasone, or propylthiouracil.
- [ ] During the post-op period, palpate behind the neck for bleeding and monitor for hematoma formation.
- [ ] Monitor post-op for symptoms of thyroid storm and hypocalcemia. Immediate treatment for a client who develops hypocalcemia and tetany after thyroidectomy is calcium gluconate.
- [ ] Treatment for a thyroid storm includes beta-adrenergic blockers (propranolol), intravenous fluids, propylthiouracil, antipyretic (acetaminophen), and humidified oxygen.
- [ ] Medical and surgical treatment can lead to permanent hypothyroidism and may require lifelong thyroid hormone replacement therapy.
- [ ] Teach clients hypothyroidism symptoms and side effects of thyroid replacement medications.

Hypothyroidism
- [ ] The thyroid gland produces low levels of T_3 and T_4 thyroid hormone.
- [ ] Symptoms include extreme fatigue, forgetfulness or confusion, cool skin, sensitivity to cold, weight gain, lethargy, decreased heart rate, hair loss, and weight gain.
- [ ] Cardiovascular assessment is essential for bradycardia and hypotension.
- [ ] Clients with hypothyroidism need lifelong replacement hormone therapy.
- [ ] Clients with hypothyroidism should be cautious taking hypnotics and sedatives until thyroid hormones are regulated.
- [ ] Assessment of therapeutic effects of thyroid replacement therapy involves assessing thyroid hormone level blood tests, heart rate, physical activity, and body temperature.
- [ ] Myxedema is hypothyroidism that has progressed to subnormal body temperatures, bradycardia, cardiac complications, and coma.
- [ ] Myxedema is treated with IV thyroid hormones, steroids, and electrolyte replacement.
- [ ] Monitor vital signs, respiratory status, and body temperature.
- [ ] Interventions include rewarming the client, protecting the client's skin, and avoiding the use of hypnotics, sedatives, and opioids.

Hyperparathyroidism

- ☐ Parathyroid glands are attached to the thyroid glands and regulate serum calcium levels.
- ☐ Hyperparathyroidism causes overproduction of parathyroid hormone.
- ☐ Clinical manifestations include elevated serum calcium, bone decalcification, renal calculi, fatigue, muscle weakness, nausea and vomiting, constipation, hypertension, and cardiac dysrhythmias.
- ☐ Due to the large range of symptoms, the client's diagnosis may be missed and the client may be thought to have a psychosomatic disease.
- ☐ Recommended management for primary hyperparathyroidism is surgery.
- ☐ Instruct the client to increase fluid intake to 2 L/day to prevent renal calculi.
- ☐ Teach the client to increase fiber, mobility, restrict calcium, and supplement phosphorus.
- ☐ Monitor for hypercalcemia and treat with IV normal saline bolus, calcitonin, and dialysis.

Hypoparathyroidism

- ☐ Thyroidectomy may lead to hypoparathyroidism if the parathyroid is also removed during surgery.
- ☐ Hypocalcemia results, causing numbness, tingling, positive Chvostek or Trousseau signs, and cramping of extremities.
- ☐ Tetany can be a life-threatening emergency.
- ☐ Therapy is aimed at increasing serum calcium levels and decreasing the symptoms of hypoparathyroidism.
- ☐ Medications include calcium gluconate IV and pentobarbital to decrease neuromuscular irritability, and parathormone may be administered.
- ☐ Provide a quiet environment with no drafts, bright lights, or sudden movement.
- ☐ Diet should be high in calcium and vitamin D and low in phosphorus.
- ☐ Monitor for tetany, seizure, respiratory difficulty, and seizure precautions.

Diabetes Mellitus

- ☐ Clinical manifestations include "three Ps," **P**olyuria, **P**olydipsia, and **P**olyphagia, weight loss, glycosuria, malaise, blurred vision, poor healing wounds, and vaginal infections.
- ☐ Laboratory results reveal a fasting blood glucose 126 mg/dL or more, random glucose greater than 200 mg/dL, a 2-hour postload glucose greater than 200 mg/dL, and >7% hemoglobin A1c (HbA1c).

- ☐ Measurement of HbA1c is used to assess blood glucose levels over a 3-month period (the life of a red blood cell).
- ☐ Higher glycosylated hemoglobin indicates the client's blood glucose level has been consistently elevated.
- ☐ Teach the client about hypoglycemia symptoms including cool, diaphoretic skin, palpitations, and decreased LOC.
- ☐ Teach hyperglycemia symptoms including hot, dry skin and dehydration.
- ☐ Unintentional increases in blood sugar can result from stress, illness, and medications such as steroids.
- ☐ Teach the client about a balanced diet, exercise, blood sugar monitoring, and medication compliance.
- ☐ Chronic complications occur as a result of blood glucose fluctuations causing microvascular and macrovascular occlusions especially in the brain, heart, eye, kidneys, and peripheral vasculature.
- ☐ To prevent complications, teach client to have at least annual eye exams with pupil dilation, annual lipid level screening, and blood pressure management.
- ☐ Teach clients to inspect their feet daily, dry feet thoroughly when wet, and to wear socks and shoes at all times.
- ☐ Clients with diabetes mellitus are also susceptible to infections due to high glucose levels.
- ☐ If hypoglycemic, give 15 to 20 g of fast-acting carbohydrate (3 to 4 glucose tabs, 120 mL juice) and retest in 15 minutes.
- ☐ In an unconscious client with hypoglycemia, give subcutaneous or IM glucagon (1 mg) or 50% dextrose solution IV.

Type 1 Diabetes Mellitus
- ☐ An absolute deficiency of insulin secretion in which clients need insulin replacement daily for life.
- ☐ A client with chronic pancreatitis may develop diabetes secondary to the pancreatitis.
- ☐ Teach client how to inject insulin, rotation sites, and side effects of insulin therapy.
- ☐ Insulin sites need to be rotated to prevent the development of lipoatrophy and hypertrophy at injection sites.
- ☐ Monitor blood glucose for hypoglycemia and other potential side effects of individual drugs.
- ☐ Clients taking insulin should eat a 15-g carbohydrate snack before moderate exercise to prevent hypoglycemia.
- ☐ Hyperglycemia can progress to diabetic ketoacidosis (DKA) in a client with type 1 diabetes mellitus.

- Clinical manifestations of DKA include Kussmaul respirations, hyperglycemia, anorexia, vomiting, thirst, polyuria, dehydration, and metabolic acidosis with ketones.
- Treat DKA with insulin, intravenous fluids, and electrolyte replacement.
- Monitor clients with DKA blood glucose, renal function and urinary output, ECG, electrolyte levels, vital signs, and lung assessments for fluid overload symptoms.
- On "sick days," teach client to test blood sugar and urine ketones every 3 to 4 hours, take in 45 to 50 g of carbohydrates every 4 hours, and report nausea, vomiting, and diarrhea and moderate ketones to practitioner.

Type 2 Diabetes Mellitus

- A relative deficiency of insulin secretion or an ineffective use of insulin by the body.
- Treated initially with diet and exercise, then oral hypoglycemic is added for clients who require greater blood sugar control.
- Monitor blood glucose for hypoglycemia and other potential side effects of individual drugs.
- Teach clients to take oral hypoglycemic at specified times and no doubling if doses are skipped.
- Hyperglycemia can progress to hyperosmolar hyperglycemia nonketotic syndrome (HHNS).
- Clinical manifestations of HHNS include hyperglycemia, polyuria, an underlying infection or acute illness, hypotension, tachycardia, profound dehydration, and hypernatremia.
- HHNS is treated similarly to DKA with giving fluids, correcting electrolyte imbalances, and insulin administration.

Diabetes Insipidus

- Diabetes insipidus is a condition in which abnormally large volumes of dilute urine are excreted as a result of deficient production of vasopressin.
- The word diabetes refers to a large amount of water being produced, but has no relation to insulin or blood sugar problems.
- Central diabetes insipidus is caused by a deficiency of antidiuretic hormone (ADH/vasopressin), causing excess urine formation and fluid loss.
- Two leading causes are hypothalamic or pituitary tumors and closed head injuries.
- Also can be caused by structural damage to the kidney (nephrogenic diabetes insipidus).

- Clinical manifestations include large quantities of pale yellow to clear concentrated urine (generally less than 1.005), extreme thirst, hypotension, tachycardia, and confusion.
- Monitor for hypovolemic shock due to increased urine output.
- A fluid deprivation test is used to diagnose diabetes insipidus.
- The fluid deprivation test involves withholding water for 4 to 18 hours and checking urine osmolality periodically.
- Central diabetes insipidus is treated with desmopressin subcutaneous, IV, or intranasal, and nephrogenic diabetes insipidus is treated with thiazide diuretics (HCTZ).
- Fluid and electrolyte replacement is critical.
- Monitor vital signs, I&O, daily weight, neuro checks, and serum electrolytes.

Addison Disease

- Addison disease is the hypofunctioning of the adrenal gland.
- Clinical manifestations include lethargy, depression, fatigue, muscle weakness, anorexia, nausea, vomiting, hypotension, and skin pigmentation that darkens.
- A definitive diagnosis of Addison disease must reflect low levels of adrenocortical hormones.
- Daily weight is an objective way to monitor fluid balance in Addison disease.
- Rapid variations in weight reflect changes in fluid volume and the need for more glucocorticoids.
- Teach clients to avoid extra potassium (salt substitutes), carry a fast-acting carbohydrate source, increase fluid intake (3,000 mL/day), and the need for lifelong steroid therapy.
- Treated with glucocorticoid replacements (hydrocortisone, cortisone, and prednisone) and mineralocorticoid replacement (fludrocortisone).
- In times of stress or illness, clients must increase steroid dose and sodium and fluid intake to prevent adrenal crisis (Addisonian crisis).
- In adrenal crisis, the uncontrolled loss of sodium and impaired mineralocorticoid function result in loss of extracellular fluid volume and possible irreversible shock.
- A client being treated for adrenal crisis should have serum sodium and potassium values monitored.
- Treat a client in adrenal crisis with hydrocortisone IV and intravenous fluids.
- Monitor vital signs, I&O, cardiac monitor, serum electrolytes, daily weight, and intake and output.

☐ Teach client to have an emergency kit at home of hydrocortisone for injection.

Cushing Disease

☐ Cushing disease is caused by an excess in mineralocorticoids and glucocorticoids from the adrenal glands.

☐ Clinical manifestations of Cushing disease include abnormal fat distribution causing an obese abdomen, buffalo hump, moon face and thin extremities, hyperglycemia, immunosuppression, and osteoporosis.

☐ In Cushing disease, increased mineralocorticoid activity causes sodium and water retention resulting in hypertension.

☐ Laboratory results reveal hypokalemia and hypernatremia and a reduction of eosinophils.

☐ Cushing disease is diagnosed with a low-dose dexamethasone suppression test.

☐ Medications include metyrapone, mitotane, and ketoconazole to block ACTH (pituitary's adrenocorticotropic hormone).

☐ If due to adrenal or pituitary tumor, a hypophysectomy or adrenalectomy will be indicated.

☐ Post-op monitor or adrenal insufficiency that could begin 12 to 24 hours post-op.

☐ Prevent an adrenal crisis with supplement hydrocortisone.

☐ Monitor vital signs, I&O, daily weight, and serum electrolytes.

Syndrome of Inappropriate Antidiuretic Hormone (SIADH)

☐ An excess of ADH is secreted causing the kidney to retain fluids causing hyponatremia and urine with low osmolality.

☐ Clinical manifestations include water retention with oliguria, edema, and weight gain.

☐ Caused by head injury, cancer, infections, and medications (vincristine, phenothiazines, tricyclics, and thiazides).

☐ Hyponatremia is a result of excess fluid rather than a deficiency of sodium.

☐ Medications include hypertonic saline to slowly increase serum sodium by 0.5 to 1 mEq/h until sodium reaches 125 to 130 mEq/L, loop diuretics (furosemide), and vasopressin receptor antagonist (conivaptan).

☐ Treatment also includes fluid restriction and seizure precautions.

☐ Monitor vital signs, I&O, daily weight, neuro checks, and serum electrolytes.

Pheochromocytoma

- ☐ Usually a benign tumor of the adrenal medulla that secrets epinephrine and norepinephrine.
- ☐ Clinical manifestations include headache, diaphoresis, palpitations, increased metabolism, hyperglycemia, and hypertension (hallmark of this tumor).
- ☐ Treatment involves surgical adrenalectomy and alpha- and beta-adrenergic blockers.
- ☐ Clients may have extreme hypertension when the tumor is manipulated during surgery.
- ☐ Clients feel anxious due to symptoms and need a calm environment and possibly benzodiazepines.

HEMATOLOGIC AND IMMUNE SYSTEMS

KEY TERMS

- ☐ **Erythrocyte** is the cellular component of blood involved in the transport of oxygen and carbon dioxide.
- ☐ **Erythropoiesis** is the process of formation of red blood cells (RBCs).
- ☐ **Erythropoietin** is the hormone produced primarily by the kidneys necessary for erythropoiesis.
- ☐ **Hematopoiesis** is a complex process of the formation and maturation of blood cells.
- ☐ **Hemostasis** is the intricate balance between clot formation and clot dissolution.
- ☐ **Leukocyte** is one of several cellular components of blood involved in defense of the body; subtypes include neutrophil, eosinophil, basophil, monocyte, and lymphocyte cells.
- ☐ **Leukopenia** means less than normal amount of white blood cells (WBCs) in circulation.
- ☐ **Lymphocyte** is a form of WBC involved in immune function.
- ☐ **Neutrophil** is a fully mature WBC capable of phagocytosis, primary defense against bacterial infection.
- ☐ **Oxyhemoglobin** is the combined form of oxygen and hemoglobin found in arterial blood.

Immune Function

- ☐ Diminished immune function in the elderly can interfere with the ability to fight infection.
- ☐ Inflammation and increased body temperature are normal immune responses to detected antigens.

TABLE 1.24	Blood Components
Component	**Characteristics**
Leukocytes	▪ Also called white blood cells, or WBCs ▪ Formed in the bone marrow and lymphatic tissue ▪ Include granulocytes and agranulocytes ▪ Provide immunity and protection from infection by phagocytosis (engulfing, digesting, and destroying microorganisms)
Plasma	▪ Liquid portion of the blood ▪ Composed of water, protein (albumin and globulin), glucose, and electrolytes
Erythrocytes	▪ Also called red blood cells, or RBCs ▪ Formed in the bone marrow and contain hemoglobin
Thrombocytes	▪ Also called platelets ▪ Formed in the bone marrow and function in the coagulation of blood

☐ Autoimmune response is one in which the immune system forms antibodies against the body's own tissues, resulting in disease.

☐ See Table 1.24 for facts covering blood components and their characteristics.

Anemia

☐ Hemoglobin or erythrocyte concentration is lower than normal due to blood loss, cell destruction, nutritional deficits, or depressed bone marrow production.

☐ There is less oxygen-carrying potential to body cells.

☐ Clinical manifestations include tachycardia, palpitations, dyspnea, dizziness, orthopnea, exertional dyspnea, numbness, and fatigue that is unrelieved by rest.

☐ The more rapidly anemia develops, the more severe its symptoms.

☐ Teach the client the importance of adhering to therapy to prevent severe cardiac complications.

☐ Teach the client to eat a healthy diet and maintain adequate amounts of iron, vitamins, and protein.

☐ Relief of fatigue may be slow as hemoglobin increases at about 1 g/dL in 1 month.

☐ The practitioner will continue oral supplementation of iron for 4 to 6 months.

Blood Transfusion

- ☐ Preparation: consented client with a large-gauge IV catheter.
- ☐ Blood must be used within 30 minutes after leaving blood bank.
- ☐ Prime IV blood tubing that includes a filter with normal saline (NS).
- ☐ Can use up to 2 units with one tubing set, but never cross tubing with different types of blood products.
- ☐ Identified client by two RNs and double-check blood compatibility.
- ☐ Infuse a small amount 5 mL/min for the first 15 minutes and then increase infusion rate as ordered.
- ☐ Check vital signs in 15 minutes after the start of the therapy.
- ☐ Blood is usually run a unit of blood over 90 minutes and has 4-hour limit for hanging blood products.
- ☐ Check hemoglobin and hematocrit in 4 to 6 hours after therapy completes.
- ☐ Assess for possible transfusion reaction symptoms including restlessness, hives, nausea, vomiting, back pain, shortness of breath, flushing, hematuria, fever, and chills, and notify the primary care provider.
- ☐ If reaction is suspected, stop the transfusion, change IV tubing to new NS line, keep the blood bag and tubing, and obtain blood and urine specimens.
- ☐ During the infusion, monitor vital signs, lung sounds, skin assessment, and urine output.
- ☐ Anticipate the need for acetaminophen, diphenhydramine, and fluids.

Diagnostic Tests

- ☐ Hematologic studies including the CBC to identify total number of blood cells (leukocytes, erythrocytes, and platelets) as well as hemoglobin, hematocrit, and RBC indices.
- ☐ Coagulation tests include INR used to monitor warfarin sodium and a PTT used to monitor intravenous heparin therapy.
- ☐ Bone marrow aspiration and biopsy are used to evaluate hematologic disorders.
- ☐ After a bone marrow biopsy, there is a risk of bleeding and infection.
- ☐ Pressure is applied to biopsy site, and site is covered with sterile dressing.

Leukemia

- ☐ Leukemia is a type of cancer of the bone marrow that specifically affects WBCs, causing abnormal cell growth and production.
- ☐ WBC or leukocyte counts are usually very high, and platelet and hemoglobin levels are low.

- Acute lymphocytic leukemia is most common in young children and in adults age 65 and older; it is more common in Caucasians than in clients with African or Asian descent.
- Bone marrow aspiration or biopsy to confirm the diagnosis.
- Clinical manifestations include bone pain, fever, night sweats, weight loss, weakness, fatigue, frequent infections, swollen lymph nodes in the neck and axilla, and bruising easily.
- Chronic lymphocytic leukemia shows a proliferation of small abnormal mature B cells and decreased antibody response.
- Uncontrolled proliferation of granulocytes occurs in myelogenous leukemia.
- The initial phase of chemotherapy for acute lymphocytic leukemia, called the induction phase, is designed to put the client into remission by giving high doses of drugs and administering doses closer together than once each month.
- A low-bacteria diet that excludes raw fruits and vegetables would be indicated for a neutropenic client with leukemia.
- During chemotherapy, tumor lysis syndrome may occur as cell destruction releases intracellular components, resulting in hyperuricemia.
- Treat tumor lysis syndrome with intravenous fluids and allopurinol.
- Monitor for signs and symptoms of infection, protect from infection and bleeding, and monitor for signs of anemia.

Thrombocytopenia

- In adults, thrombocytopenia is indicated when the platelet count is less than 100,000/microliter.
- The classic symptoms for thrombocytopenia are petechiae and bruising.
- Idiopathic thrombocytopenic purpura and disseminated intravascular coagulation cause platelet aggregation and bleeding.
- Heparin-associated thrombocytopenia may be suspected when a decrease in platelet count from 230,000/microliter to 5,000/microliter is noted in a client who has had coronary artery bypass graft surgery.

Thalassemia

- A chronic, inherited microcytic anemia characterized by defective hemoglobin synthesis and ineffective erythropoiesis.
- Thalassemia occurs primarily in people of Italian, Greek, African, Asian, Middle Eastern, East Indian, and Caribbean descent.
- Treatment includes chronic lifelong need for blood transfusions.

Sickle Cell Anemia

- Inherited disorder (inherit sickle hemoglobin) primarily in clients of African descent.

- ☐ A triggering event (usually deoxygenation) causes formation of sickle-shaped hemoglobin.
- ☐ Resulting in microvascular occlusion, ischemia, and infarction primarily in the bone, hands and feet, liver, and kidney.
- ☐ Sequestration of the sickle-shaped hemoglobin in the liver and a hyperhemolytic crisis increased destruction of RBCs.
- ☐ Clinical manifestations include chronic anemia, pain, jaundice, thrombosis, disability, organ damage, increased risk of infection, and possible early death.
- ☐ Assess for symptoms of acute vasoocclusive crisis causing tissue necrosis, tissue hypoxia, and inflammation.
- ☐ Teach the client about crisis triggers including stress, exercise, dehydration, elevation, and any condition that decreases oxygen.
- ☐ Hematopoietic stem cell transplant may be curative if a donor match can be found.
- ☐ Treat a crisis with narcotic analgesia, antibiotics, oxygen, hydration, steroids, blood transfusions, and arginine to enhance availability of the vasodilator nitric oxide.
- ☐ Preventative medications include hydroxyurea to prevent sickling.
- ☐ Folic acid is also given daily to enhance erythropoiesis.
- ☐ Assess for acute chest syndrome: manifested by fever, respiratory distress, and new infiltrates in the chest X-ray.
- ☐ Also, monitor liver and kidney laboratory results, LOC, and I&O.

Hemophilia

- ☐ Is an inherited bleeding disorder.
- ☐ Hemophilia A results from a deficiency of factor VIII.
- ☐ Christmas disease is also called hemophilia B and results from a factor IX deficiency.
- ☐ Assess occult bleeding (urine, stool, and joints).
- ☐ Treatment includes infusion of factor VIII or X (whatever the deficiency).
- ☐ Client and family teaching involves teaching the administration of factor concentrate at home.
- ☐ Clients must avoid agents that interfere with platelet aggregation and clotting such as NSAIDs, herbals, and alcohol.
- ☐ Teach client to watch for bleeding from nose, gums, urine, stool, and excessive menstrual flow.
- ☐ Client should wear a medical alert bracelet.
- ☐ Teach to seek emergency care for a sudden, severe headache, neuro changes, and respiratory distress.

Disseminated Intravascular Coagulation (DIC)

☐ A systemic disorder where platelets and clotting factors are consumed, resulting in microthrombi and excessive bleeding.

☐ The laboratory finding most consistent with disseminated intravascular coagulation is a low platelet count.

☐ Clinical manifestations include unusual bleeding in body orifices, petechiae, ecchymosis, hematoma formation, tachycardia, tachypnea, and change in LOC.

☐ Complications include hemorrhage, shock, and multisystem organ failure.

☐ Monitor for cardiovascular, neuro, renal, hepatic, and pulmonary status, vital signs, pulse oximetry, and cardiac monitor.

☐ Administer oxygen, intravenous fluids, and blood products.

☐ Limit invasive procedures and needle sticks.

Multiple Myeloma

☐ Characterized by malignant plasma cells that produce an increased amount of immunoglobulin that is not functional.

☐ As more malignant plasma cells are produced in multiple myeloma, there's less space in the bone marrow for red blood cell production, and anemia develops.

☐ Clinical manifestations include bone pain usually in the back or ribs, increasing during the day with movement and decreasing with rest.

☐ Laboratory results reveal elevated monoclonal protein level in the serum.

☐ Evidence of end organ damage: **C**alcium elevation, **R**enal insufficiency, **A**nemia, **B**one lesions (CRAB) assists in the diagnosis of myeloma.

☐ Diagnosis confirmed by bone marrow biopsy.

☐ Treated with dexamethasone, cyclophosphamide, and thalidomide.

☐ Radiation therapy useful in strengthening the bone at a lesion.

☐ NSAIDs given for pain and bisphosphonates used to strengthen bones and reduce bone pain.

☐ Teach the client that activity restrictions such as lifting no more than 10 pounds to prevent fractures are necessary.

☐ Teach the client to assess temperature as antibody function is impaired and infections are common and can be life-threatening.

Function of the Immune System

☐ Natural immunity is nonspecific and provides a broad spectrum of defense against and resistance to infection.

☐ Cells involved are monocytes, macrophages, dendrite cells, natural killer cells, basophils, eosinophils, and granulocytes.

☐ In cell-mediated immunity, T cells respond directly to antigens (foreign substances such as bacteria or toxins that induce antibody formation).

☐ Cell-mediated immunity involves destruction of target cells—such as virus-infected cells and cancer cells—through secretion of lymphokines (lymph proteins).

☐ Examples of cell-mediated immunity are rejection of transplanted organs and delayed immune responses that fight disease.

☐ Assessing for immune dysfunction should include fever, cough, chills and sweats, shortness of breath, stiff neck, burning with urination, increased urination, diarrhea, and new onset of soreness and pain.

☐ There are three main types of T cells: killer, helper, and suppressor T cells.

☐ T cells probably originate from stem cells in the bone marrow; the thymus gland controls their maturity, and in the process, a large number of antigen-specific cells are produced. Killer T cells bind to the surface of the invading cell, disrupt the membrane, and destroy it by altering its internal environment.

☐ Helper T cells stimulate B cells to mature into plasma cells, which begin to synthesize and secrete immunoglobulin (proteins with known antibody activity).

☐ Suppressor T cells reduce the humoral response.

☐ B cells are responsible for humoral- or immunoglobulin-mediated immunity.

☐ Neutropenia occurs when the absolute neutrophil count falls below 1,000/microliter, reflecting a severe risk for infection.

Rh-Positive Blood

☐ People with the D antigen have Rh-positive blood type.

☐ If Rh-positive blood is administered to an Rh-negative person, the recipient develops anti-Rh agglutinins.

☐ Subsequent transfusions with Rh-positive blood to an Rh-negative person may cause serious reactions with clumping and hemolysis of red blood cells.

Immunoglobulin

☐ Five major classes of immunoglobulin exist. (See Table 1.25 for classes and characteristics of immunoglobulins.)

☐ Intravenous immunoglobulin (IVIG) is an important treatment for a variety of disease states that are characterized by deficient production of antibodies.

TABLE 1.25	Classes of Immunoglobulins
Class	Characteristics
Immunoglobulin G	■ Makes up about 80% of plasma antibodies ■ Appears in all body fluids ■ The major antibacterial and antiviral antibody
Immunoglobulin M	■ First immunoglobulin produced during an immune response ■ Too large to easily cross membranes ■ Usually present only in the vascular system
Immunoglobulin A	■ Found mainly in body secretions, such as saliva, sweat, tears, mucus, bile, and colostrum ■ Defends against pathogens on body surfaces, especially those that enter the respiratory and GI tracts
Immunoglobulin D	■ Present in plasma ■ Easily broken down ■ Predominant antibody on the surface of B cells ■ Mainly an antigen receptor
Immunoglobulin E	■ Antibody involved in immediate hypersensitivity reactions or allergic reactions that develop within minutes of exposure to an antigen

☐ IVIG is administered to treat DiGeorge syndrome, common variable immunodeficiency disease, and idiopathic thrombocytopenia purpura.

☐ IV doses of 200 to 800 mg/kg/body weight administered every 3 to 4 weeks.

Human Immunodeficiency Virus (HIV)

☐ A negative HIV antibody test means that HIV antibodies weren't in the client's blood at the time the test was performed; if antibodies to HIV are present, the test result is positive.

☐ Antibodies to HIV may take 3 weeks to 6 months or longer to develop; however, the client is still infectious during this time.

☐ A diagnosis of AIDS is made if a client tests positive for HIV, has a $CD4^+$ T-cell count below 200 cells/microliter, and has one or more specific opportunistic infections or cancers along with the HIV infection.

☐ HIV is most easily transmitted in blood, semen, and vaginal secretions and has also been found in urine, feces, saliva, tears, and breast milk.

- ☐ Teach clients about safe sexual practices to decrease the risk of transmitting HIV infection to sexual partners.
- ☐ Consistent and correct use of condoms is the only effective method to decrease the risk of sexual transmission of HIV infection.
- ☐ Standard precautions must be utilized in the health care setting to prevent the risk of exposure.
- ☐ Postexposure prophylaxis includes zidovudine (ZDV) and lamivudine (3TC) or emtricitabine (FTC). Follow up with postexposure testing at 1 month, 3 months, and 6 months and possibly 1 year.
- ☐ Treatment and protocols are continually evolving to treat HIV/AIDS.
- ☐ Antiretroviral agents block the change from RNA-DNA in replication. These include reverse transcriptase inhibitors, nucleoside reverse transcriptase inhibitors (NRTIs), and nonnucleoside reverse transcriptase inhibitors (NNRTIs).
- ☐ Protease inhibitors (PIs) interfere with an enzyme that HIV uses to create infectious viral particles.
- ☐ Integrase inhibitors block insertion of DNA into host cell.
- ☐ Entry/fusion inhibitors block HIV's entry into healthy cells.
- ☐ Teach clients to take medications as prescribed to prevent drug resistance.
- ☐ Assess physical and psychosocial status, and identify potential risk factors: IV drug abuse and risky sexual practices.
- ☐ Monitor immune system function, nutritional status, skin integrity, respiratory and neurologic status, and fluid and electrolyte balance.

Rheumatoid Arthritis (RA)

- ☐ Rheumatic disease encompasses autoimmune, degenerative, inflammatory, and systemic conditions that affect the joints, muscle, and soft tissues.
- ☐ Clinical manifestation is inflammation, stiffness and pain in the joints, immobility, fatigue, and sleep disturbance.
- ☐ Degenerative joint disease is due to noninflammatory wear and tear on joints and is often seen in athletes.
- ☐ Screening tests include CBC, ESR, and rheumatoid factor and are also used to monitor the progress of RA or response to therapy.
- ☐ Treatment includes NSAIDs for mild and moderate pain, immune modulators (infliximab), steroids (prednisone), and disease-modifying antirheumatic drugs (DMARDs; sulfasalazine) to slow disease progression.

□ Head to toe assessment is essential as symptoms can show in all body systems.

□ Adequate sleep can improve pain management; low-dose antidepressant medications such as amitriptyline may be prescribed.

□ Teach client pain management techniques, good body mechanics, relaxation techniques, adequate nutrition, and coping mechanisms.

Systemic Lupus Erythematosus (SLE)

□ Is a chronic, inflammatory, autoimmune disorder that affects connective tissue throughout the body.

□ Affects women eight times more often than men; usually strikes during childbearing age.

□ Head to toe assessment of clients is essential to determine the extent of involvement.

□ Body affects include CAD, vasculitis, pneumonitis, lupus nephritis, CKD, end-stage renal disease, and vasculitis of the brain.

□ Kidney failure is the most common cause of death.

□ Clinical manifestations include a butterfly rash (superficial lesions over the cheeks and nose), other skin rashes, photosensitivity, oral ulcers, joint pain, renal problems, blood disorders, infections, and neurologic problems including seizure.

□ Pancytopenia (anemia, thrombocytopenia, leukopenia, and neutropenia) and elevated antinuclear antibody titer support the diagnosis of SLE.

□ Pain management includes NSAIDs, corticosteroids, antimalarial agents (hydroxychloroquine), and cytotoxic agents (methotrexate).

□ DMARDs (belimumab) suppress immune response.

□ Teach the client about infection symptoms, rest periods, smoking cessation, bleeding precautions, and skin protection from sun and harsh chemicals.

Hodgkin Lymphoma

□ Cancer of the lymphatic system spreading throughout the body.

□ In stage I of Hodgkin disease, symptoms include a single enlarged lymph node (usually), unexplained fever, night sweats, malaise, and generalized pruritus.

□ Clinical manifestations include swollen cervical, axilla, and groin lymph nodes, fatigue, unintended weight loss, fever, and night sweats.

□ Diagnosed with lymph node biopsy revealing Reed-Sternberg cells.

□ Laboratory tests may reveal mild anemia and elevated ESR.

☐ Herpes zoster infection is a common secondary infection.

☐ Treatment involves 2 to 4 months of chemotherapy and radiation therapy.

☐ Standard pharmacologic therapy includes doxorubicin, bleomycin, vinblastine, and dacarbazine (ABVD therapy).

☐ Client teaching about chemotherapy side effects is essential and the possible development of secondary cancers later in life.

REVIEW QUESTIONS ▐▐▐▐▐▐▐

1. A nurse is assessing a client with heart failure. The breath sounds commonly auscultated in clients with heart failure are:
  1. tracheal.
  2. fine crackles.
  3. coarse crackles.
  4. friction rubs.

2. When suctioning the respiratory tract of a client, it is recommended that the suctioning period not exceed how many seconds?
  1. 5 seconds.
  2. 10 seconds.
  3. 15 seconds.
  4. 20 seconds.

3. A client with chronic renal failure is receiving hemodialysis three times a week. To protect the fistula, the nurse should:
  1. keep the fistula at heart level.
  2. apply an elastic bandage to the fistula site.
  3. palpate for a thrill and auscultate for a bruit over the fistula.
  4. start an IV in the fistula site for dialysis use.

4. A nurse is obtaining assessment data on a client diagnosed with acute kidney injury. Which finding warrants calling the health care provider?
  1. Respiratory rate of 16 breaths per minute
  2. Sodium level 145 mEq/L
  3. Blood urea nitrogen (BUN) 25 mg/dL
  4. Peaked T waves on electrocardiogram

5. Which of the following is a risk factor for the development of pressure ulcers?
  1. Ambulating less than twice a day
  2. An indwelling urinary catheter
  3. Decreased serum albumin level
  4. Elevated white blood cell count

Chapter References

Baranoski, S., & Ayello, E. (2015). *Wound care essentials* (4th ed.). Philadelphia, PA: Wolters Kluwer.

DeVita, V., Lawrence, T., & Rosenberg, S. (Eds.). (2015). *Cancer principles and practice of oncology.* (10th ed.). Philadelphia, PA: Wolters Kluwer.

Farrell, M., & Dempsey, J. (2013). *Smeltzer & Bare's textbook of medical-surgical nursing* (3rd ed.). Philadelphia, PA: Wolters Kluwer.

Hinkle, J. L., & Cheever, K. H. (2013). *Brunner & Suddarth's textbook of medical-surgical nursing* (13th ed.). Philadelphia, PA: Lippincott Williams & Wilkins.

Taylor, C., Lillis, C., & Lynn, P. (2014). *Fundamentals of nursing: The art and science of person-centered nursing* (8th ed.). Philadelphia, PA: Wolters Kluwer.

2

Maternal-Neonatal Care

ANTEPARTUM CARE

KEY TERMS

- [ ] **Antepartum care** refers to care of a mother before childbirth.
- [ ] **Zygote** refers to a fertilized egg.
- [ ] **Linea nigra** is a pigmented line extending from the symphysis pubis to the top of the fundus during pregnancy.
- [ ] **Striae gravidarum**, or stretch marks, are slightly depressed streaks that commonly occur over the abdomen, breast, and thighs during the second half of pregnancy.
- [ ] **Gravida** refers to the number of times a woman has been pregnant.
- [ ] **Para** refers to the number of pregnancies completed after 20 weeks' gestation regardless of whether neonates were alive.
- [ ] **Braxton Hicks contractions** are painless uterine contractions that occur throughout pregnancy.
- [ ] **Quickening** refers to fetal movement felt as fluttering in the abdomen; it is distinguishable between 16 and 22 weeks' gestation.
- [ ] **Ballottement**—on pelvic examination, if the lower uterine segment is tapped sharply by the lower examining hand, the fetus is felt to bounce in the amniotic fluid up against the top examining hand.
- [ ] **Oligohydramnios** is less than the normal amount of amniotic fluid.
- [ ] **Hydramnios** is more than the normal amount of amniotic fluid.

Early Pregnancy

- [ ] Fertilization occurs in the fallopian tube when the nuclei of a sperm and ovum unite.
- [ ] The fertilized egg is called a zygote and contains 23 pairs of chromosomes (22 pairs of autosomal chromosomes and 1 pair of sex chromosomes).

TABLE 2.1	GTPAL
Letter	Indicates
G	Gravida—The number of times a woman has been pregnant
T	Term—The number of term pregnancies completed at 37 weeks' gestation or after
P	Preterm—The number of preterm pregnancies completed between 20 and 37 weeks' gestation
A	Abortion—The number of pregnancies ending before 20 weeks' gestation
L	Living—The number of children currently living

☐ The zygote undergoes rapid cell division as it migrates to the endometrium of the fundal region of the uterus, where it implants about 7 to 9 days after fertilization.

☐ After implantation, the endometrium is called the decidua.

☐ To calculate the estimated date of birth with Nägele's rule, determine the first day of the last menstrual period, subtract 3 months, and add 7 days.

☐ See Table 2.1 for more information on GTPAL.

☐ See Table 2.2 for common signs of pregnancy.

TABLE 2.2	Common Signs of Pregnancy	
Presumptive	Probable	Positive
■ Breast changes ■ Amenorrhea ■ Nausea/vomiting ■ Uterine enlargement ■ Quickening ■ Striae/linea nigra	■ Positive pregnancy tests (urine and/or blood) ■ Chadwick sign—color change of the vagina from pink to violet ■ Goodell sign—softening of the cervix ■ Hegar sign—softening of the lower uterine segment	■ Ultrasound visualization of fetus ■ Positive FHR ■ Fetal movements felt by the examiner

TABLE 2.3	Fetal Membranes
Membrane	Description
Chorion	■ Closest to the uterine wall ■ Gives rise to the placenta
Amnion	■ The thin, tough, inner fetal membrane that lines the amniotic sac

Embryonic/Fetal Structures and Functions
☐ See Table 2.3 for facts covering fetal membranes.

Embryonic Germ Layers
☐ The embryonic germ layers generate fetal tissue. (See Table 2.4 for more information on embryonic germ layers.)

Umbilical Cord
☐ The umbilical cord serves as the lifeline from the embryo to the placenta.

☐ The umbilical cord contains two arteries, one vein, and Wharton's jelly (which prevents kinking of the cord in utero).

Amniotic Fluid
☐ Amniotic fluid prevents heat loss, preserves constant fetal body temperature, cushions the fetus, and facilitates fetal growth and development.

☐ Oligohydramnios (less than the normal amount of amniotic fluid) may be associated with variable decelerations due to decreased cushion for the umbilical cord.

TABLE 2.4	Embryonic Germ Layers
Embryonic Germ Layer	Purpose
The ectoderm (outer)	■ Generates the epidermis, nervous system, pituitary gland, salivary glands, optic lens, lining of the lower portion of the anal canal, hair, and tooth enamel
The endoderm (inner)	■ Generates the epithelial lining of the larynx, trachea, bladder, urethra, prostate gland, auditory canal, liver, pancreas, and alimentary canal
The mesoderm (middle)	■ Generates the connective and supporting tissues; the blood and vascular system; the musculature; teeth (except enamel); mesothelial lining of the pericardial, pleural, and peritoneal cavities; and kidneys and ureters

- Amnioinfusion may be used to provide additional fluid, decreasing cord compression and the severity of variable decelerations.
- Hydramnios (more than the normal amount of amniotic fluid) may be associated with uterine rupture or cord accidents.

Placenta
- The placenta is an organ attached to the uterine wall that provides the fetus with oxygenation, nutrients, and waste removal.
- The umbilical cord attaches from the placenta to the fetus.

Human Chorionic Gonadotropin
- Human chorionic gonadotropin (HCG) is a glycoprotein hormone produced in pregnancy that is made by the developing embryo after conception and later by the placenta.
- HCG increases in a woman's blood and urine to fairly large concentrations until the 15th week of pregnancy.

Physiologic Changes of Pregnancy
- A pregnant woman breathes deeper, which increases the tidal volume of gas moved in and out of the respiratory tract with each breath.
- The oxygen consumption in the pregnant woman is greater than in the nonpregnant state.
- During pregnancy, there is a slight increase in respiratory rate.
- Pregnancy creates an increase in intravascular volume and workload of the heart.
- Benign systolic murmurs are heard in up to 90% of pregnant clients; the murmur disappears soon after birth.
- Approximately 40% of a woman's cardiac output is delivered to the uterus; therefore, blood loss can occur quite rapidly in the event of uncontrolled bleeding.
- Heart rate may increase up to 15 beats/minute by the end of pregnancy.
- Systolic and diastolic blood pressures may decrease slightly by the end of pregnancy.
- As pregnancy advances, the apical pulse may be found slightly higher than the fourth intercostal space because of uterine displacement of the diaphragm.
- The white blood cell count rises slightly in pregnancy.
- Physiologic anemia occurs when hemoglobin and hematocrit values decrease during pregnancy due to the increase in plasma volume exceeding the increase in red blood cell production.
- The linea nigra is a pigmented line extending from the symphysis pubis to the top of the fundus during pregnancy.

- Striae gravidarum, or stretch marks, are slightly depressed streaks that commonly occur over the abdomen, breast, and thighs during the second half of pregnancy.
- Breasts enlarge and begin to produce colostrum by the 16th week.
- The uterus grows at a consistent rate. Fundal height is measured in centimeters from the symphysis pubis to the top of the uterus.
- Fundal height correlates roughly with the week of gestation and is one way to assess fetal growth over the course of the pregnancy.
- At 20 weeks' gestation, fundal height should be at about the umbilicus.

Common Pregnancy Discomforts

- Nausea and vomiting should subside by the end of the first trimester; if they don't, the nurse should suspect an undiagnosed problem, such as hyperemesis gravidarum or other factors that may be exacerbating the nausea and vomiting. Dehydration must be corrected.
- Leukorrhea, increased vaginal discharge, generally occurs during the first trimester and decreases at the end of this period.
- Leg cramps, ankle edema, heart burn, and shortness of breath are normal during the second and third trimesters.
- Eating small, frequent meals will place less pressure on the esophageal sphincter, reducing the likelihood of esophageal reflux.

Vena Cava Syndrome

- As the enlarging uterus increases pressure on the inferior vena cava, it compromises venous return, which can cause dizziness, light-headedness, and pallor when the client is supine.
- Vena cava syndrome could impair blood flow to the uterus, possibly decreasing oxygen to the fetus.
- The nurse can relieve symptoms of dizziness, light-headedness, and pallor in the supine maternity client by turning the client on her left side, which relieves pressure on the vena cava and restores venous return.

PREGNANCY SURVEILLANCE

- When assessing a pregnant client, remember that although the mother and fetus have separate and distinct needs, they have an interdependent relationship.
- Factors that influence the mother's health can also affect the fetus, and changes in fetal well-being can influence the mother's physical and emotional health.
- The first prenatal visit includes a physical exam, blood serum studies, detailed history, risk identification, and health promotion and education.
- The blood pressure, urine protein, weight, fundal height, fetal heart rate, and fetal movements are monitored during all prenatal visits.

- ☐ In healthy pregnancy, prenatal visits occur monthly through 28 weeks, every 2 weeks until 36 weeks, and then weekly until 40 weeks.
- ☐ Daily fetal movement counts are an easy way for pregnant women to monitor fetal well-being.
- ☐ Ultrasounds are used during pregnancy to ensure healthy anatomy, measure amniotic fluid, determine fetal growth, assess the placenta, and identify risks.
- ☐ Teach pregnant women to report danger signs: decreased fetal movement, bleeding, fluid leaking, contractions, and fever.

Ectopic Pregnancy

- ☐ Ectopic pregnancy occurs when a pregnancy implants outside of the uterus.
- ☐ The most common site of an ectopic pregnancy is the fallopian tube.
- ☐ An ectopic pregnancy is more likely in women with a history of pelvic inflammatory disease or previous ectopic pregnancy.
- ☐ Clinical manifestations of ectopic pregnancy include bleeding referred shoulder pain, and unilateral stabbing abdominal pain.
- ☐ If ectopic pregnancy is suspected, an ultrasound will be performed to confirm the diagnosis.
- ☐ Ectopic pregnancy may spontaneously end, but may require interventions such as methotrexate injections or laparoscopic surgery to prevent rupture.
- ☐ A ruptured ectopic pregnancy causes severe hemorrhage and requires emergency life-saving surgery to remove the pregnancy. Clients will likely require volume support with blood transfusions.

Gestational Trophoblastic Disease (Hydatidiform Mole)

- ☐ Gestational trophoblastic disease occurs when there is rapid deterioration of trophoblastic cells that fill with fluid. The embryo fails to develop.
- ☐ Ultrasound is the technique of choice in diagnosing gestational trophoblastic disease.
- ☐ Clinical manifestations of gestational trophoblastic disease include bleeding during the first half of pregnancy, hyperemesis, hypertensive disorders of pregnancy, absent fetal heart tones, and rapidly enlarging uterus.
- ☐ Bleeding with gestational trophoblastic disease is often dark brown (resembles prune juice) and may occur erratically for weeks or months.
- ☐ There is a risk of choriocarcinoma following gestational trophoblastic disease, which requires monitoring.
- ☐ Treatment for gestational trophoblastic disease is a dilation and curettage (D&C) to remove the abnormal cells, and clients may require volume support with blood transfusions.

TABLE 2.5 TORCH Infections	
Teratogen	Prevention
Toxoplasmosis	■ Avoid cat feces ■ Cook all food to appropriate temperatures
Others ■ Syphilis, Hepatitis, HIV ■ Varicella ■ Parvovirus B19	■ Practice safe sex, no IV drug use, and get proper screening for disease ■ Vaccination ■ Avoid people infected with illness
Rubella	■ Vaccination ■ Avoid people infected with illness
Cytomegalovirus	■ Avoid people infected with illness
Herpes simplex virus	■ Practice safe sex

☐ Monitor for blood loss and grief, and ensure client has serial monitoring of HCG levels to monitor for development of choriocarcinoma.

TORCH Infections

☐ TORCH is an acronym for a group of diseases that cause congenital conditions if a fetus is exposed. Pregnant women should be counseled on prevention, and providers should monitor for development of any TORCH conditions to ensure proper care. (See Table 2.5 for more information on TORCH infections.)

Group B Beta-Hemolytic Strep Infection (GBS)

☐ GBS are normal skin bacteria.

☐ Pregnant women who carry GBS are at risk to pass the bacteria to neonates during the birth process.

☐ GBS infection is associated with neonatal sepsis and death.

☐ Screen all pregnancies for GBS at 35 to 36 weeks' gestation with a vaginal/rectal culture.

☐ Clients with positive GBS screens will be treated during labor with IV penicillin to prevent transition of the bacteria to the neonate during birth.

☐ Neonates will be monitored for development of sepsis.

Gestational Diabetes

☐ All pregnant clients are screened for gestational diabetes at 24 to 28 weeks. High-risk clients may have an early screen.

☐ The screen is a 1-hour glucose tolerance test.

☐ If the screen is positive, gestational diabetes is diagnosed with a 3-hour glucose tolerance test.

☐ A woman with diabetes has an increased risk for perinatal complications, including hypertension, preeclampsia, and neonatal hypoglycemia.

☐ During pregnancy of a diabetic client, the fetus secretes high levels of insulin to counteract the high maternal glucose levels, which may result in severe hypoglycemia after birth.

☐ Clients should monitor and record blood glucose levels fasting, 2 hours after meals, and before bedtime.

☐ Clients with gestational diabetes are usually managed by diet alone to control their glucose intolerance. If glucose levels cannot be controlled, oral medication or insulin may be used.

☐ Teach the client about an American Diabetic Association (ADA) diet, blood glucose monitoring, and monitoring fetal movement.

Hypertensive Disorders

☐ Gestational hypertension refers to elevated blood pressure without proteinuria in a woman after 20 weeks' gestation; blood pressure levels return to normal in these clients postpartum.

☐ Criteria for diagnosing preeclampsia include a blood pressure of either:

○ A blood pressure of ≥140 mm Hg systolic or ≥90 mm Hg diastolic PLUS the presence of proteinuria *OR*

○ An increase in prepregnancy baseline of ≥30 mm Hg systolic or ≥15 mm Hg diastolic *PLUS* the presence of proteinuria

☐ Preeclampsia is a syndrome defined by hypertension and proteinuria that may be associated with other signs and symptoms, such as edema, visual disturbances, headache, increased deep tendon reflexes, and epigastric pain.

☐ The incidence of preeclampsia in obese clients is about seven times greater than that in nonobese pregnant clients.

☐ Eclampsia occurs when the pregnant woman develops seizures or coma in the presence of symptoms of preeclampsia.

☐ Women with preeclampsia may develop peripheral edema and increased deep tendon reflexes.

☐ Women with severe preeclampsia may develop HELLP syndrome (**H** = hemolysis; **EL** = elevated liver enzymes; **LP** = low platelet count), a multiple organ failure syndrome that may lead to death if untreated.

☐ Treatment for gestational hypertension includes bed rest lying left lateral position, low environmental stimuli, monitoring for worsening symptoms, and increased fetal surveillance.

☐ If oral medications are required to treat hypertension, labetalol, nifedipine, or hydralazine is used.

☐ Teach the client to maintain bed rest and monitor for severe headache, visual changes, epigastric/right upper quadrant pain, increased edema/weight gain, and daily fetal kick counts.

Magnesium Sulfate

☐ Magnesium sulfate may be administered to pregnant clients with preeclampsia/eclampsia to prevent seizures and lower blood pressure.

☐ The anticonvulsant mechanism of magnesium is believed to depress seizure foci in the brain and peripheral neuromuscular activity.

☐ Monitor the client closely for respiratory depression, decreased urine output, severely diminished deep tendon reflexes, level of consciousness, respiratory function, and magnesium toxicity.

☐ Calcium gluconate is the antidote for magnesium toxicity and should be at the bedside.

Human Immunodeficiency Virus (HIV)

☐ A mother can transmit HIV to her child transplacentally at various gestational ages, perinatally through maternal blood and body fluids, and postnatally through breast milk.

☐ Administration of zidovudine antiretroviral therapy to HIV-positive pregnant women significantly reduces the risk of transmission to the fetus.

☐ Teach the client to monitor fetal movement and take prescribed antiretroviral therapy.

Rh Isoimmunization

☐ Rh isoimmunization occurs when Rh-positive fetal blood cells cross into the maternal circulation of an Rh-negative woman and stimulate maternal antibody production.

☐ In subsequent pregnancies with Rh-positive fetuses, maternal antibodies may cross back into the fetal circulation and destroy the fetal blood cells in Rh isoimmunization.

☐ $Rh_o(D)$ immune globulin (RhoGAM) is given prophylactically around 28 weeks to pregnant women with Rh-negative blood to prevent antibody formation from Rh-positive conceptions. It is also given anytime they experience bleeding during pregnancy.

☐ Teach all pregnant women with Rh-negative blood to seek their providers anytime they experience bleeding during pregnancy.

Acute Pyelonephritis

☐ Pyelonephritis is infection of the kidney and is a serious condition in a pregnant client.

☐ Clinical manifestations include fever, nausea, vomiting, malaise, unilateral flank pain, and costovertebral angle tenderness.

☐ A urinalysis will reveal RBCs, WBCs, and bacteria. Collect blood and urine cultures.

- Medications include a dose of IV antibiotics and then switching to PO, analgesia, antipyretics, and IV fluids.
- Monitor I & O, urine color and clarity, vital signs, and pain level.
- Encourage increased fluids and rest.
- Teach the client to return if she becomes more lethargic, cannot keep food or fluids down, or has increased pain, vaginal bleeding, contractions, or decreased fetal movement.

Placental Abnormalities

- See Table 2.6 for facts covering placenta previa and placental abruption.
- A marginal placenta previa is characterized by implantation of the placenta in the margin of the cervical os, not covering the os.
- In a partial placenta previa, the placenta partially occludes the cervical os.
- In a total placenta previa, the internal cervical os is completely covered by the placenta.
- In clients with placenta previa, fetal surveillance through ultrasound examination every 2 to 3 weeks is indicated to evaluate fetal growth, amniotic fluid, and placental location.

TABLE 2.6	Placenta Previa and Placental Abruption	
	Placenta Previa	Placental Abruption
Definition	Placenta is implanted in the lower part of the uterus and occludes the cervix	Premature separation of the placenta
Risk factors	■ Increased parity ■ Advanced maternal age ■ Past cesarean birth	■ Increased parity ■ Advanced maternal age ■ Short umbilical cord ■ Hypertension ■ Trauma ■ Cocaine abuse
Symptoms	■ Painless bright red bleeding	■ Painful bright red bleeding, rigid abdomen
Treatment	■ Monitor for blood loss ■ Monitor fetal well-being (heart tones, ultrasounds for growth) ■ No cervical exams ■ Cesarean birth ■ May require volume support	■ Immediate cesarean birth (high risk of death for fetus and mother) ■ May require volume support

- ☐ Placenta accreta/percreta/increta is the abnormal attachment of the placenta too deeply in the uterus. It may attach to or through the myometrium of the uterus and even into other tissue.

Multiple Gestation

- ☐ Twins can be monozygotic (identical) or dizygotic (fraternal).
- ☐ Pregnancies with multiple gestation are considered high risk.
- ☐ Multiple gestation requires more frequent monitoring and fetal surveillance.
- ☐ Multiple gestations have higher risk for hypertension, preterm labor, and cesarean section.
- ☐ Antenatal steroids may be given to clients between 24 and 34 weeks' gestation to enhance fetal lung maturity in conditions that may require early birth.
- ☐ With a twin or other multiple gestations, the fetuses can be in several presentation combinations: both vertex, both breech, one vertex and one in transverse lie, or one vertex and one breech.

Nonstress Test

- ☐ The nonstress test is the preferred antepartum heart rate screening test for pregnant clients in the third trimester with complications. It is performed with an electronic fetal monitor.
- ☐ A reactive nonstress test is two or more fetal heart rate (FHR) accelerations that exceed the baseline by at least 15 beats/minute lasting 15 seconds within a 20-minute period in the presence of fetal movement.
- ☐ A nonstress test is based on the theory that a healthy fetus will have transient FHR accelerations in response to fetal movement.
- ☐ Teach clients that there is no preparation required. Clients will be connected to an external fetal monitor for at least 20 minutes and the test is interpreted in the provider office or hospital.

Fetal Heart Rate (FHR) Variability

- ☐ Baseline FHR variability refers to fluctuations in the baseline FHR that are irregular in amplitude and frequency. (See Table 2.7 for more information on FHR variability.)

Fetal Heart Rate (FHR) Decelerations

- ☐ A variable deceleration is an abrupt decrease in FHR of 15 beats/minute or greater, lasting 15 seconds or more, and less than 2 minutes in duration.
- ☐ An early deceleration is a gradual decrease in FHR lasting ≥30 seconds, with lowest point of deceleration occurring with the peak of a contraction.

TABLE 2.7 Fetal Heart Rate Variability

Variability	Interpretation
Absent variability	No baseline fluctuation.
Minimal variability	Baseline fluctuates by 5 beats/minute or fewer.
Moderate or normal variability	Baseline fluctuates from 6 to 25 beats/minute.
Marked variability	Baseline fluctuates >25 beats/minute.

☐ A late deceleration is a gradual decrease in FHR lasting ≥30 seconds, with the onset of the deceleration occurring after the beginning of the contraction and the lowest point of the contraction occurring after the peak of the contraction.

☐ A prolonged deceleration of the FHR is a visually apparent decrease from the baseline that is 15 beats/minute or more, lasting 2 minutes or more but less than 10 minutes.

☐ If a FHR deceleration lasts longer than 10 minutes, it is considered a baseline change. (See Table 2.8 for more information on FHR decelerations.)

TABLE 2.8 Fetal Heart Rate Decelerations

VEAL CHOP (Acronym for Fetal Heart Rate Deceleration Patterns)				Nursing Action
V	Variable deceleration	**C**	Cord compression	■ Position change ■ If no improvement/severe, apply oxygen at 10 L/min by mask ■ Stop oxytocin ■ Contact provider ■ May require amnioinfusion
E	Early deceleration	**H**	Head compression	■ Document ■ Check cervical status
A	Acceleration	**O**	OK and normal	■ Document
L	Late deceleration	**P**	Placental insufficiency/problem	■ Position change ■ Apply oxygen at 10 L/min by mask ■ Stop oxytocin ■ Contact the provider

INTRAPARTUM CARE

KEY TERMS

- [ ] **Intrapartum care** refers to care of the client during labor.
- [ ] **Fetal station** or **fetal descent** is the relationship of the fetal presenting part to the pelvic ischial spines.
- [ ] **Cervical dilation** is the increasing of the size of the cervical os from 0 to 10 cm.
- [ ] **Cervical effacement** is cervical thinning and shortening, which is measured from 0% (thick) to 100% (paper thin).

Fetal Attitude

- [ ] Fetal attitude refers to the relationship of the fetal parts (such as the chest, chin, or arms) to one another during the passage through the birth canal.
- [ ] Flexion is the normal fetal attitude (the fetal position).
- [ ] Extension could make birth difficult.
- [ ] See Figure 2.1 for an illustration of fetal station.

Fetal Lie

- [ ] The relationship of the long axis of the fetus to the long axis of the mother refers to fetal lie. (See Fig. 2.2 for an illustration of fetal lie.)
- [ ] There are three possible fetal lies: longitudinal, transverse, and oblique.
- [ ] See Table 2.9 for Leopold Maneuvers.

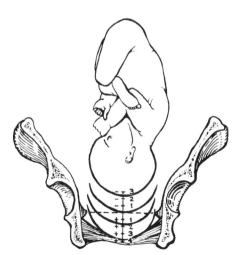

Figure 2.1 Fetal station is the relationship of the fetal presenting part to the pelvic ischial spines. It is designated by centimeters above (−) or below (+) the ischial spines. When the presenting part is even with the ischial spines (0), the fetus is said to be engaged.

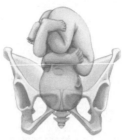

A. Longitudinal lie

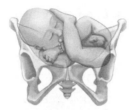

B. Transverse lie

Figure 2.2 Fetal lie. Fetal lie is the relationship of the long axis of the fetus to the long axis of the mother. **A.** Longitudinal lie occurs when the long axis of the fetus is parallel to that of the mother (fetal spine to maternal spine side-by-side). **B.** Transverse lie occurs when the long axis of the fetus is perpendicular to the long axis of the mother (fetal spine lies across the maternal abdomen and crosses her spine).

Assessing Fetal Heart Tones

☐ Fetal heart tones are best auscultated over the back fetal shoulder. Leopold maneuver assists in placement of the Doppler.

☐ When the fetus is in the breech position, fetal heart tones are heard at or above the level of the umbilicus.

TABLE 2.9	Leopold Maneuvers
Maneuver	Action
First	Palpate the fundus to determine consistency, shape, and mobility of the fetus.
Second	Palpate both sides of the abdomen to determine the direction the fetal back is facing.
Third	Palpate the symphysis pubis to determine the part of the fetus engaged in the inlet.
Fourth	The fourth maneuver will help to determine flexion or extension of the fetal head and neck.

☐ Fetal tachycardia and excessive fetal activity are the first signs of fetal hypoxia.

☐ Accelerations in the FHR strip indicate normal oxygenation, whereas decelerations in the FHR sometimes indicate abnormal fetal oxygenation.

☐ A normal FHR is 120 to 160 beats/minute.

☐ Baseline fetal tachycardia is an FHR greater than 160 beats/minute.

☐ Baseline fetal bradycardia is an FHR less than 110 beats/minute.

Cardinal Movements

☐ As the fetus moves through the birth canal, it goes through position changes to ensure that the smallest diameter of fetal head presents to the smallest diameter of the birth canal.

☐ Termed the cardinal mechanisms or movements of labor, these position changes occur in the following sequence: descent, flexion, internal rotation, extension, external rotation, and expulsion.

Fetal Presentation

☐ Fetal presentation refers to the relationship of the fetus to the cervix.

☐ Fetal presentation is assessed through vaginal examination, abdominal inspection and palpation, sonography, or auscultation of fetal heart tones.

☐ Fetal presentation indicates which part of the fetus will pass through the cervix first during birth.

☐ Cephalic fetal presentations are head presentations that include vertex, brow, sinciput, and mentum. (See Fig. 2.3 for cephalic fetal presentations.)

☐ A vertex presentation (flexion of the fetal head) is the optimal presentation for passage through the birth canal.

☐ A breech presentation is when the presenting part is not the head. (See Fig. 2.4 for breech presentations.)

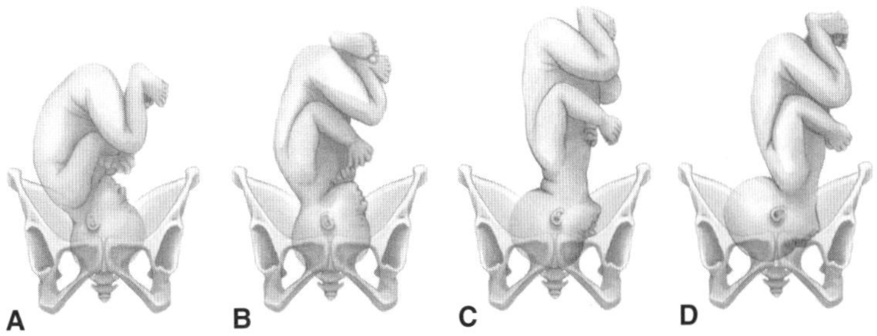

Figure 2.3 Cephalic presentations. **A.** Vertex. **B.** Sinciput. **C.** Brow. **D.** Mentum (face).

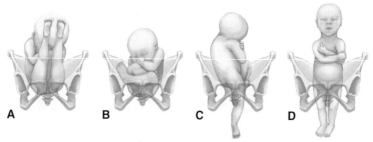

Figure 2.4   Breech presentations. **A.** Complete breech. **B.** Frank breech. **C.** Single footling. **D.** Double footling.

Fetal Position

☐ Fetal position is the relationship of the presenting part of the fetus to a specific quadrant of the mother's pelvis.

☐ Fetal position influences the progression of labor and helps determine whether surgical intervention is needed. Occiput anterior positioning is ideal for vaginal birth.

☐ During a vaginal examination of a client in labor, if the nurse palpates the fetus's larger, diamond-shaped fontanel toward the anterior portion of the client's pelvis, the fetal position is occiput posterior.

☐ Occiput posterior position of the fetus commonly produces intense back pain during labor.

☐ Positioning the client on her side can facilitate the rotation from occiput posterior to occiput anterior position.

☐ Posterior positioning of the fetal head can make it difficult for the head to pass under the maternal symphysis pubis bone.

Cervix

☐ Cervical dilation is the increasing of the size of the cervical os from 0 to 10 cm.

☐ Cervical effacement is cervical thinning and shortening, which is measured from 0% (thick) to 100% (paper thin).

Uterine Contractions

☐ Oxytocin is the hormone responsible for stimulating uterine contractions.

☐ Oxytocin may be administered to augment or induce uterine contractions and requires electronic monitoring and more frequent assessment.

☐ True contractions are regular and predictable, increasing in frequency and intensity, causing cervical effacement and dilation.

☐ True contractions are felt initially in the lower back and radiate to the abdomen in a wavelike motion.

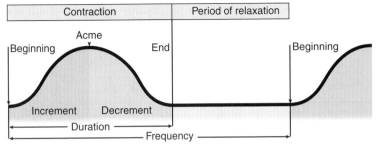

Figure 2.5 Phases of a uterine contraction. The increment is the building up of the contraction. The acme is the contraction's highest point or peak intensity and the decrement is the decreasing intensity of the contraction. A period of relaxation normally follows the contraction.

- □ Contractions are measured by duration, intensity, and frequency (DIF). (See Fig. 2.5 for the phases of a uterine contraction.)
- □ Contraction duration is measured from the beginning of the increment of the contraction to the end of the decrement of the contraction.
- □ Contraction duration averages 30 seconds early in labor and 60 to 90 seconds later in labor.
- □ Contraction frequency is measured from the beginning of one contraction to the beginning of the next.
- □ Contraction frequency averages 5 to 30 minutes apart early in labor and 2 to 3 minutes apart later in labor.
- □ Contraction intensity is assessed during the acme phase and can be measured with an intrauterine catheter or by palpation.
- □ It is important that the uterus has at least 60 seconds of rest between contractions.

Labor
- □ During labor, cervical dilation and effacement occur.
- □ Labor progress can be directly assessed only through cervical examination.
- □ A report of rectal pressure usually indicates a low presenting fetal part, signaling imminent birth.
- □ See Tables 2.10 and 2.11 for more information on the stages of labor and the phases in the first stage of labor.

Amniotomy
- □ An amniotomy is an artificial rupture of membranes by a trained practitioner.
- □ When the amniotic membranes are ruptured, the umbilical cord may enter the birth canal with the gush of fluid and the presenting part may cause cord compression.

TABLE 2.10   Stages of Labor

First Stage	Second Stage	Third Stage	Fourth Stage

▪ Period from the onset of true labor to complete dilation of the cervix
▪ Broken into three phases: latent, active, and transitional
▪ Primiparous: from 6 to 18 h
▪ Multiparous: from 2 to 10 h
	▪ Period from complete dilation to birth
	▪ Primiparous:
	   ● 40 min (20 contractions)
	▪ Multiparous:
	   ● 20 min (10 contractions)
		▪ Period from birth of the neonate to expulsion of the placenta and lasts from 5 to 30 min	▪ Period from 1 to 4 h after birth

☐ The most important assessment with amniotomy is FHR. A sudden drop in FHR is indicative of prolapsed cord.

☐ Amniotic fluid should be clear and free from debris and odor. Green/brown/yellow-stained fluid may indicate infection or meconium.

☐ After amniotomy, contractions may intensify.

☐ Monitor fetal heart tones, contractions, and maternal temperature after an amniotomy is performed.

☐ Provide pericare and limit cervical exams.

Epidural Anesthesia

☐ The client should be placed on her left side or sitting upright, with her shoulders parallel and legs slightly flexed, for an epidural block.

TABLE 2.11   Phases in the First Stage of Labor

Latent	Active	Transitional
▪ Cervix is dilated 0-3 cm. ▪ Contractions are irregular. ▪ Cervical effacement is almost complete. ▪ Client may experience anticipation, excitement, or apprehension.	▪ Cervix is dilated 4-7 cm. ▪ Cervical effacement is complete. ▪ Contractions are about 5-8 min apart and last 45-60 s with moderate-to-strong intensity.	▪ Cervix is dilated 8-10 cm. ▪ Contractions are about 1-2 min apart and last 60-90 s with strong intensity.

□ The client's back shouldn't be flexed for an epidural block because this position increases the possibility that the dura may be punctured and the anesthetic will accidentally be given as spinal, not epidural, anesthesia.

□ One of the major adverse effects of epidural administration is hypotension. Administering a bolus of IV fluid prior to placement of epidural can decrease the risk for hypotension.

Amniocentesis

□ An amniocentesis is the withdrawal of amniotic fluid through the abdomen with assistance of ultrasound.

□ The procedure is done to collect diagnostic information on the fetus or to analyze the amniotic fluid.

□ Before amniocentesis, the client should void to empty the bladder to reduce the risk of bladder perforation.

□ Risks of amniocentesis include PROMs fetal injury, infection, and Rh isoimmunization.

□ Monitor for fetal well-being, contractions, and fluid leaking.

□ Rh-negative clients will need prophylactic $Rh_o(D)$ immune globulin.

Advanced Fetal Monitoring

□ A contraction stress test measures the fetal response to uterine contractions on an electronic fetal monitor.

□ A biophysical profile combines a nonstress test with ultrasound imaging to determine fetal well-being.

□ A score ranges from 0 to 10, with 10 being a perfect score.

○ A score of 8 to 10 is considered normal.

○ A score of 6 is considered borderline.

○ A score of 5 and under requires immediate intervention and possible birth.

Cephalopelvic Disproportion (CPD)

□ Narrowing of the birth canal at the inlet, midpelvis, or outlet causes a disproportion between the size of the fetal head and the pelvic diameters, or cephalopelvic disproportion (CPD).

□ CPD results in failure of labor to progress and necessitates a cesarean birth.

□ Monitor the client's vital signs, contractions, and any signs and symptoms of fetal distress.

□ Prepare the client for probable cesarean birth.

Preterm Labor

□ Preterm labor is onset of labor before 37 weeks' gestation.

- ☐ Medical attempts to stop labor are attempted if the fetus is not in distress, the membranes are intact, and the cervix has not had advanced dilation.
- ☐ Tocolytics are used to stop labor contractions.
- ☐ Terbutaline is a common tocolytic that may cause maternal pulmonary edema and tachycardia.
- ☐ Magnesium sulfate is sometimes used as a tocolytic for its neuromuscular effect on uterine contractions. (See gestational hypertension for monitoring info.)
- ☐ Corticosteroids may be administered to mothers between 24 and 34 weeks' gestation to aid fetal lung maturity if preterm birth is impending.
- ☐ Maintain the client on bed rest and pelvic rest.
- ☐ Teach clients to report any decrease in fetal movement, increase in contractions, increased pelvic pressure, vaginal bleeding, or fluid leaking.

Meconium
- ☐ Meconium in the amniotic fluid is a sign of fetal distress and is not a normal finding, even during a prolonged birth.
- ☐ Amnioinfusion may be used during labor to thin meconium.
- ☐ Suctioning the neonate's mouth and nose as soon as the head is delivered is necessary to prevent aspiration.
- ☐ Meconium aspiration is meconium aspirated into the lungs during birth.
- ☐ Monitor neonate's APGAR score, lung sounds, cyanosis, and signs of respiratory distress.
- ☐ Neonate will be transferred to the neonatal intensive care unit (NICU) for respiratory assistance, antibiotics, and careful monitoring of vital signs and oxygenation.

Premature Rupture of Membranes (PROMs)
- ☐ PROM is the rupture of membranes beyond 37 weeks' gestation but before the onset of labor.
- ☐ With preterm premature rupture of membranes (PPROMs) in a client under 37 weeks' gestation, cervical examinations are contraindicated to reduce the incidence of infection.
- ☐ Confirmation of ruptured amniotic membranes is done with nitrazine paper and a positive ferning test.
- ☐ Rupture of membranes increases the risk of infection. Nursing care should include fetal monitoring, pericare, more frequent temperature monitoring, and limiting cervical exams.

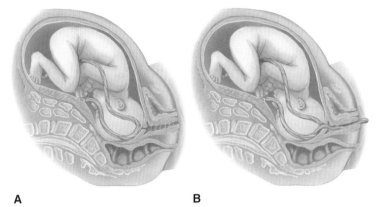

A   **B**

Figure 2.6   Umbilical cord prolapse. **A.** The cord is prolapsed but still remains in the uterus. **B.** The cord is visible at the vulva.

Prolapsed Umbilical Cord

- ☐ When the umbilical cord precedes the fetal presenting part, it's known as a prolapsed cord. (See Fig. 2.6 for an illustration of umbilical cord prolapse.)
- ☐ Cord prolapse is more likely in clients who have rupture of membranes before fetal head engagement (head in negative station) and have malpositioned fetuses.
- ☐ When membranes rupture, the cord can be swept through with the amniotic fluid.
- ☐ With a negative station, there is room between the fetal head and the maternal pelvis for the cord to slip through.
- ☐ In a breech presentation, the fetal head is in the fundus, and smaller portions of the fetus settle into the lower portion of the uterus, allowing the cord to lie beside the fetus.
- ☐ A small (low-birth-weight fetus) fetus is more mobile within the uterus and the cord can rest between the fetus and the inside of the uterus or below the fetal head.
- ☐ If the presenting part compresses against the cord, there will be severe bradycardia and possible fetal demise.
- ☐ In umbilical prolapse, the protruding umbilical cord should never be pushed back into the uterus because this could damage the cord, obstruct the flow of blood through the cord to the fetus, or introduce infection into the uterus.
- ☐ Prolapsed cord requires an emergency cesarean birth.
- ☐ Nursing interventions include manually elevating the fetal head off the cord, placing the client in knee-chest or Trendelenburg position

to have gravity aid in relieving cord compression, and preparing for emergency cesarean birth.

Abnormal Fetal Heart Rate (FHR)

☐ Abnormal FHR patterns include fetal bradycardia, fetal tachycardia, decreased variability, and FHR decelerations.

☐ Position the client left lateral, apply oxygen, stop contraction induction, perform cervical exam, increase IV fluids as needed, and contact the practitioner.

POSTPARTUM CARE

KEY TERMS

☐ **Lochia** is the discharge from the sloughing of the uterine decidua.

☐ **Mastitis** is an infection of the breast characterized by flulike symptoms, along with redness and tenderness in the breast.

Postpartum Assessment

☐ A focused physical assessment should be performed every 15 minutes for the first 1 to 2 hours postpartum, including assessment of the bladder, uterus, breast, bowel, lochia, episiotomy/perineum, extremities, vital signs, and incision.

☐ Postpartum women are at increased risk of deep vein thrombosis (DVT) because of changes in clotting mechanisms to control bleeding at birth.

☐ Assess calves for redness, unilateral edema, and tenderness.

☐ In the early postpartum period, the glomerular filtration rate rises and progesterone levels drop, resulting in rapid diuresis.

☐ Assess for signs and symptoms of dehydration. Encourage PO intake of fluids.

Postpartum Uterus

☐ Monitor uterine tone, cramping, urine output, and lochia.

☐ The uterus should be palpable at the level of the umbilicus from 1 hour after birth and for about the next 24 hours.

☐ When a nurse is assessing the fundus of a postpartum client and finds that the fundus is boggy, the nurse should first massage the uterus to stimulate it to contract.

☐ A full bladder may displace the uterine fundus above the umbilicus to the left or right side of the abdomen and increase pain. This prevents the uterus from contracting.

☐ The fundus will continue to descend (involution) about 1 cm/day until it isn't palpable above the symphysis pubis.

☐ The uterus shrinks to its prepregnancy size by 5 to 6 weeks after birth.

☐ Teach the client to void often to prevent urinary retention.

Postpartum Teaching

☐ The client should wipe from front to back after urination or a bowel movement to avoid contaminating the perineal area.

☐ Perineal pads should be changed when they are soiled to keep the perineum clean.

☐ Sitz baths help decrease inflammation and tension in the perineal area.

☐ Ice should only be applied to the perineum for the first 24 hours after birth to decrease edema and provide pain relief.

☐ The client should cleanse the perineal area after urinating or a bowel movement using a spray or peribottle with warm water.

☐ Kegel exercises result in increased blood flow, which brings oxygen and other nutrients to the perineal area to aid in healing.

Lochia

☐ Lochia is the discharge from the sloughing of the uterine decidua. (See Table 2.12 for the types of lochia.)

Postpartum Adaptation

☐ Talking, cooing, and cuddling are positive signs of mother-infant attachment.

☐ Eye contact, touching, and speaking help establish attachment with a neonate.

☐ Feeding a neonate is an important role of a new mother and facilitates attachment.

☐ Encouraging the partner to hold the neonate will facilitate attachment.

TABLE 2.12	Types of Lochia
Type	Characteristics
Lochia rubra	■ Has a fleshy odor and is bloody with small clots ■ Occurs for the first 2 to 3 d after birth
Lochia serosa	■ Pinkish or brown with a serosanguinous consistency and fleshy odor ■ Occurs during days 3 through 9 postpartum
Lochia alba	■ Yellow to white discharge ■ Usually begins about 10 d after birth; it may last from 2 to 6 wk

TABLE 2.13	Rubin's Theory of Maternal Role Attainment
Phase	**Action**
Taking-in phase	Usually lasts 2–3 d Mother is passive and dependent and expresses her own needs rather than the neonate's needs
Taking-hold phase	Usually lasts from days 3 to 10 postpartum Mother strives for independence and autonomy The mother is ready to take responsibility for her own care as well as her infant's
Letting-go phase	Begins several weeks later, when the mother incorporates the new infant into the family unit

☐ During this taking-in phase, the client may ask the nurse to help her with self-care, wants to talk about the birth experience, and lets others make decisions for her.

☐ During the taking-in phase, the mother is concerned with her own needs and requires support from staff and relatives.

☐ See Table 2.13 for Rubin's theory of maternal role attainment.

Breast-Feeding

☐ Breast-feeding offers the best nutrition for human infants.

☐ Breast-feeding provides protection from the most common childhood illnesses.

☐ Decreases development of allergies.

☐ Decreases the risk of sudden infant death syndrome (SIDS).

☐ Provides numerous emotional and physical benefits.

☐ Breast-feeding mothers have less postpartum bleeding, enhanced postpartum weight loss, protection from diseases, and enhanced emotional benefits.

☐ Prolactin is the hormone responsible for milk production, while oxytocin produces the let-down reflex.

☐ The breasts normally produce colostrum for the first few days after birth.

☐ Milk production begins 1 to 3 days postpartum.

☐ Breast-feeding should be initiated as soon after birth as possible.

☐ When breast-feeding after a cesarean birth, the client should be encouraged to use the football hold to avoid incisional discomfort.

☐ The mother should be encouraged to breast-feed her infant every 2 to 3 hours throughout the night as well as during the day to increase the milk supply.

- ☐ The nipples should be allowed to air-dry after breast-feeding to keep them dry and prevent irritation.
- ☐ Only water should be used to wash the nipples because soap removes natural oils and dries out the nipples.
- ☐ The breast-feeding client should consume an additional 500 calories/day, increase protein intake, and eat foods high in vitamins and minerals.
- ☐ Increased fluid intake is also important to maintaining supply.
- ☐ When breast-feeding, the baby should grasp both the nipple and areola with his mouth.
- ☐ Because HIV can be transmitted to the baby through breast milk, the HIV-positive client should not breast-feed.

Formula Feeding
- ☐ Commercially available formulas provide adequate nutrition for neonates.
- ☐ Formula-fed infants should be fed every 3 to 4 hours.

Postpartum Blues
- ☐ The term "postpartum blues" refers to a transient mood alteration that arises during the first 3 weeks postpartum and is typically self-limiting.
- ☐ Postpartum blues affects 50% to 80% of postpartum clients.
- ☐ The client with postpartum blues experiences crying and sadness, generally between 3 to 5 days postpartum, but this condition resolves itself quickly.
- ☐ Assess maternal stress and dissatisfaction, stressors, self-esteem, and amount of support.
- ☐ Provide a therapeutic and open conversation about the client's feelings and moods.
- ☐ Provide the client with resources, including appropriate referral if necessary.

Postpartum Hemorrhage
- ☐ Postpartum hemorrhage is excessive bleeding following birth. (See Table 2.14 for more information on postpartum hemorrhage.)
- ☐ Bleeding is considered excessive when a woman saturates a sanitary pad in 1 hour.
- ☐ A firm uterus helps control postpartum hemorrhage by clamping down on uterine blood vessels.
- ☐ Continuous seepage of blood may be due to cervical or vaginal lacerations if the uterus is firm and contracting.
- ☐ Because magnesium sulfate relaxes smooth muscle and can increase the risk of postpartum hemorrhage, the uterus should be assessed for uterine atony in a client who experienced preeclampsia.

TABLE 2.14	Postpartum Hemorrhage		
Occurrence	Causes	Treatment	Risk Factors
Early (≤24 h after birth)	▪ Uterine atony (no. 1 cause) ▪ Tissue trauma	▪ Massage fundus ▪ Repair tissue ▪ Medications (oxytocin, methylergonovine, carboprost tromethamine) ▪ Volume replacement	▪ Multiple gestation ▪ Hydramnios ▪ Large baby ▪ Operative birth ▪ Placental abnormalities ▪ Magnesium sulfate use ▪ Advanced maternal age ▪ High parity
Late (24 h to 6 wk after birth)	▪ Retained placenta ▪ Uterine infection ▪ Fibroids	▪ Surgery ▪ Antibiotics ▪ Volume replacement	▪ Cesarean birth ▪ Operative birth ▪ Advanced maternal age ▪ High parity ▪ Placental abnormalities ▪ Manual extraction of placenta

☐ Women who deliver twins are at a higher risk for postpartum hemorrhage due to overdistention of the uterus, which causes uterine atony.

⌖ ☐ Retained placental fragments and uterine atony may cause subinvolution of the uterus, making it soft, boggy, and larger than expected.

☐ Monitor vital signs continuously or at least every 10 to 15 minutes, until the client's condition stabilizes.

Postpartum Depression

☐ Postpartum depression occurs in approximately 10% to 15% of all postpartum women.

☐ Clinical manifestations include disabling feelings of inadequacy and an inability to cope that can last up to 3 years.

☐ The client is often tearful and despondent with postpartum depression.

☐ All postpartum women should be screened for emotional disturbances.

☐ Postpartum depression requires treatment that may consist of therapy and pharmacologic methods.

Postpartum Neurosis/Psychosis

- ☐ Postpartum neurosis includes neurotic behavior during the initial 6 weeks after birth.
- ☐ Clinical manifestations include hallucinations, delusions, and phobias.
- ☐ A more severe mood alteration, seen in approximately 20% of clients, involves changes that occur within a few days after birth and may last for a few days to more than 1 year.
- ☐ Postpartum psychosis is linked with suicide and infanticide and requires immediate treatment with psychiatric care and pharmacotherapy.

Rh Isoimmunization

- ☐ A positive Coombs test means that the Rh-negative woman is now producing antibodies to the Rh-positive blood of the neonate.
- ☐ Administering $Rh_o(D)$ immune globulin to the Rh-negative client who gave birth to an Rh-positive neonate within 72 hours of birth prevents formation of antibodies that can destroy fetal blood cells in the next pregnancy.
- ☐ $Rh_o(D)$ immune globulin is not given to the baby.

Infections

- ☐ Postpartum women must be monitored for signs of infection in the urinary tract, perineum, incisions, uterus, and breasts (mastitis). Teach clients to monitor temperature, foul-smelling lochia, urinary frequency, dysuria, incisional erythema, incisional drainage, and severe pain in breasts, uterus, bladder, back, incisions, or perineum.

Diabetes Mellitus

- ☐ Postpartum insulin requirements are usually significantly lower than prepregnancy requirements.
- ☐ Clients with diabetes have decreased insulin needs for the first few days postpartum.
- ☐ Clients with gestational diabetes do not require treatment postpartum, but they are at an increased risk to develop type 2 diabetes mellitus in the future.
- ☐ Teach clients to maintain healthy lifestyles and healthy diets and to have diabetes screening with providers.

Mastitis

- ☐ Mastitis is an infection of the breast characterized by flulike symptoms, along with redness and tenderness in the breast.
- ☐ Mastitis is more likely in a breast-feeding mother. The most common cause of mastitis is *Staphylococcus aureus*, transmitted from the neonate's mouth.

- ☐ Encourage breast-feeding on the affected side first, increase PO intake of fluids, and complete emptying of the affected breast with each feeding, expressing milk by hand or using a pump, if necessary.
- ☐ Affected mothers will need oral antibiotics and antipyretics.
- ☐ Teach clients to discuss breast-feeding with providers prior to taking any medications.

Pulmonary Embolism (PE)

- ☐ A PE develops when a thrombus (stationary blood clot) from a vein becomes an embolus (moving clot) that lodges in the pulmonary circulation.
- ☐ Pregnant women may experience an embolus of amniotic fluid (amniotic fluid embolus).
- ☐ Clinical manifestations include sudden dyspnea, along with diaphoresis and confusion.
- ☐ Shortness of breath in the client on anticoagulant therapy for DVT should be reported immediately because it may be a symptom of PE. (See *Chapter 1 Adult Care* for DVT monitoring and care.)

NEONATAL CARE

KEY TERMS

- ☐ **Convection** heat loss is the flow of heat from the body surface to cooler air.
- ☐ **Conduction** is the loss of heat from the body surface to cooler surfaces in direct contact.
- ☐ **Evaporation** is the loss of heat that occurs when a liquid is converted to a vapor.
- ☐ **Radiation** is the loss of heat from the body surface to cooler solid surfaces not in direct contact but in relative proximity.
- ☐ **Acrocyanosis**, a normal finding, also called peripheral cyanosis, is a bluish discoloration of the hands and feet in the neonate and shouldn't last more than 24 hours after birth.
- ☐ **Polydactyly** refers to more than five digits on an extremity.
- ☐ **Syndactyly** refers to two or more digits fused together.
- ☐ **Vernix caseosa** is a white, cheesy material that may be present on the neonate's skin at birth.
- ☐ **Lanugo** is the fine soft hair that may cover the neonate.
- ☐ **Milia** are small raised white bumps on the facial skin that resolve without intervention.
- ☐ **Caput succedaneum** is a boggy edematous swelling present at birth that crosses the suture line and most commonly occurs in the occipital area.
- ☐ **Cephalhematoma** is a collection of blood between the skull and periosteum that doesn't cross cranial suture lines.

Neonate Admission Procedures

☐ For an uncomplicated birth at term, there is benefit in delaying umbilical cord clamping for a minimum time ranging from 1 minute until the cord stops pulsating after birth.

☐ Aquamephyton injection is administered because neonates have coagulation deficiencies due to a lack of organisms that help produce vitamin K in the intestines, which helps the liver synthesize clotting factors.

☐ Erythromycin ointment is administered in both eyes prophylactically almost immediately after birth because both chlamydia and gonorrhea are common causes of neonatal conjunctival infections.

☐ Most neonates will begin their Hepatitis B vaccination in the neonatal period.

Apgar

☐ The Apgar scoring system provides a way to evaluate the neonate's cardiopulmonary and neurologic status using assessments performed at 1 and 5 minutes after birth and repeated every 5 minutes until the infant stabilizes. (See Table 2.15 for more information on Apgar parameters.)

☐ Heart rate, respiratory effort, muscle tone, reflex irritability, and color of the neonate are assessed to measure the Apgar score.

☐ Each of the signs in the Apgar score is assigned a score of 0, 1, or 2, with the highest possible total score being a 10.

TABLE 2.15 Apgar Parameters

The Apgar Score Measures 5 Parameters		0 pts	1 pt	2 pts
A	Appearance (color)	Blue/pale all over	Blue extremities, pink torso	Pink all over
P	Pulse (heart rate)	None	<100	≥100
G	Grimace (reflex irritability)	None	Weak	Cries, pulls away
A	Activity (muscle tone)	None	Some flexion of arms	Arms flexed, legs resist extension
R	Respiratory (respiratory effort)	None	Weak cry, irregular	Strong cry

□ An Apgar score of 8 to 10 indicates that the neonate is in no apparent distress; a score below 8 indicates that resuscitative measures may be needed. An Apgar score of 5 or less indicates a need for resuscitative efforts.

Neonatal Vital Signs
□ Normal neonatal apical heart rate is 120 to 160 beats/minute.
□ Normal neonatal respirations are 30 to 60 breaths/minute.
□ A neonate's temperature is about 99°F (37.2°C) at birth and should remain at least 97°F (36.1°C).
□ Normal neonatal blood pressure reading ranges from 60/40 to 90/45 mm Hg.
□ Auscultation of the precordium should be the primary means to assess heart rate in a neonate.
□ Heart rate assessment should be the primary vital sign by which to assess the need for resuscitation in a neonate.
□ The chest compression-ventilation ratio should be 3:1 for neonates.

Thermoregulation
□ Convection heat loss is the flow of heat from the body surface to cooler air.
□ Conduction is the loss of heat from the body surface to cooler surfaces in direct contact.
□ Evaporation is the loss of heat that occurs when a liquid is converted to a vapor.
□ Radiation is the loss of heat from the body surface to cooler solid surfaces not in direct contact but in relative proximity.
□ If a neonate's environment is too cold, his metabolism must increase to warm his body cells, resulting in increased oxygen demand with resultant hypoxia.
□ If a neonate's environment is too warm, his metabolism must decrease to cool his body.
□ Neonates use nonshivering thermogenesis to increase body temperature.
□ Immediately drying the neonate after birth decreases evaporative heat loss from his moist body.
□ Placing the neonate on a warm, dry towel decreases conductive heat losses.
□ Preterm neonates are not able to thermoregulate due to the lack of brown fat; the more preterm the infant, the more immature the thermoregulation system is.
□ The increased metabolic rate with cold stress leads to the use of glycogen stores and produces hypoglycemia with symptoms including hyperactivity, twitching, jitteriness, and shrill cry.

Neonatal Assessment

- ☐ Conjunctival hemorrhages are commonly seen in neonates secondary to the cranial pressure applied during the birth process.
- ☐ Epstein pearls, found in the mouth, are similar to facial milia.
- ☐ Soft, smooth skin in a neonate is a sign of adequate hydration.
- ☐ A sunken fontanel and no urine output in the first 24 hours of life are signs of abnormal hydration.
- ☐ A neonate's pupils normally react to light in the same way as an adult's.
- ☐ A neonate's lacrimal glands are immature, resulting in tearless crying for up to 2 months.
- ☐ Greenish brown stools at 48 hours are normal and indicate that the neonate is eliminating digested liquid instead of meconium.
- ☐ Acrocyanosis, a normal finding also called peripheral cyanosis, is a bluish discoloration of the hands and feet in the neonate and shouldn't last more than 24 hours after birth.
- ☐ Bronchopulmonary dysplasia is a complication common in neonates who receive prolonged mechanical ventilation at birth.
- ☐ Esophageal atresia is a structural defect in which the esophagus and trachea communicate with each other.
- ☐ Neonates may have polydactyly (more than five digits on an extremity) or syndactyly (two or more digits fused together).

Common Neonatal Skin Findings

- ☐ Vernix caseosa, which protects the fetus in utero, is a white, cheesy material that may be present on the neonate's skin at birth.
- ☐ Lanugo, fine soft hair covering the neonate, may be present.
- ☐ Milia are small raised white bumps on the facial skin that resolve without intervention.
- ☐ A port-wine stain (nevus flammeus) is a capillary angioma located below the dermis and is commonly found on the face.
- ☐ A strawberry hemangioma (nevus vasculosus) is a capillary angioma located in the dermal and subdermal skin layers, indicated by a rough, raised, sharply demarcated birthmark.
- ☐ A telangiectatic hemangioma (stork bite) is a salmon pink coloration found at the nape of the neck, eyelids, or forehead.
- ☐ A Mongolian spot, a large macule/patch that is gray or blue, is commonly found over the lumbosacral area in neonates of Black, Asian, Latin American, or Native American origin and is due to the deposition of melanocytes.
- ☐ Erythema toxicum neonatorum causes a transient maculopapular rash—a normal finding in all neonates.

Neonatal Reflexes

☐ The full-term neonate's neurologic system should produce equal strength and symmetry in responses and reflexes.

☐ Diminished or absent reflexes in a neonate may indicate a serious neurologic problem, and asymmetrical responses may indicate trauma during birth, including nerve damage, paralysis, or fracture.

☐ The sucking reflex is elicited when a nipple is placed in the neonate's mouth and stimulus is placed on the roof of the neonate's mouth.

☐ The rooting reflex is elicited when the neonate's cheek is stroked; the neonate turns his head in the direction of the stroke.

☐ The Moro reflex (startle reflex) is elicited when the neonate is lifted above the crib and suddenly lowered, or after a loud noise; the arms and legs symmetrically extend and then abduct while the fingers spread to form a "C."

☐ The tonic neck (fencing position) reflex is elicited when the neonate's head is turned while the neonate is lying supine; the extremities on the same side straighten while those on the opposite side flex.

☐ To elicit a plantar grasp reflex, which usually disappears around age 9 months, the nurse would touch the sole of the foot near the base of the digits, causing flexion or grasping.

☐ The palmar grasp reflex is elicited when a finger is placed in each of the neonate's hands; fingers grasp tightly enough to be pulled to a sitting position.

☐ A positive Babinski sign (plantar reflex) is elicited stroking of the lateral aspect of the sole of the foot; the neonate's toes fan. This reflex is present in infants until approximately age 1.

☐ The dancing or stepping reflex is elicited when the neonate is held upright with the feet touching a flat surface; the neonate exhibits dancing or stepping movements.

☐ The trunk incurvature reflex (Galant reflex) is elicited when a finger is run laterally down the neonate's spine; the trunk flexes and the pelvis swings toward the stimulated side.

Neonatal Skull

☐ The neonatal skull has two fontanels: a diamond-shaped anterior fontanel and a triangular-shaped posterior fontanel. (See Fig. 2.7 for an illustration of fontanels.)

Fetal Abstinence Syndrome

☐ A neonate experiencing drug withdrawal should be swaddled to prevent him from flailing and stimulating himself; he should be moved to a quiet area of the nursery to minimize environmental stimuli.

☐ Medications, such as phenobarbital, should be given as needed to neonates experiencing drug withdrawal.

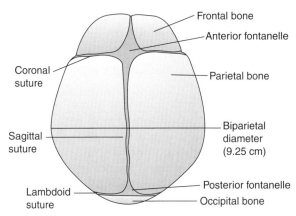

Figure 2.7 The fontanels. The anterior fontanel is shaped like a diamond, normally measures 4 to 5 cm at its widest point, and is formed by the junction of the sagittal, frontal, and coronal sutures. The posterior fontanel is shaped like a triangle, normally measures 1 to 2 cm at its widest point, and is formed by the junction of the sagittal and lambdoidal sutures. (From Pillitteri, A. (2003). *Maternal and child nursing* (4th ed.). Philadelphia, PA: Lippincott Williams & Wilkins.)

Fetal Alcohol Syndrome

☐ Distinctive facial dysmorphology of children with fetal alcohol syndrome most commonly involves the eyes (microphthalmia).

☐ Microcephaly is generally seen with fetal alcohol syndrome, as are short palpebral fissures and an abnormally developed philtrum.

☐ Neonates may have significant central nervous system problems.

☐ Nursing considerations are based on the effects of fetal alcohol syndrome on the neonate and may include NICU care, referral to social work, carefully monitoring vital signs and intake/output, and developmental care.

Hyperbilirubinemia

☐ Increased bilirubin levels result from the impaired conjugation and excretion of bilirubin and difficulty clearing bilirubin from plasma.

☐ Clinical jaundice arising before age 24 hours or lasting beyond 14 days, or serum bilirubin level increasing by more than 5 mg/dL/day (85.52 µmol/L), suggests pathologic jaundice.

☐ Physiologic jaundice occurs within the first 3 to 4 days.

☐ Jaundice usually appears in a cephalocaudal progression from head to feet.

☐ The neonate with an ABO blood incompatibility with its mother would have a positive Coombs test result and will have pathologic jaundice.

☐ If untreated, it could progress to neurologic sequelae. (See *Chapter 3 Pediatric Care* for additional details.)

Phototherapy

☐ Phototherapy employs a fluorescent light to decompose bilirubin through skin.

☐ The neonate's eyes and genitalia must be covered with eye patches to prevent damage from phototherapy.

☐ The temperature of a neonate receiving phototherapy should be monitored at least every 2 to 4 hours because of the risk of hypothermia with phototherapy. A warmer may be necessary.

☐ Monitor temperature, weight, intake and output, irradiance levels, and skin condition.

Infection

☐ The neonate's color commonly changes with an infectious process and generally becomes ashen or mottled.

☐ The neonate with an infection will usually show a decrease in activity level or lethargy.

☐ Temperature instability, especially when it results in a low temperature in the neonate, may be a sign of infection.

☐ Transmission of group B beta-hemolytic streptococci (GBS) to the fetus results in respiratory distress that can rapidly lead to septic shock.

Neonates with Diabetic Mothers

☐ Neonates of mothers with diabetes are at risk for hypoglycemia due to increased insulin levels because the neonate's liver can't initially adjust to the changing glucose levels after birth.

☐ Hypoglycemia in a neonate is expressed as jitteriness, lethargy, diaphoresis, and a serum glucose level below 40 mg/dL (2.22 mmol/L).

☐ Neonates of mothers with diabetes are at increased risk for macrosomia (excessive fetal growth) as a result of the combination of the increased supply of maternal glucose and an increase in fetal insulin.

☐ Neonates of diabetic mothers are at risk for respiratory distress syndrome, hypocalcemia, hyperbilirubinemia, and congenital anomalies.

☐ Carefully monitor blood glucose levels before feedings, I&O and vital signs, and for complications.

Respiratory Distress Syndrome

☐ Nasal flaring and audible grunting are signs of respiratory distress in a neonate.

- Tachypnea and retractions are other signs of respiratory distress in a neonate.

Transient Tachypnea of the Newborn

- Transient tachypnea of a newborn is caused by a delay in removing excessive amounts of lung fluid.
- Nursing care includes supporting oxygenation, careful monitoring of vital signs, oral/nasal suction with a bulb syringe, and monitoring I&O.
- Respiratory distress may require admission to the NICU and ventilation support.

Small or Preterm Neonates

- The small-for-gestational age/preterm neonate is at risk for developing polycythemia due to chronic hypoxia during intrauterine life.
- The small-for-gestational age/preterm neonate is at risk for hypoglycemia and hypothermia due to decreased glycogen stores.
- Preterm birth is the single most important risk factor for developing respiratory distress syndrome.

Nutrition for At-Risk Neonates

- Studies have proven that breast milk provides preterm neonates with better protection from infection, such as necrotizing enterocolitis (NEC), because of the antibodies contained in the milk.
- Breast milk feedings can be started as soon as the neonate is stable.

Circumcision

- Circumcision is the surgical removal of the foreskin from the penis.
- A yellow-white exudate around the glans of the neonate's penis 2 days after circumcision is a normal finding. It is part of the granulation process for a healing penis after circumcision; it shouldn't be removed.
- Risks include hemorrhage, infection, urethral complication, and adhesions. Petroleum gauze is applied to the circumcision site for the first 24 hours to prevent the skin edges from sticking to the diaper.
- Monitor for bleeding, infection, urinary function, and pain following the procedure.
- Teach parents to clean area twice a day with warm water and monitor for signs and symptoms of infection.

Variations in Head Size

☐ Caput succedaneum is a boggy edematous swelling present at birth that crosses the suture line; it most commonly occurs in the occipital area and usually resolves within 3 to 4 days.

☐ A cephalhematoma is a collection of blood between the skull and periosteum that doesn't cross cranial suture lines and resolves in 3 to 6 weeks.

☐ Microcephaly is usually the result of congenital cytomegalovirus or congenital rubella virus infection.

☐ Molding refers to the overlapping of cranial sutures that occurs as the fetus passes through the birth canal, which causes the neonate's head to appear cone shaped.

☐ Hydrocephalus is an increase in the size of the entire head as a result of increased cerebrospinal fluid volume.

Lung Maturity

☐ Surfactant works by reducing surface tension in the lung and allows the lung to remain slightly expanded, decreasing the amount of work required for inspiration.

☐ Lecithin and sphingomyelin are phospholipids that help compose surfactant in the lungs; lecithin peaks at 36 weeks' gestation, and sphingomyelin concentrations remain stable. The ratio of lecithin and sphingomyelin, or the L/S ratio, can be measured to determine lung maturity.

☐ Chronic fetal stress tends to increase lung maturity.

Postterm Neonate

☐ Lanugo, fine hair covering the body of the fetus, disappears as pregnancy progresses, with very little remaining on the postterm neonate. Postdate fetuses lose the vernix caseosa, and the epidermis may become dry and desquamated.

☐ A postterm neonate would have a well-developed breast bud of 5 to 10 mm in diameter.

☐ Sole creases increase in number and depth with gestational age; a postterm neonate would have deep sole creases and a preterm neonate would have no sole creases.

☐ Postterm fetuses are at increased risk for meconium aspiration.

☐ There is an increased risk for hypoglycemia in postterm neonates. Monitor the infant for signs and symptoms of hypoglycemia— jitteriness, high-pitched cry, ineffective thermoregulation, and lethargy.

REVIEW QUESTIONS ▐▐▐▐▐▐▐▐▐

1. A primiparous client at 4 hours after a vaginal birth and manual removal of the placenta voids for the first time. The nurse palpates the fundus, noting it to be 1 cm above the umbilicus, slightly firm, and deviated to the left side, and notes a moderate amount of lochia rubra. The nurse notifies the physician based on the interpretation that the assessment indicates:
   1. perineal lacerations.
   2. retained placental fragments.
   3. cervical lacerations.
   4. urine retention.

2. While the nurse is caring for a multiparous client in active labor at 36 weeks' gestation, the client tells the nurse, "I think my water just broke." What should the nurse do **first**?
   1. Turn the client to the right side.
   2. Assess the color, amount, and odor of the fluid.
   3. Assess the fetal heart rate pattern.
   4. Check the client's cervical dilation.

3. The primary health care provider orders an amnioinfusion for a primigravid client at term who is diagnosed with oligohydramnios. Which should the nurse include in the client's teaching plan about the purpose of this procedure?
   1. To decrease the frequency and severity of variable decelerations
   2. To minimize the possibility of fetal metabolic alkalosis
   3. To increase the fetal heart rate accelerations during a contraction
   4. To raise the amniotic fluid index to more than 15 cm

4. Which factors in the client's history place her at greater risk for cord prolapse? Select all that apply.
   1. −2 station
   2. Low-birth-weight infant
   3. Rupture of membranes
   4. Breech presentation
   5. Prior abortion
   6. Low-lying placenta

5. For which finding should the nurse assess in a preterm neonate suffering from cold stress?
   1. Yellowish undercast to the skin color
   2. Increased abdominal girth
   3. Hyperactivity and twitching
   4. Slowed respirations

Chapter References

AWHONN. (2008). The role of the nurse in postpartum mood and anxiety disorders. https://www.awhonn.org/awhonn/binary.content.do?name=Resources/Documents/pdf/5_PMAD.pdf

Butkus, S. (Ed). (2015). *Maternal-neonatal nursing made incredibly easy* (3rd ed.). Philadelphia, PA: Lippincott Williams & Wilkins.

Pillitteri, A. (2014). *Maternal and child health nursing: Care of the childbearing and childrearing family* (7th ed.). Philadelphia, PA: Lippincott Williams & Wilkins.

Ricci, S. C. (2013). *Essentials of maternity, newborn, and women's health nursing* (3rd ed.). Philadelphia, PA: Lippincott Williams & Wilkins.

Pediatric Care

GROWTH AND DEVELOPMENT

KEY TERMS

- [ ] **Neonate** or **newborn** is birth to age 1 month.
- [ ] **Toddler** is a child of ages 1 to 3 years.
- [ ] **Preschool child** is a child of ages 3 to 5 years.
- [ ] **School-age child** is a child of ages 5 to 12 years.
- [ ] **Adolescent** is a child of ages 13 to 18 years.

Birth to 1 Month

- [ ] Neonate can hold head momentarily.
- [ ] Neonate has a strong grasp reflex.
- [ ] Neonate's hands remain mostly closed in a fist.

Infant 2 to 4 Months

- [ ] The instinctual smile appears at 2 months and the social smile at 3 months.
- [ ] At 2 months, the infant can lift head 45 degrees when prone.
- [ ] At 4 months, the infant can lift head 90 degrees when prone.
- [ ] At 2 months, the infant can track objects up to 180 degrees.
- [ ] By the end of 4 months, the infant holds head erect and displays only slight head lag.
- [ ] At 3 months, the infant reaches out and at 4 months can grasp objects with both hands.
- [ ] At 3 months, the most primitive reflexes begin to disappear, except for the protective and postural reflexes (blink, parachute, cough, swallow, and gag reflexes), which remain for life.

Infant 5 to 6 Months

- [ ] At 5 months, the infant rolls over from stomach to back.
- [ ] At 6 months, the infant rolls over from back to stomach.
- [ ] At 6 months, the infant cries when the parent leaves, attempts to crawl when prone, and voluntarily grasps and releases objects.

☐ Teething usually begins around age 6 months; therefore, offering a teething ring is appropriate at this age.

☐ At age 6 months, the infant voluntarily grasps and releases objects.

☐ At 6 months, the infant sits with support.

☐ At 6 months, the infant displays good head control and there is no head lag.

Infant 7 to 9 Months

☐ At 7 to 9 months, the infant can self-feed crackers and a bottle.

☐ At 7 months, the infant can transfer objects from hand to hand and "rakes" objects.

☐ At 8 months, object permanence is exhibited by the infant looking for objects that have been hidden from sight.

☐ At 8 months, the infant can sit alone without support.

☐ Fear of strangers appears to peak during the 8th month of age.

☐ At 8 months, the infant has beginning pincer grasp.

☐ At 9 months, the infant can pull himself to a standing position.

Infant 10 to 12 Months

☐ At 10 months, the infant can move from a prone position to sitting.

☐ At 11 months, the infant can hold on to furniture while walking (cruising) and may walk with one hand held by 12 months.

☐ At 10 to 12 months, birth weight triples and birth length increases about 50%.

☐ At 10 months, the infant can say "mama" and "dada" and responds to his own name at age 10 months.

☐ At 10 months, the infant can say about five words but understands many more.

☐ By 12 months, the infant can say a few words, with more words and short phrases being added each month.

☐ An infant takes his first steps at 12 months.

Child 16 Months

☐ At 16 months, a child engages in solitary play and has little interaction with other children.

Toddler

☐ The toddler period includes ages 1 to 3 and is a slow growth period with a weight gain of 4 to 9 pound (2 to 4 kg) over 2 years.

☐ The toddler's normal pulse rate is 100 beats/minute, normal respiratory rate is 26 breaths/minute, and normal blood pressure is 99/64 mm Hg.

☐ The toddler uses at least 400 words as well as two- to three-word phrases and comprehends many more by age 2; the toddler uses about 11,000 words by age 3.

Preschool Child
☐ In the preschool child, ages 3 to 5 years, the normal pulse rate is from 90 to 100 beats/minute, normal respiratory rate is 25 breaths/minute, and normal blood pressure ranges from 85/60 to 90/70 mm Hg.

☐ Preschoolers see death as temporary, a type of sleep or separation.

☐ Magical thinking and fantasy play are more characteristic during the preschool years.

☐ A preschooler typically asks for a bandage after having blood drawn because he has poorly defined body boundaries and believes he will lose all of his blood from the hole the needle has made.

School-Age Child
☐ In the school-age child, ages 5 to 12 years, the normal pulse rate is from 75 to 115 beats/minute, normal blood pressure ranges from 106/69 to 117/76 mm Hg, and normal respiratory rate ranges from 20 to 25 breaths/minute.

☐ Accidents are a major cause of death and disability in children ages 5 to 12.

☐ A school-age child might ask why his friends don't visit because peers become important by that age.

Adolescent
☐ An adolescent might be upset about a surgical scar because he's concerned about body image.

☐ Thinking about the future is typical of an adolescent facing death.

☐ Ages 12 to 18 years encompass the adolescent period, which is a period of rapid growth characterized by puberty-related changes in body structure and psychosocial adjustment.

Piaget
☐ Recognizing that a ball of clay is the same object even when flattened out is an example of the theory of conservation, which occurs during Piaget's concrete operational stage in early school-age children (ages 7 to 11).

☐ According to Piaget's theory of cognitive development, an 8-month-old child will look for an object after it disappears from sight to develop the cognitive skill of object permanence.

Socialization
☐ During the school-age years, the most important social interactions typically are those with peers, and children socialize more frequently with friends than with parents.

- ☐ Peer-to-peer interactions lead to the formation of intimate friendships between same-sex children.
- ☐ Friendships with opposite-sex children are uncommon during the school-age years.
- ☐ Interest in peers of the opposite sex generally doesn't begin until ages 10 to 12.

Gross Motor Skills

- ☐ At age 3, gross motor development and refinement in hand-eye coordination enable a child to ride a tricycle.
- ☐ Gross motor skills of the 6-month-old infant include rolling from front to back and back to front.

Chest Circumference

- ☐ Chest circumference is most accurately measured by placing the measuring tape around the infant's chest with the tape covering the nipples.
- ☐ If chest circumference is measured above or below the nipples, a false measurement is obtained.

Tanner's Stages

- ☐ Sexual maturity in males and females is classified according to Tanner's stages, named after the original researcher on sexual maturity.
- ☐ In Tanner stage 1, males and females are in the prepubertal stage.
- ☐ In Tanner stage 2, female breast buds appear with elevation of breast and papilla. The areola is slightly widened and appears as a small mound. In males, the testicles enlarge and scrotum thins. In both males and females, there is sparse growth of hair.
- ☐ In Tanner stage 3, in females, further enlargement of the breast and areola occurs. In males, there is enlargement of the penis. In both males and female, hair darkens and becomes coarse.
- ☐ In Tanner stage 4, in females, the breast enlarges and the nipple and papilla protrude and appear as a secondary mound. In males, increased size of the penis (width) occurs. The testes and scrotum enlarge as well. Hair is adult like but covering smaller area for both male and female.
- ☐ In Tanner stage 5, mature stage with hair adult in type with spread to medial surface of the thighs.

Fontanels

- ☐ The diamond-shaped anterior fontanel normally closes between ages 9 and 18 months.
- ☐ The triangular posterior fontanel normally closes between ages 2 and 3 months.

Reflexes

- ☐ The palmar grasp reflex disappears around age 3 to 4 months.
- ☐ The plantar grasp reflex disappears at age 6 to 8 months.
- ☐ The Moro reflex disappears around age 4 months.

CARDIOVASCULAR SYSTEM

KEY TERMS

- ☐ **Pulmonary atresia** is a narrowing or malformation of the pulmonic valve.
- ☐ **Tricuspid atresia** is a narrowing or malformation of the tricuspid valve.
- ☐ **Acyanotic heart defects** cause shunting of blood from left to right.
- ☐ **Cyanotic heart defects** cause shunting of blood from right to left.
- ☐ **Aortic stenosis** is a narrowing of the aortic valve.
- ☐ **Coarctation of the aorta** is a narrowing of the aorta.
- ☐ **Pulmonic stenosis** is a narrowing of the entrance of the pulmonary artery.
- ☐ **Tricuspid stenosis** is failure of the tricuspid valve to develop.
- ☐ **Mitral stenosis** is failure of the mitral valve to develop.

Key Considerations

- ☐ In response to surgery and cardiopulmonary bypass, the body secretes aldosterone and antidiuretic hormone.
- ☐ Aldosterone and antidiuretic hormone increase sodium levels, decrease potassium levels, increase water retention, and decrease urine output.
- ☐ When the heart stretches beyond efficiency, an extra heart sound, or S_3 gallop, may be audible.
- ☐ Hypotension and bradycardia are considered a late sign of shock in children.
- ☐ Infants and children with heart defects tend to have poor nutritional intake and weight loss, indicating poor cardiac output, heart failure, or hypoxemia.
- ☐ A neonate's vascular system changes with birth; certain factors help to reverse the flow of blood through the ductus arteriosus and ultimately favor its closure.
- ☐ Ductus arteriosus closure typically begins within the first 24 hours after birth and ends within a few days after birth.
- ☐ At birth, oxygenated blood normally causes the ductus arteriosus to constrict, and the vessel closes completely by age 6 weeks.

Heart Sounds

☐ The first heart sound (S_1) can best be heard at the fifth intercostal space, left midclavicular line in a 2-year-old child.

☐ The second heart sound (S_2) is heard at the second intercostal space in a 2-year-old child.

☐ The third heart sound (S_3) is heard with the stethoscope bell at the apex of the heart in a 2-year-old child.

☐ The fourth heart sound (S_4) can be heard at the third or fourth intercostal space in a 2-year-old child.

☐ The fourth heart sound (S_4) is heard late in diastole and may be a normal finding in children.

Heart Murmurs

☐ A grade 1 heart murmur is commonly difficult to hear and softer than the heart sounds.

☐ A grade 2 murmur is usually equal to the heart sounds.

☐ A grade 4 murmur is associated with a precordial thrill.

☐ A grade 6 murmur can be heard with the naked ear or with the stethoscope off the chest.

Arrhythmias

☐ Premature atrial contractions are common in fetuses, neonates, and children.

☐ Atrial fibrillation is an uncommon arrhythmia in children that arises from a disorganized state of electrical activity in the atria.

☐ Bradyarrhythmias are congenital, surgically acquired, or caused by infection.

☐ Premature ventricular contractions are more common in adolescents.

☐ Sinus tachycardia is commonly seen in children with a fever.

☐ Sinus arrhythmia is a common occurrence in childhood and adolescence.

☐ Sinus block, sinus bradycardia, and sinus tachycardia are respiration-independent arrhythmias.

☐ Sinus arrest may occur in children when vagal tone is increased, such as during Valsalva maneuver elicited when vomiting, gagging, or straining during a bowel movement.

Heart Rate

☐ A heart rate of 100 beats/minute is a normal finding for a 1-year-old child.

☐ A heart rate of around 180 beats/minute in a 1-year-old child may represent sinus tachycardia.

☐ A heart rate of less than 80 beats/minute in a 1-year-old child can be characterized as sinus bradycardia.

Cardiac Catheterization

☐ In the immediate postcatheterization phase, the child should avoid raising the head, sitting, straining the abdomen, or coughing.

☐ The pulse below the catheterization site should be strong and equal to the pulse in the unaffected extremity.

☐ A weakened pulse below the cardiac catheterization site may indicate vessel obstruction or perfusion problems.

Congenital Heart Disease

☐ Congenital heart disease can be divided into cyanotic and acyanotic defects.

☐ Acyanotic defects cause shunting of blood from left to right. Oxygenated blood shunts back to the lungs.

☐ Cyanotic defects cause shunting of blood from right to left, thus causing decreased pulmonary blood flow. Unoxygenated blood shunts away from the lungs. Degree of cyanosis depends on the degree of obstruction to the pulmonary blood flow.

Acyanotic Defects

☐ Ventricular septal defect (VSD) occurs when there is an opening between ventricles.

☐ Atrial septal defect (ASD) occurs when there is an opening between atriums.

☐ Patent ductus arteriosus (PDA) occurs when the neonate's ductus arteriosus fails to close after birth resulting in a shunting of blood between the aorta and the pulmonary artery.

☐ Obstructive lesions can cause obstructed blood flow.

☐ Aortic stenosis is a narrowing of the aortic valve.

☐ Coarctation of the aorta is a narrowing of aorta.

☐ See Table 3.1 for more information on acyanotic heart defects.

Cyanotic Heart Defects

☐ Tetralogy of Fallot is a cyanotic heart defect and includes a VSD, pulmonic stenosis, an overriding aorta, and right ventricular hypertrophy.

☐ Transposition of the great arteries (TGA) is a cyanotic heart defect and occurs when the aorta arises off the right ventricle and the pulmonary artery arises from the left ventricle, which leaves no communication between pulmonary and systemic circulation.

TABLE 3.1	Acyanotic Heart Defects		
Defect	Characteristics	Symptoms	Treatment
Atrial septal defect (ASD)	■ Infants and young children usually asymptomatic ■ Most close spontaneously	■ Moderate-to-large ASD ■ Tachycardia ■ Tachypnea ■ Retractions ■ Diaphoresis ■ Poor feeding and weight gain ■ Tire easily ■ Murmur ■ Heart failure	■ Surgery to close or patch if it has not closed by 4 y of age ■ May require treatment for heart failure such as diuretics
Patent ductus arteriosus (PDA)	■ Common in preterm infants ■ Mostly resolve within 6 mo ■ Most often asymptomatic	■ Tachycardia ■ Tachypnea ■ Retractions ■ Diaphoresis ■ Poor feeding and weight gain ■ Tire easily ■ Murmur ■ Heart failure	■ Indomethacin to close ■ Surgery to close at 1–2 y ■ Heart failure treatment

Tetralogy of Fallot

☐ A child with tetralogy of Fallot may exhibit clubbing of fingers or may squat or assume a knee-chest position to reduce venous blood flow from the lower extremities and to increase systemic vascular resistance, which diverts more blood flow into the pulmonary artery.

☐ The arterial oxygen saturation of infants with TOF can suddenly drop markedly; called a "tetralogy spell or 'tet spell,'" this usually results from a sudden increased constriction of the outflow tract to the lungs, which further restricts the pulmonary blood flow.

☐ Treatments are focused on reducing cardiac workload, treating congestive heart failure, and supporting growth and development.

☐ Providing shunts to decrease pulmonary blood flow and cardiac surgery to repair anomaly. Some mild heart defects may not require intervention.

☐ Medications include digoxin and diuretics.

Transposition of the Great Arteries (TGA)

☐ Clinical manifestations include heart failure, murmur, hypoxia, decreased cardiac output, and poor growth and development.

☐ Higher pressures in the upper extremities and weak pulses are characteristic of coarctation of the aorta.

☐ In treating TGA, prostaglandin E_1 is necessary to maintain the patency of the ductus arteriosus and improve systemic arterial flow in children.

☐ For small VSDs, a stitch closure is performed; larger VSDs may be repaired by sewing a patch over the defect.

☐ Preterm neonates having PDA may receive oral indomethacin, a prostaglandin inhibitor, to encourage ductal closure. If indomethacin isn't effective in closing a PDA, surgery is suggested.

☐ Patent foramen ovale, PDA, and VSD are associated defects related to TGA.

☐ Assess for clinical manifestations of respiratory distress, heart failure, hypoxia, and hypoxemia, and infection.

☐ Assess degree of cyanosis, vital signs, pulses, and oxygen saturation.

☐ Check for allergies to iodine or shellfish if cardiac catheterization is required.

☐ Teach parents about the signs and symptoms of respiratory distress, congestive heart failure, and infection.

☐ Teach parents how to administer medications: digoxin and diuretics.

☐ Prophylactic antibiotics may be administered prior to dental procedures.

☐ See Table 3.2 for more information on cyanotic heart defects.

Endocarditis

☐ Endocarditis is an acquired not congenital heart disease.

☐ Infective endocarditis is usually caused by the bacteria *Streptococcus viridans*, gram-negative bacilli.

☐ Bacteria in endocarditis may grow into adjacent tissues and may break off and embolize elsewhere, such as the spleen, kidney, lung, skin, and central nervous system.

☐ It is common in children with congenital heart defects.

☐ Clinical manifestations include low-grade intermittent fever, fatigue, tachycardia, anorexia, weight loss, and decreased activity level.

☐ Treatment will require antibiotics (penicillins or macrolides) and possibly a valve replacement.

☐ Teach parents about the signs and symptoms of infection.

☐ Teach about the need for prophylactic antibiotics with dental procedures.

TABLE 3.2 Cyanotic Heart Defects

Defect	Characteristics	Symptoms	Treatment
Tetralogy of Fallot (TOF)	▪ Includes four defects: pulmonic stenosis, right ventricular hypertrophy, VSD, and an overriding aorta ▪ Oxygen poor blood flows from the right ventricle to the aorta	▪ Tachycardia ▪ Tachypnea ▪ Dyspnea ▪ Diaphoresis ▪ Feeding difficulty ▪ Poor weight gain ▪ Murmur ▪ Cyanosis/mottling ▪ Clubbing ▪ Polycythemia ▪ Tet spells ▪ Squatting (toddlers)	▪ Prostaglandin E to maintain PDA and increase pulmonary blood flow ▪ Management of tet spells (knee-chest position, morphine, propranolol, O_2) ▪ Surgery before 6 mo if having tet spells ▪ Palliative shunt procedure in stages to allow child to grow and improve outcome
Transposition of the great vessels	▪ Aorta rises from the right ventricle ▪ Pulmonary artery rises from the left ventricle	▪ Severe cyanosis and respiratory distress at birth ▪ Progresses to hypoxia and acidosis	▪ Prostaglandin E to maintain PDA to sustain life ▪ Arterial switch surgery before 1 wk of age

Kawasaki Disease

☐ Kawasaki disease is an acquired heart disease.

☐ Kawasaki disease is considered a multisystem vasculitis leading to inflammation of the pharynx and oral mucosa to which the cause is unknown.

☐ With Kawasaki disease, there is a risk of coronary artery involvement and possible aneurysm.

☐ Clinical manifestations include a red, cracked lips and a "strawberry" tongue, fever for more than 5 days, and an elevated erythrocyte sedimentation rate (ESR) and WBC.

☐ Also, it may include abdominal pain, vomiting, and pain in the joints and desquamation of the hands and feet.

☐ The most serious complication of Kawasaki disease is cardiac involvement.

☐ Medications include aspirin therapy and may also require intravenous immunoglobulin administration. Monitor cardiac status, vital signs, I&O, and daily weights.

☐ Provide symptom relief for fever, rash, and oral care.

☐ Monitor for seizures and provide seizure precautions.

☐ It will require periodic follow-up with echocardiography and electrocardiography.

Acute Rheumatic Fever

☐ Acute rheumatic fever is an inflammatory disorder of connective tissue that follows an episode of group A beta-hemolytic streptococci.

☐ Clinical manifestations include fever, chills, myalgia and arthralgia, shortness of breath, murmur, weakness, leukocytosis, and elevated ESR.

☐ Monitor for clinical manifestations of heart failure.

☐ It will have a positive antistreptolysin-O (ASLO) titer, and blood cultures would be positive for *Streptococcus* organisms.

☐ Medications include penicillin or erythromycin and aspirin.

☐ Maintain the child on bed rest, and monitor for clinical manifestations of heart failure.

☐ Teach parents how about following up with cardiologist and antibiotic prophylaxis for dental procedures.

HEMATOLOGIC AND IMMUNE SYSTEMS

KEY TERMS

☐ **Hypochromia** is a decreased hemoglobin concentration.

☐ **Naturally acquired active immunity** occurs after exposure to a disease.

☐ **Naturally acquired passive immunity** occurs during placental transfer of antibodies.

Immunity

☐ In naturally acquired active immunity, the immune system makes antibodies after exposure to disease. This requires contact with the disease.

☐ In naturally acquired passive immunity, no active immune process is involved; antibodies are passively received through placental transfer by immunoglobulin G (the smallest immunoglobulin) and breast-feeding (colostrum).

Human Immunodeficiency Virus (HIV)

☐ The incidence of HIV in the adolescent population has increased since 1995, even though more information about the virus is targeted to reach the adolescent population.

☐ Because of passive antibody transmission, all infants born to HIV-infected mothers test positive for antibodies to HIV up to about age 18 months; confirmation of diagnosis during this time requires detection of the HIV antigen.

☐ When a neonate is born to HIV-infected mom, the neonate will receive the polymerase chain reaction (PCR) test at 48 hours, in 1 to 2 months, in 3 to 6 months, and then at 15 to 18 months.

☐ The HIV has a much shorter incubation period in children than in adults; children who receive the virus by placental transmission are usually HIV positive by age 6 months and develop clinical signs by age 3.

Hemophilia

☐ Hemophilia is a group of genetic disorders leading to a deficiency of blood clotting factors, primarily in males.

☐ Hemophilia is an X-linked recessive disorder.

☐ There are two types: hemophilia A is called factor VIII deficiency or classic hemophilia and hemophilia B is also called factor IX deficiency or Christmas disease.

☐ Clinical manifestations include painful joints, bruising, bleeding from any orifice, and hemarthrosis.

☐ Laboratory values reveal a prolonged PT and decreased clotting factors.

☐ Clinical management of hemophilia includes administration of clotting factors. Desmopressin acetate (DDAVP) tablets and fresh frozen plasma may be needed.

☐ Assess for bleeding including occult blood.

☐ Involve school nurse in the child's care.

☐ Avoid IM injections and rectal temperature.

☐ Teach the child to avoid rigorous contact sports, administration of clotting factors, and use of a soft toothbrush.

Iron Deficiency Anemia

☐ Iron deficiency anemia is a common cause of nutritional anemia during childhood that is characterized by poor red blood cell production.

☐ In iron deficiency anemia, insufficient body stores of iron lead to depleted red blood cell mass, decreased hemoglobin concentration (hypochromia), and decreased oxygen-carrying capacity of the blood.

☐ Peak incidence of iron deficiency anemia occurrence is at age 12 to 18 months.

☐ Clinical manifestations include pallor, fatigue, cardiac murmur, and tachycardia.

☐ Laboratory results reveal decreased hemoglobin and RBC levels, an increased total iron-binding capacity and reticulocyte count.

☐ Clinical management of iron deficiency anemia includes a diet high in iron and supplemental iron administration.

☐ Teach the parents about giving cow's milk only after the child is 1 year of age, the side effects of iron therapy, and to instruct the child to rinse the mouth after taking iron to prevent staining of teeth.

Leukemia

☐ Leukemia results from bone marrow failure and proliferation of immature WBCs, which infiltrate the bone marrow–replacing stem cells that produce RBCs, WBCs, and platelets ("crowds out" normal cells) resulting in pancytopenia: anemia, thrombocytopenia, and neutropenia.

☐ In children, the most common type of leukemia is acute lymphocytic leukemia (ALL).

☐ In adolescents, acute myelogenous leukemia (AML) is more common and is believed to result from a malignant transformation of a single stem cell.

☐ Children between ages 3 and 7 have the best prognosis for ALL.

☐ Clinical manifestations include fever, pallor, increased bruising, petechiae, lethargy, enlarged liver, lymphadenopathy, and bone and joint pain.

☐ Laboratory values reveal anemia, thrombocytopenia, and neutropenia (pancytopenia).

☐ Bone marrow aspiration will reveal leukemic blasts greater than 25%.

☐ Treatment includes radiation, chemotherapy, and stem cell transplant.

- ☐ Children may need infusion of blood products during course of treatment.
- ☐ Monitor for side effects of chemotherapy and radiation, bleeding, infection, and anemia.
- ☐ Place child on infection precautions.
- ☐ Teach the parents and child signs and symptoms of infection.

Sickle Cell Anemia

- ☐ Sickle cell anemia is an autosomal recessive condition that causes a defect in the hemoglobin molecule, which changes the shape of red blood cells, altering their oxygen-carrying capacity.
- ☐ The hemoglobin in sickle cell anemia is referred to as hemoglobin S as the red blood cells acquire a sickle shape.
- ☐ Clinical manifestations of sickle cell anemia include periodic, painful attacks called sickle cell crises, which may be triggered or intensified by dehydration, deoxygenation, or acidosis.
- ☐ Children with sickle cell anemia may also display fever, arthralgia, chest pain, shortness of breath, and abdominal pain.
- ☐ Laboratory values reveal decreased hemoglobin and increased reticulocyte count.
- ☐ Clinical management includes pain control with opioid analgesics, hydration, and oxygen therapy.
- ☐ Child may require blood transfusion.
- ☐ Critical nursing care includes pain management and monitoring oxygenation.
- ☐ Teach the child to avoid conditions that increase incidence of dehydration, illness, or increased altitude.

RESPIRATORY SYSTEM

KEY TERMS

- ☐ **Myringotomy** is a surgical incision into the eardrum.
- ☐ **Tympanostomy** is an incision of the tympanic membrane.
- ☐ **Tympanostomy tube** is a small plastic tube inserted into the eardrum to keep the middle ear aerated.

Pulmonary Anatomy in the Child

- ☐ Lungs aren't fully developed at birth and alveoli continue to grow and increase in size through age 8.
- ☐ A child's respiratory tract has a narrower lumen than an adult's until age 5; the narrow airway makes the young child prone to airway obstruction and respiratory distress from inflammation, mucus secretion, or a foreign body.

- ☐ The American Academy of Pediatrics endorses placing infants faceup in their cribs (or "back to sleep") as a way to reduce sudden infant death syndrome (SIDS).
- ☐ The usual lying-down position of infants favors the pooling of fluid such as formula in the pharyngeal cavity.

Sudden Infant Death Syndrome (SIDS)

- ☐ There is an increased risk of SIDS with prematurity, low birth weight, maternal smoking, and multiple births and in subsequent siblings of two or more SIDS victims.
- ☐ Infants with apnea, central nervous system disorders, or respiratory disorders have a higher risk of SIDS.
- ☐ Peak age for SIDS is age 2 to 4 months.
- ☐ Teach parents the A, B, C's of sleeping. Place infant in Alone, on Back, and in Crib.
- ☐ Avoid plush pillows, stuffed animals, and no cosleeping.

Croup

- ☐ Croup is a viral syndrome that affects the larynx, trachea, and bronchi to the degree that can cause airway obstruction. More common in children age 6 months to 3 years.
- ☐ Clinical manifestations of croup include a seallike cough, inspiratory stridor, tachypnea, copious secretions, and retractions.
- ☐ Chest X-ray (AP and lateral) will reveal "steeples sign."
- ☐ Monitor airway and for symptoms of respiratory distress and assess respiratory effort, breath sounds, and oxygen saturation.
- ☐ Provide oxygen and nasal bulb suction as needed.
- ☐ Medication therapy includes racemic epinephrine, nebulized albuterol, and budesonide.
- ☐ Occasionally, systemic prednisone (Decadron) is used.

Epiglottitis

- ☐ Epiglottitis is an inflammation of the epiglottis (bacterial) caused by *Streptococcus* A, B, or C and *Streptococcus pneumoniae, Haemophilus influenza type b*, and *Staphylococcus aureus.*
- ☐ Epiglottitis is a medical emergency because of rapid airway obstruction.
- ☐ Clinical manifestations include suddenly illness with high fever (higher than 102.2°F [39°C]), intense sore throat, stridor, and the 3Ds (dysphagia [difficulty swallowing], dysphonia [hoarseness], and drooling).
- ☐ The child may assume a tripod position and refuse to lie down.
- ☐ Lateral neck X-ray reveals a narrowed airway and enlarged epiglottis.
- ☐ Keep the head of bed elevated or in upright position.

- Give oxygen and prepare for intubation.
- Medications include antibiotics, hydration, and antipyretics (for fever and pain).
- Nursing actions include respiratory assessment to recognize respiratory distress promptly and have emergency equipment readily available.
- The child with epiglottitis shouldn't be allowed anything by mouth during the initial phases of the infection to prevent aspiration.
- Tongue blades or throat swabs are contraindicated with acute epiglottitis and may cause the epiglottis to spasm.

Cardiopulmonary Resuscitation (CPR)

- The assessment sequence of airway, breathing, and compressions needs to be followed when a child is found unresponsive.
- A compression-ventilation ratio of 30:2 is recommended for the lone rescuer performing CPR on infants and children.
- For health care providers performing 2-rescuer CPR on infants and children, a compression-ventilation ratio of 15:2 is recommended.
- If a tracheal tube is in place when performing CPR on an infant or child, compressions should not be interrupted for ventilations.
- When performing chest compressions, the depth of compressions corresponds to about 1½ inches (4 cm) in an infant and 2 inches (5 cm) in most children.

Choking

- After the airway is open in an unconscious choking 10-month-old infant, the nurse should check for a foreign object and remove it with a finger sweep if it can be seen.
- If ventilation is unsuccessful in the unconscious choking 10-month-old infant, the nurse should then give five back blows and five chest thrusts in an attempt to dislodge the object.
- Blind finger sweeps should never be performed in an infant or child because this may push the object further back into the airway.
- A child between ages 1 and 8 years should receive abdominal thrusts to help dislodge the object.
- Infants younger than age 1 year should receive back blows before chest thrusts and should never receive abdominal thrusts.

Tonsillectomy/Postoperative Care

- Offer soft foods or cool nonacidic fluids. No red colored popsicles or drinks.
- For pain control, offer acetaminophen and a gargle baking soda and water (1/2 tsp in 240 mL of water).

☐ Assess for bleeding, increased swallowing, and infection.

☐ Referred ear pain 4 to 8 days after surgery or a sore throat for 7 to 10 postsurgery is expected.

☐ Advise the parents of no vigorous exercise for 1 week after surgery.

☐ After surgery, the child should remain prone with their head turned to the side to allow the blood and other secretions to drain from the mouth and pharynx, reducing the risk of aspiration.

Chronic Otitis Media (OM)

☐ Chronic OM is an inflammation of the middle ear that is either viral or bacterial in origin usually preceded by an upper respiratory infection.

☐ Children with chronic OM commonly require surgery for a myringotomy and ear tube placement.

☐ In an infant or child, the eustachian tubes are short, wide, and straight and lie in a horizontal plane, allowing them to be more easily blocked by conditions such as large adenoids and infections.

☐ Cartilage lining is underdeveloped in the 1-year-old child, making the eustachian tubes more distensible and more likely to open inappropriately.

☐ The tympanic membrane may present as bright red or yellow, bulging or retracted. While a dull gray membrane fluid is consistent with chronic OM.

☐ Clinical manifestations include displaced light reflex, ear pain (acute onset), fever, pulling at ear, and vomiting and diarrhea.

☐ Pharmacology includes penicillin (amoxicillin) as first-line treatment for 10 days. Other alternatives are as follows: cephalosporin (cefuroxime [Ceftin] or cefdinir [Omnicef]).

☐ Alternative (may be viral) will require conservative treatment: to manage symptoms including acetaminophen/ibuprofen.

☐ ENT referral is recommended.

☐ Myringotomy and tympanostomy tubes are treatment for recurrent infections.

☐ Monitor the child for eardrum perforation. This is the most common complication that is signified by sudden relief of pain.

☐ Monitor for conductive hearing loss and speech problems.

☐ Teach parents to complete the entire prescription of antibiotics, eliminate secondhand smoke exposure, and encourage breast-feeding and no bottle to bed.

Eardrops

☐ For infants receiving eardrops, the parent should be told to gently pull the earlobe down and back to visualize the external auditory canal.

☐ For children receiving eardrops over age 3 and for adults, the earlobe is gently pulled slightly up and back.

Bronchopulmonary Dysplasia

☐ Persistence of lung disease following preterm birth and respiratory support provided in the neonatal period secondary to high oxygen birth/positive pressure ventilation.

☐ The infant with bronchopulmonary dysplasia will have impaired gas exchange related to retention of carbon dioxide and borderline oxygenation secondary to fibrosis of the lungs.

☐ Thermoregulation is important for the infant with bronchopulmonary dysplasia because both hypothermia and hyperthermia will increase oxygen consumption and may increase oxygen requirements.

☐ Clinical manifestations include respiratory distress (tachypnea, dyspnea, increased work or breathing, and wheezing).

☐ Maintain airway with gentle ventilation and may require tracheostomy.

☐ Medications include surfactant, diuretics, bronchodilators, and steroids.

☐ Provide chest physiotherapy and monitor oxygen saturation.

☐ Monitor for growth retardation, developmental delays, pulmonary hypertension, and respiratory infections.

Tracheostomy Tube

☐ Before and after suctioning a tracheostomy tube, provide hyperventilation to the child to prevent hypoxia.

☐ When suctioning a tracheostomy tube, insert the catheter 0.5 cm beyond the tracheostomy tube.

Bronchiolitis

☐ Bronchiolitis is caused by a virus (50% are caused by respiratory syncytial virus [RSV]).

☐ The peak age for infection is 2 to 6 months of age.

☐ Bronchiolitis is preceded by an upper respiratory infection (nasal stuffiness, rhinitis, cough, and fever).

☐ Clinical manifestations of bronchiolitis include wheezing or crackles, flaring, retractions, tachypnea, and problems feeding which can lead to cyanosis.

☐ Bronchiolitis caused by infection with RSV will be confirmed by a nasal swab.

☐ Manage airway, assess lung and heart sounds, apply oxygen, and perform chest physiotherapy and aspiration with bulb syringe.

☐ Medications include bronchodilators and nebulized epinephrine.

- ☐ Encourage hydration.
- ☐ When caring for a child with RSV infection, gowns, gloves, and masks should be worn to prevent the spread of infection.
- ☐ It's essential for parents of infants with bronchiolitis to be able to recognize signs of increasing respiratory distress and know how to count the respiratory rate.

Pertussis

- ☐ Pertussis (whooping cough) is an upper respiratory infection that is caused by the *Bordetella pertussis* bacteria spread by droplet and direct contact.
- ☐ Client is communicable for 4 to 6 weeks, and the disease has a duration of 6 weeks.
- ☐ Begins with mild respiratory symptoms. In the 2nd week, symptoms progress to paroxysmal cough with inspiratory whoop that is sometimes followed by vomiting.
- ☐ Pertussis is diagnosed by a nasal swab.
- ☐ Medications include antibiotics (macrolides), corticosteroids, and albuterol nebulizers.
- ☐ Encourage rest, fluids, and humidified air.
- ☐ Assess child's hydration status, respiratory status, and oxygen saturation.
- ☐ Maintain droplet precautions until 5 to 7 days after antibiotics are initiated.
- ☐ Monitor for complications especially pneumonia.
- ☐ Pertussis is a reportable disease.
- ☐ Teach parents that immunization is important in the prevention of pertussis.

Foreign Body Aspiration

- ☐ For a child with a possible foreign body aspiration, a cough with stridor and changes in phonation would occur if the foreign body were in the larynx.
- ☐ For a child with a possible foreign body aspiration, asymmetrical breath sounds indicate that the object may be located in the bronchi.
- ☐ Bronchoscopy can give a definitive diagnosis of the presence of foreign bodies and is also the best choice for removal of the object with direct visualization.
- ☐ Chest X-ray and lateral neck X-ray may also be used to detect foreign bodies, but findings vary.
- ☐ Some X-ray films may appear normal or show changes such as inflammation related to the presence of the foreign body.

- ☐ Fluoroscopy is valuable in detecting and localizing foreign bodies in the bronchi.

Cystic Fibrosis

- ☐ Cystic fibrosis (CF) is an autosomal recessive disorder of exocrine glands causing a malabsorption of fat and increased loss of chloride in sweat (greater than 60 mEq/L [60 mmol/L]).
- ☐ It also causes alterations in the respiratory and gastrointestinal system.
- ☐ Meconium ileus is commonly a presenting sign of CF.
- ☐ CF affects the pancreatic ducts reducing enzymes needed to digest fat and proteins. Food is also poorly digested because of the thick mucus in bowels.
- ☐ Diagnosis is performed using genetic testing and newborn screening. Also, the sweat chloride test and pulmonary function tests are performed.
- ☐ Clinical manifestations of CF include thick and sticky mucus, greasy stools (steatorrhea) that are frothy and foul smelling, productive cough, shortness of breath, and frequent respiratory infections.
- ☐ Medications include bronchodilators, pancreatic enzymes, and water-soluble forms of vitamins A, D, E, and K.
- ☐ Encourage a high-calorie, high-protein diet, and consume higher than usual amounts of fluids and sodium. Child may need additional tube feedings.
- ☐ Perform chest physiotherapy to break up mucus.
- ☐ Monitor for respiratory infection and intestinal obstruction. Apply supplemental oxygen if needed.

NEUROSENSORY SYSTEM

Head Trauma

- ☐ A finding of dilated and nonreactive pupils in a child who has sustained trauma may indicate that anoxia or ischemia of the brain has occurred.
- ☐ After a trauma, if the pupils are fixed (don't move) in addition to being dilated and nonreactive, herniation of the brain stem has occurred.

Concussion

- ☐ Concussion is a transient impairment of consciousness often resulting from blunt head trauma.
- ☐ It occurs frequently with sports such as hockey, football, and soccer.
- ☐ It results in no loss or brief loss of consciousness.

- ☐ Clinical manifestations include mild headache, slowness in thinking, memory problems, loss of balance, and unsteady gait.
- ☐ Monitor over several hours for decreased level of consciousness.
- ☐ Prepare parents and teachers to expect altered behavior during weeks to months of recovery.
- ☐ Recommend no sports until resolved.

Myelomeningocele (Spina Bifida)

- ☐ A neural tube defect in which the spinal cord and nerves protrudes through a vertebral defect usually in the thoracic and lumbar regions of the spine.
- ☐ Common issues include seizures, bowel and bladder incontinence, and hydrocephalus.
- ☐ Clinical manifestations include visualization of vertebral defect. However, spina bifida occulta will show as a tuft of hair or dimple at the sacrum.
- ☐ Clinical management includes surgery within 24 to 48 hours of birth and child may require shunt for hydrocephalus.
- ☐ Monitor or observe for increased intracranial pressure.
- ☐ Before surgical repair, ensure sac integrity by applying sterile saline dressing.
- ☐ Position child in the prone position.
- ☐ Teach parents urinary catheterization, bowel training (fiber, suppositories), and skin care.
- ☐ Beware of latex allergy with these children.
- ☐ Promote mobility, and encourage PT/OT.
- ☐ Myelomeningocele may be prevented with prenatal folic acid.

Hydrocephalus

- ☐ Hydrocephalus is caused by an alteration in circulation of the cerebrospinal fluid (CSF), causing an increase in CSF and intracranial pressure.
- ☐ In noncommunicating hydrocephalus, an obstruction occurs in the free circulation of CSF, causing increased pressure on the brain or spinal cord.
- ☐ In most cases, congenital hydrocephalus is noncommunicating.
- ☐ Communicating hydrocephalus involves the free flow of CSF between the ventricles and the spinal cord; increased pressure on the spinal cord is caused by defective absorption of CSF.
- ☐ Clinical manifestations include eyes deviate downward (the "setting-sun sign"), high-pitched cry, bulging fontanel, and vomiting.
- ☐ Cushing triad: decrease in respirations, an increase in blood pressure, and a decrease in pulse rate.

- [ ] Monitor airway and keep head of bed at 20 to 30 degrees.
- [ ] Medications include osmotic diuretics (mannitol), corticosteroids, loop diuretics, hypertonic saline, and anticonvulsants.
- [ ] Surgical intervention includes a ventriculostomy to allow the ventricles to drain and placement of a shunt.
- [ ] After shunt insertion, the child should be placed flat in bed to avoid rapid decompression of CSF, and on the left side or on their back to avoid occlusion of the shunt and blockage of the drainage of CSF.
- [ ] After ventriculoperitoneal shunt placement for hydrocephalus, the child should be placed on the side opposite the surgical site to prevent pressure on the shunt valve.

Seizures

- [ ] Abnormal electrical discharges from the brain that cause involuntary movement and behavior and sensory alterations.
- [ ] Various seizure types classified as general or partial seizures.
- [ ] The etiology includes hypoxia, brain trauma/tumor/infection, hypoglycemia, hyponatremia, and acute febrile state.
- [ ] Child is at increased risk for a febrile seizure from 3 months to 5 years as a result of rapid temperature rise greater than 102°F (38.9°C).
- [ ] Clinical management includes maintain airway and have prepared suction available and IV access.
- [ ] Document seizure type, description, aura, duration, and level of consciousness.
- [ ] Care during postictal state includes vital signs, neuro assessment, sidelying, and maintaining airway with suction and oxygen.
- [ ] Institute seizure precautions by keeping bed low and padding side rails.
- [ ] Medications for emergent seizures include diazepam (Valium) IV/rectal or lorazepam (Ativan) IV.
- [ ] Anticonvulsants include phenytoin (Dilantin), carbamazepine (Epitol), and valproic acid (Depakene). They should be given with food.
- [ ] Surgical treatment is done occasionally to remove tumor/lesion or removal of a portion of the brain causing seizure activity.
- [ ] Teach parents that during a seizure, they should ease the child to the floor to prevent falling and unnecessary injury.
- [ ] Teach parents not to put anything in the child's mouth during a seizure.
- [ ] Teach parents to recognize triggers such as flashing lights, bright lights, and too much stimulation.
- [ ] Teach that close follow-up with practitioner will be necessary especially for laboratory monitoring.
- [ ] See Table 3.3 for more types and manifestations of seizures.

TABLE 3.3 Seizures

Seizure Type	Clinical Manifestation
Absence seizure (petit mal)	■ Decreased level of consciousness (LOC) for 5–10 s, mistaken for daydreaming, and eyelids twitching; blank staring
Tonic-clonic (grand mal seizure)	■ Abrupt onset and loss of consciousness for 1–2 min. Preceded by aura and includes a postictal state ■ Tonic: stiff and rigid muscles, cyanosis, may stop breathing, bite tongue, bowel and bladder incontinence ■ Clonic: alternating contraction and relaxation and drooling
Complex partial seizure	■ Decreased LOC for several minutes, automatisms (such as lip smacking), and amnesia about seizure
Simple partial seizure	■ Maintaining consciousness but child has unusual sensations with autonomic sensations (changes in heart rate, offensive smell) ■ May also have unilateral abnormal extremity movement
Febrile seizure	■ Include eyes rolling, limb stiffening, and stiff muscle contraction for 1–2 min

Meningitis

☐ Acute inflammation of the meninges caused by viral or bacterial organisms.

☐ As the organisms invade the meninges, the CSF spreads the infectious agent to the brain.

☐ Clinical manifestations include abrupt onset of flulike symptoms: rash, fever, chills, malaise, stiff neck, maculopapular rash, vomiting, bulging fontanels, and headache.

☐ Neonates may especially have subnormal temperatures, irritability, and decreased appetite.

☐ Neurologic signs such as nuchal rigidity drowsy, disorientation, hallucinations, and convulsions.

☐ Positive Brudzinski and Kernig sign.

☐ The CSF reveals an increased WBC count, decreased glucose (increased with viral), and elevated protein levels.

☐ Prepare child for a lumbar puncture.

☐ Medications include penicillin or cephalosporin, antipyretics, and intravenous fluids.

☐ Monitor vital signs, neuro assessment, and respiratory status.

☐ Place on contact and droplet precautions.

☐ Decreased environmental stimulation (low lights, low sound).

☐ Monitor for seizures, shock, hypotension, disseminated intravascular coagulation, and coma.

Attention Deficit Hyperactivity Disorder (ADHD)

☐ There are two types: inattention and inattention and impulsivity and hyperactivity (most common).

☐ Boys are four times more likely than girls to have ADHD, and ADHD affects 6% to 9% of all school-age children.

☐ Clinical manifestations include inattention to rules, poor listener, inability to sustain attention to complete tasks, forgetfulness, loses things, disorganized, easily distracted, excessive talking, and impulsivity.

☐ Medications include administration of stimulants such as methylphenidate (Concerta).

☐ Other treatments include biofeedback.

☐ Parenting support includes a highly structured environment without excessive stimulation with a calm and firm approach.

☐ Parents should also praise for acceptable behavior, cooperation, and attention.

☐ Teach parents to set limits for acceptable behavior and role model behaviors.

☐ Provide physical activities for children to expend energy.

☐ Make sure all stimulants are given before 4 PM to avoid disruption in sleep cycle.

☐ Monitor appetite, weight, blood pressure, heart rate, and psychological status while taking stimulants.

Cerebral Palsy

☐ Chronic impairment of motor control and muscle tone for which the severity varies.

☐ Risk factors: preterm birth, maternal rubella infection, and birth trauma.

☐ Clinical manifestations include visual, hearing, and speech impairments, developmental delays, seizures, hypotonia, hypertonia, lack of coordination, and gait disturbance.

☐ Medications include muscle relaxants and anticonvulsants (if seizures).

☐ PT, OT, and speech therapy evaluations.

☐ Treatment may include braces and splints.

☐ Encourage follow-up care and coordination of care in school.

☐ Promote optimal nutrition for growth and development.

☐ Coordinate care with PT, OT, and speech therapy services to promote optimal function.

☐ Monitor skin and joint range of motion.

☐ Teach parents measures to prevent pressure ulcers and contractures.

Lumbar Puncture

☐ For a lumbar puncture, the nurse should position the child on their side with their back curved, avoiding flexion of the neck onto the chest.

☐ Curving the back maximizes the space between the lumbar vertebrae, facilitating needle insertion.

Hearing

☐ By ages 5 to 6 months, the infant can localize sounds presented on a horizontal plane and begins to imitate selected sounds.

☐ By ages 7 to 12 months, the infant can localize sounds in any plane.

☐ By age 18 months, the child can hear and follow a simple command without visual cues.

☐ Children who have difficulty with language development by age 18 months should have their hearing evaluated.

Down Syndrome

☐ Down syndrome or trisomy 21 occurs when there is all or part of a third copy of chromosome 21.

☐ Down syndrome is characterized by intellectual disability, dysmorphic facial features, and other distinctive physical abnormalities attributed to a chromosomal aberration.

☐ Clinical manifestations include mild to moderate intellectual disability, short stature with pudgy hands, Simian crease of hand, small head, and upward slanting eyes.

☐ Common to have congenital heart defects, gastroesophageal reflux, and upper respiratory infections and are at increased risk for leukemia.

☐ Coordinate speech therapy and PT and OT as indicated to promote optimal functioning.

☐ Teach parents proper hand hygiene and infection control to prevent respiratory infections.

☐ Encourage genetic counseling for the family.

MUSCULOSKELETAL SYSTEM

Duchenne Muscular Dystrophy

- ☐ Duchenne muscular dystrophy is an X-linked genetic disorder that occurs only in males.
- ☐ Usually inherited by males from their mother.
- ☐ It is marked by muscular deterioration due to a lack of production of dystrophin that progresses throughout childhood, and they usually lose their ability to walk independently by age 12.
- ☐ There is an absence of dystrophin that results in breakdown of muscle fibers; muscle fibers are replaced with fatty deposits and collagen in muscles.
- ☐ Death occurs by early adulthood usually from respiratory failure.
- ☐ Usually presents by age 5 with developmental milestones in sitting and standing not being met.
- ☐ Clinical manifestations include falling frequently and muscle weakness that inhibits ability to do typical age-appropriate activities such as running, riding a bicycle, or climbing stairs.
- ☐ Laboratory results reveal an increased serum creatinine level.
- ☐ Coordinate services PT and OT to maintain physical function as long as possible.
- ☐ Maintain respiratory function.
- ☐ Assess and maintain nutritional status.
- ☐ Surgery may be done to correct contractures, but it doesn't change the course of the disease.
- ☐ Encourage genetic counseling for the family.

Casting

- ☐ After hip spica cast application, a child is at risk for peripheral neurovascular dysfunction due to compartment syndrome.
- ☐ For the infant with a hip spica cast, the infant's body and cast should be at a 180-degree angle.
- ☐ Assessing neurovascular status, circulation, and motion is necessary in all children with a cast.
- ☐ The child with a full body cast may exhibit signs and symptoms of anxiety most likely caused by the feeling of being claustrophobic.
- ☐ Foul odors from the cast may be a sign of infection and should be reported to the practitioner immediately.
- ☐ Capillary refill of less than 3 seconds is a normal finding in a casted extremity.

- [ ] During the first 24 hours, the child may feel warmth under the cast as it dries.
- [ ] For itching under the cast, cool air from a hair dryer may soothe the itch.
- [ ] Elevating the cast above the heart and application of ice helps reduce swelling.
- [ ] To prevent foot drop in a casted leg, the foot should be supported with 90 degrees of flexion.
- [ ] Monitor for compartment syndrome with casted extremities. Unrelieved pain is the primary indicator with also decreased pulse, pallor, and unable to move extremities.

Traction

- [ ] Buck traction is a form of skeletal traction that pulls directly on the skeleton using a pin placed into the bone.
- [ ] The child's position should be changed every 2 hours to prevent skin breakdown when using Buck traction.
- [ ] Bryant traction is the usual method for treating a simple fracture of the femur in a child younger than age 3 and weighing less than 35 pound (15.9 kg). In Bryant traction, both legs are suspended 90 degrees off the bed, even though only one is fractured, with the child's body weight providing the countertraction.
- [ ] Pin site care involves cleaning the insertion sites to reduce the risk of infection and observing the site for signs and symptoms of infection.
- [ ] To prevent venous stasis after skeletal traction application, antiembolism stockings or an intermittent compression device is used on the unaffected leg.
- [ ] For the child in traction, all joints, except those immediately proximal and distal to the fracture, should be placed through range of motion every shift.

Scoliosis

- [ ] Scoliosis is a lateral curvature of the spine that is commonly identified at puberty and throughout adolescence. Greater than 10 degrees curvature is abnormal.
- [ ] There are three causes: idiopathic (most cases are girls 10 to 13 years), congenital, and those related to neuromuscular disorders.
- [ ] Clinical manifestations include uneven hips and shoulders, one-sided rib hump, rib asymmetry, and a prominent scapula.
- [ ] Treatment for a mild or 10 to 20 degrees curvature includes exercises and X-rays every 6 months to monitor.
- [ ] Treatment for a moderate or 20 to 40 degrees curvature is braces and spinal fusion.

- ☐ Treatment for a curvature greater than 40 degrees a Harrington rod placement is needed.
- ☐ Postoperative care includes pulmonary and neurovascular assessments, pain, log rolling, head of bed flat, and skin care.
- ☐ Monitor for complications, which can include hemorrhage, infection, and ileus.
- ☐ Child will wear a brace after surgery and is usually placed on bed rest and ordered to lie flat.

Crutches
- ☐ To walk down the stairs with crutches, the crutches are first placed on the lower step, and then the affected leg is lowered, followed by the unaffected leg.

Weightbearing
- ☐ Touchdown weightbearing prevents the child from putting weight on the extremity, but the child may touch the floor with the affected extremity.
- ☐ Full weightbearing allows for full weightbearing on the affected extremity.
- ☐ Partial weightbearing allows for only 30% to 50% weightbearing on the affected extremity.
- ☐ Nonweight bearing is no weight on the extremity, and the extremity must remain elevated.

Bone Healing
- ☐ Bone healing occurs much faster in a child than in an adult because the child's bones are still growing.
- ☐ The younger the child, the faster the bone heals.
- ☐ Bone healing takes approximately 1 week for every year of life up to age 10.

Fractures
- ☐ The most common fractures in the child are clavicular fractures and greenstick fractures.
- ☐ Greenstick fractures of the long bones are related to the increased flexibility of the young child's bones; the compressed side of the bone bends while the side under tension fractures.
- ☐ After casting for a fracture of the radius, pain over a bony prominence, such as in the wrist or elbow, signals an impending pressure ulcer and requires prompt attention.
- ☐ Avascular necrosis is common with fractures to the subcapital region, secondary to possible compromise of blood supply to the femoral head.

☐ For a femur fracture to heal properly, it usually requires traction before casting.

☐ A greenstick fracture occurs when the bone is bent beyond its limits, causing an incomplete fracture.

☐ A plastic deformation or bend occurs when there is a microscopic fracture line where the bone bends.

☐ A buckle fracture occurs due to compression of the porous bone, causing a raised area or bulge at the fracture site.

☐ A complete fracture is one in which the bone is broken into separate pieces.

Clubfoot

☐ Congenital anomaly of the foot and lower leg that is twice as likely in males. (See Fig. 3.1 for clubfoot variations.)

☐ Some suspect intrauterine positioning or a possible genetic link as a cause.

☐ Clinical manifestations include the foot or feet turning inward and can be rigid and difficult to move.

☐ Treatment begins right after birth with serial casting.

☐ Cast is changed weekly for 4 to 6 weeks and may include bracing after casting series.

☐ If casting fails, the child will require surgery and after surgery, 2 to 3 months of castings follow.

☐ Braces or corrective shoes may be used to maintain the correction.

Developmental Dysplasia of the Hip

☐ Abnormal connection between the femoral head and the acetabulum, leading to instability and abnormal movement. The femoral head is improperly aligned causing hip instability, dislocation, and or dysplasia.

☐ Commonly diagnosed in the neonate or later in infancy.

☐ Clinical manifestations include unequal leg length, asymmetry of the thigh and gluteal folds, and limited abduction of hip.

☐ Also demonstrates Allis sign (one knee higher at flexed position) and Barlow-Ortolani signs (hip click and hard to abduct).

☐ In the older child, signs are more obvious. Observe posture and gait may be limping or level of the pelvis may be unequal.

☐ A positive Trendelenburg sign will show an unstable hip due to weakened muscles.

☐ Treatment in infants younger than 6 months is to keep hips flexed and abducted using the Pavlik harness for 3 to 5 months.

☐ Treatment in children older than 6 months will be to apply Bryant skin traction or surgery and application of a hip spica cast.

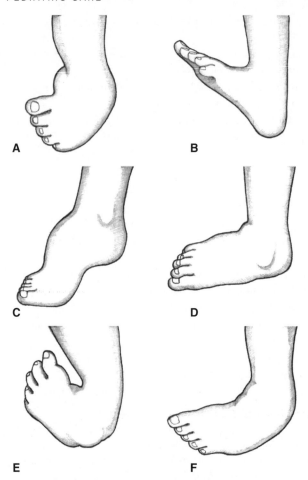

Figure 3.1   Clubfoot variations. Clubfoot can occur in many different variations. **A. Talipes equinovarus** in which the infant's foot is inverted. **B. Talipes calcaneus** or dorsiflexion of the foot, as if the infant is walking on his heel. **C. Talipes equinus** or plantar flexion, as if the infant is pointing his toes. **D. Talipes valgus** or eversion of the ankles, when the infant's feet are turning out. **E. Talipes calcaneovarus** in which the infant's feet are dorsiflexed, inverted, and adducted. **F. Talipes varus** or inversion of the ankles, with the soles of the infant's feet facing each other.

☐   Assess neurovascular status, the lung, and bowel sounds.

☐   Maintain traction, provide cast care, and control pain. It is critical to maintain in the abduction position to encourage repair and healing.

☐   Teach parents how to care for cast and the maintenance of hip abduction.

Juvenile Rheumatoid Arthritis

- Chronic autoimmune inflammatory disease of the connective tissue characterized by joint inflammation, which limits movement in one or more joints or other body systems.
- Occurs before 16 years of age.
- Seventy percent of children experience full remission by adulthood.
- Diagnosis is made by ruling out other possible disorders.
- Clinical manifestations include joint swelling with decreased joint mobility and pain, lethargy, poor appetite, flulike symptoms, rash, and skin nodules.
- Young children may present with limping.
- There are no specific lab tests; however, ESR and WBC may be elevated, and rheumatoid factor and antinuclear antibody may be positive.
- Medications include nonsteroidal anti-inflammatory drugs (NSAIDs) like aspirin and if no response corticosteroids and methotrexate are used.
- Assess pain and inflammation.
- Provide comfort measures including application of moist heat, relaxation, and positioning.
- Promote normal growth and development.
- Encourage physical therapy (PT) and occupational therapy (OT) to promote mobility.

GASTROINTESTINAL SYSTEM

KEY TERMS

- **Gastroschisis** is a herniation of the bowel through an abnormal opening in the abdominal wall.
- **Necrotizing enterocolitis** is an ischemic disorder of the gut.
- **Meconium ileus** is failure to pass meconium by 24 hours of age.
- **Steatorrhea** is fatty, foul-smelling, frothy, bulky stools caused by reduced absorption of fat by the intestine.

Key Considerations

- The extrusion reflex (or tongue-thrust reflex), which protects the infant from food substances that their system is too immature to digest, persists to ages 3 to 4 months.
- The neonate has immature muscle tone of the lower esophageal sphincter and low volume capacity of the stomach, which cause the neonate to "spit up" frequently.
- Increased myelination of nerves to the anal sphincter allows for physiologic control of bowel function, usually around age 2.

- ☐ The liver's slow development of glycogen storage capacity makes the infant prone to hypoglycemia.
- ☐ Diarrhea in infants can rapidly lead to dehydration and electrolyte imbalances, especially hyponatremia and hypokalemia.

Celiac Disease

- ☐ Malabsorption syndrome characterized by intolerance of the gluten protein gliadin found in grains, such as wheat, rye, oats, and barley—which cause poor food absorption.
- ☐ Clinical manifestations include chronic diarrhea, steatorrhea, abdominal pain, vomiting, and weight loss.
- ☐ Diagnosis is made with the laboratory test revealing positive Antigliadin antibodies.
- ☐ Children are managed with a lifelong low gluten diet.
- ☐ Teach parents to read ingredient labels to ensure gluten free foods.

Stools

- ☐ Steatorrhea (fatty, foul-smelling, frothy, bulky stools) is common with celiac disease because of the inability to absorb fat.
- ☐ Clay-colored stools are characteristic of a decrease or absence of conjugated bilirubin.
- ☐ Red currant jelly stool is an indication of intussusception.

Cleft Lip

- ☐ Cleft lip is a congenital anomaly caused by a malformation that occurs during fetal development. Can extend from lip to nasal area and be unilateral or bilateral.
- ☐ Cleft lip can be identified in utero via ultrasound and on physical exam.
- ☐ Infants with cleft lip will have problems sucking.
- ☐ Surgical repair of cleft lip occurs around 1 to 3 months of age.

Cleft Palate

- ☐ Cleft palate is a congenital anomaly that affects the soft palate or the soft and hard palate and can occur with cleft lip.
- ☐ Cleft palate is associated with dental malformations and delayed speech development.
- ☐ Cleft palate is identified by assessing the roof of the infant's mouth to determine condition.
- ☐ The infant with cleft palate may also choke and cough with feedings and have problems sucking.
- ☐ Surgical repair of cleft palate is usually performed at 8 months of age.

Cleft Lip and Palate Repair

- ☐ After the repair, keep the head of the bed elevated and the child supine or sidelying. Do not allow to the child to lie on the suture line.

☐ Perform suture line care and prohibit pacifiers to protect the suture line.

☐ The child may require soft elbow restraints to keep their hands out of the mouth.

☐ For cleft lip repair, progress diet from clear liquids, to half strength formula, and to full strength formula.

☐ For cleft palate repair, progress the diet from clear liquids to a soft diet.

☐ Assess the child for sucking problems and provide flanged nipples.

☐ Monitor the child for pain, infection, and aspiration.

☐ Monitor the child's growth and development patterns.

☐ Monitor the child for dental or speech problems.

☐ Teach childbearing women about folic acid supplementation to prevent cleft lip.

Esophageal Atresia with Tracheoesophageal Fistula

☐ Esophageal atresia with tracheoesophageal fistula occurs when either the distal end of the esophagus ends in a blind pouch and the proximal end of the esophagus is linked to the trachea via a fistula or the proximal end of the esophagus ends in a blind pouch and the distal portion of the esophagus is connected to the trachea via a fistula.

☐ Both esophageal atresia and tracheoesophageal fistula are congenital conditions.

☐ Clinical manifestations include drooling cyanosis, choking, coughing, and an inability to pass a feeding tube.

☐ Monitor the infant for an increased risk for aspiration pneumonia.

☐ This condition is a surgical emergency and is corrected in stages.

☐ Post-op care includes keeping the airway patent, elevate the head of the bed, monitor vital signs and oxygen saturation, and perform a pulmonary assessment.

☐ Weigh the child daily and monitor for infection.

☐ May require gastrostomy tube feedings and parents will need education regarding tube feedings.

Diaphragmatic Hernia

☐ Diaphragmatic hernia is an abnormal opening in the diaphragm where the abdominal organs may herniate into the chest that causes respiratory problems.

☐ Clinical manifestations include respiratory distress at birth, irregular chest movements, lack of breath sounds on the side with the hernia, and bowel sounds that are heard in the chest.

- ☐ Be prepared for resuscitation at birth if already identified in utero via ultrasound.
- ☐ Surgical emergency because of life-threatening problems.
- ☐ Immediate transfer to NICU for immediate respiratory support is essential.
- ☐ Positioning the infant with a diaphragmatic hernia on the affected side lets the lung on the unaffected side expand, making breathing easier.

Pyloric Stenosis

- ☐ Pyloric stenosis is hypertrophy of the pyloric sphincter muscle, which causes stenosis and obstruction.
- ☐ The exact cause of pyloric stenosis is unknown but is more common in males.
- ☐ The diagnosis of pyloric stenosis is usually made by 2 months of age.
- ☐ In infants 2 to 8 weeks after birth, symptoms include projectile vomiting 30 to 60 minutes after feeding.
- ☐ Other clinical manifestations include failure to gain weight, a palpable olive-shaped epigastric mass in the right upper quadrant, and visible peristaltic waves.
- ☐ Diagnosis is made with an upper GI series of X-rays or abdominal ultrasound.
- ☐ Pyloric stenosis is surgically corrected with a pyloromyotomy.
- ☐ Monitor the child for dehydration and fluid and electrolyte imbalances.
- ☐ Progress slowly with fluids within 6 hours of surgery and then progress slowly with diluted fluids.
- ☐ Monitor daily weights.
- ☐ Even with successful surgery, most infants will have some vomiting during the first 24 to 48 hours after the surgical repair.

Poisoning

- ☐ In the recovery phase following ingestion of drain cleaner, scar tissue develops as the burn from ingestion heals leading to esophageal strictures.
- ☐ Be prepared to assist with performing a tracheostomy.
- ☐ Home administration of syrup of ipecac is no longer recommended by the American Academy of Pediatrics for poisoning.
- ☐ Elevating the head and legs to the level of the heart will promote venous drainage and decrease the chance of the child going into shock after poisoning.
- ☐ The most common pain medications accidentally ingested are acetaminophen-containing (Tylenol-containing) drugs, nonsteroidal anti-inflammatory drugs, and opioids.

Hydrocarbon Poisoning

- ☐ Hydrocarbons are naturally occurring in petroleum, natural gas, and coal.
- ☐ If a child ingests poisonous hydrocarbons, keeping the child calm and relaxed will help prevent vomiting, which can damage the esophagus from regurgitation of the gastric poison.
- ☐ The risk of chemical pneumonitis exists if vomiting occurs in a child who has ingested poisonous hydrocarbons.
- ☐ Chemical pneumonitis is the most common complication of ingestion of a hydrocarbon, such as kerosene.
- ☐ Child may require intubation and mechanical ventilation. Prepare for gastric lavage.
- ☐ Monitor vital sign, cardiac rhythm, and oxygen saturation.

Salicylate Poisoning

- ☐ After ingestion of poisonous amounts of salicylates, there's usually a delay of 6 hours before evidence of toxicity is noted.
- ☐ Gastric lavage is used in the immediate treatment for salicylate poisoning because the stomach contents and salicylates will move from the stomach to the remainder of the GI tract, where vomiting will no longer result in the removal of the poison.
- ☐ Clinical manifestations of salicylate toxicity include tinnitus, hyperventilation, Kussmaul respiration, and nausea and vomiting.

Acetaminophen Poisoning

- ☐ Acetaminophen poisoning damages the liver, leading to elevated serum alanine aminotransferase and aspartate aminotransferase levels.
- ☐ After therapy with acetylcysteine is started for acetaminophen poisoning, liver enzymes should begin to fall.
- ☐ During the first 12 to 24 hours after ingestion, profuse sweating is a significant sign of acetaminophen poisoning.
- ☐ Weak pulse, hypothermia, and decreased urine output are common findings with acetaminophen poisoning.
- ☐ If the child is seen within 4 hours of ingestion, activated charcoal should be given to prevent absorption of acetaminophen.
- ☐ Gastric lavage is recommended only if the child is seen within 1 hour of ingestion in acetaminophen poisoning.

Lead Poisoning

- ☐ In older homes that contain lead-based paint, paint chips may be eaten directly by the child or they may cling to toys or hands that are then put into the mouth.
- ☐ Ingested lead is initially absorbed by bone; X-rays reveal a characteristic "lead line" at the epiphyseal line.

- ☐ Chronic ingestion of lead produces effects on the central nervous, renal, and hematologic systems.
- ☐ Lead is dangerously toxic to the biosynthesis of heme, and the reduced amounts of heme molecule in red blood cells cause anemia.
- ☐ Paralysis may occur in lead toxicity as toxic damage to the brain progresses.
- ☐ Lead intoxication produces damage to the central nervous system that is difficult to repair.
- ☐ One diagnostic characteristic of lead poisoning is a gingival or Burton line, which refers to black lines along the gums.
- ☐ Chelation therapy is the main treatment for lead poisoning and involves the removal of metal by combining it with another substance.
- ☐ Sometimes, exchange transfusions may be needed to remove the lead from the blood quickly.
- ☐ A calcium-chelating agent is used for the treatment of lead poisoning, resulting in hypocalcemia.

Appendicitis

- ☐ Caused by an obstruction of the appendiceal lumen leading to bacterial proliferation and edema causing the vascular supply to be compromised. Rupture results from increasing ischemia and necrosis.
- ☐ Most common emergency abdominal surgery in children.
- ☐ Clinical manifestations include periumbilical pain shifting to right lower quadrant pain at McBurney point, fever, nausea and vomiting, guarding, and rebound tenderness.
- ☐ Child may also be motionless or assume a sidelying position with knees flexed.
- ☐ Laboratory tests reveal elevated WBC count.
- ☐ Goal is early identification, pain management, and surgical removal.
- ☐ The sudden cessation of abdominal pain in the child with appendicitis may indicate perforation or infarction of the appendix, requiring emergency surgery.
- ☐ Post-op care includes monitoring for infection and pain control.
- ☐ Assess gastrointestinal status including bowel sounds, flatus, and bowel movement.

Gastroenteritis

- ☐ Young children with gastroenteritis are at high risk for developing a fluid volume deficit because their intestinal mucosa allows for more fluid and electrolytes to be lost when they have gastroenteritis.

- [ ] The main goal of the health care team in young children with gastroenteritis should be to rehydrate the infant; deficient fluid volume is life threatening.
- [ ] Allowing only clear liquids while recovering from gastroenteritis gives the intestine time to heal, but the fluids should be reintroduced slowly to determine the child's ability to tolerate and retain them.

Pinworms

- [ ] Intestinal parasitic worm infection where child is infected by swallowing the worm eggs. Worms can migrate to the vagina.
- [ ] Children in crowded conditions are at higher risk.
- [ ] Clinical manifestations include intense anal itching and irritation.
- [ ] Cellophane tape is placed near the anal edge to capture the eggs it and can assist in diagnosing.
- [ ] Medications include mebendazole and pyrantel pamoate.
- [ ] Teach strict proper hand hygiene to prevent reinfection and spread.

GENITOURINARY SYSTEM

KEY TERMS

- [ ] **Hypospadias** means the urethra is located on the ventral surface of the penis.
- [ ] **Epispadias** means the urethra is located on the dorsal surface of the penis.

Acute Glomerulonephritis

- [ ] Autoimmune process that involves inflammation of the glomeruli of the kidneys.
- [ ] Characterized by antigen–antibody complexes that obstruct glomeruli secondary to a beta-hemolytic streptococcal infection. Frequently, this occurs 10 to 21 days after infection.
- [ ] Can be asymptomatic but usual signs and symptoms include abrupt onset flank or midabdominal pain, malaise, fever, decreased urine output, dysuria, periorbital edema, costovertebral angle tenderness, and hypertension.
- [ ] Urinalysis findings: specific gravity less than 1.030, proteinuria, hematuria, and the presence of red blood cell casts.
- [ ] Laboratory results reveal elevated WBC and a positive ASLO titer (recent pharyngeal strep infection).
- [ ] Monitor fluid status, vital signs, laboratory results, weight, I&O, and edema.

- ☐ Children with acute glomerulonephritis can develop severe hypertension requiring treatment.
- ☐ Monitor respiratory status including oxygen saturation.
- ☐ Medications include antihypertensives, diuretics, and penicillin.
- ☐ Place child on bed rest, and monitor skin for breakdown.
- ☐ Monitor for complications such as acute hypertension, infection, and acute renal failure.
- ☐ Teach parents to complete all antibiotics for streptococcal infections.

Hypospadias and Epispadias
- ☐ Hypospadias and epispadias are congenital anomalies with an abnormal urethral opening on the penis.
- ☐ In hypospadias, the urethra is located on the ventral surface of the penis.
- ☐ In epispadias the urethra is located on the dorsal surface of the penis.
- ☐ These children are not circumcised and will have surgical correction during first year of life.
- ☐ Post-op care includes assessment of I&O, pain, and bladder spasms and for bleeding and infection.
- ☐ Urine may be blood tinged for several days.
- ☐ Medications for bladder spasms are anticholinergics (oxybutynin).
- ☐ Complete incision care and use a double diapering technique if stents are placed.
- ☐ Teach parent to not allow their child straddle toys and avoid tub baths until incisions heal and stents are removed. They should limit the child's activity for 2 weeks.
- ☐ Instruct parents on incision care and report symptoms of infection, complete all antibiotics, and encourage child to drink plenty of fluids.

Urinary Tract Infection (UTI)
- ☐ Infection of the upper or lower urinary tract that can be caused by the bacteria *Escherichia coli*, urinary stasis (neurogenic bladder), vesicoureteral reflux, or genitourinary defect.
- ☐ In vesicoureteral reflux, urine flows back up the ureter, past the incompetent valve, and back into the bladder after the child has finished voiding resulting in incomplete emptying of the bladder and stasis of urine, providing a good medium for bacterial growth and subsequent infection.
- ☐ Upper UTI (pyelonephritis) affects the ureters, renal pelvis, and renal parenchyma.
- ☐ Lower UTI (cystitis) affects the bladder/urethra.

- Signs of lower UTI include frequency, dysuria, strong urine, cloudy, hematuria, abdominal pain, and enuresis.
- Signs of upper UTI are the same as lower UTI with addition of high fever, chills, and costovertebral tenderness.
- Signs and symptom in newborns include unexplained fever, poor feeding, V/D, and decreased urine output.
- A urinalysis may show RBCs, WBCs, and bacteria.
- Medications include antibiotics (sulfamethoxazole, trimethoprim [Bactrim], and fluoroquinolones).
- Children with pyelonephritis are usually hospitalized.
- Surgical correction if there is a structural defect.
- Consider potential for sexual abuse or sexual activity with recurrent UTIs.
- Monitor for signs and symptoms of lower UTI worsening to pyelonephritis.
- Teach children to wipe front to back, wear cotton underwear, practice regular voiding, and avoid bubble baths.

Urine Specimens
- The most accurate test to analyze bacterial content in the urine of a child less than 2 years old is properly performed bladder catheterization.
- Bagged urine specimen, clean-catch urine specimen, and first-voided urine specimen have a high incidence of contamination not related to infection.
- When collecting a clean-catch urine specimen, the first-voided specimen of the day should never be used because of urinary stasis; this also applies after a nap.
- The clean-catch urine specimen should be collected midstream, not at the beginning or end of urination.

Neuroblastoma
- A neuroblastoma is a malignancy that occurs in the adrenal gland or in the sympathetic nervous system of the abdomen, head, neck, pelvis, or chest.
- Most neuroblastomas have metastasized at time of diagnosis.
- Abdominal clinical manifestations include a firm nontender mass in the abdomen and bowel and bladder dysfunction.
- Bone and spinal cord lesion signs and symptoms include pain, limping, and weakness and problems with mobility.
- Metastasis is common to the bone marrow, organs, and lymph nodes.
- Laboratory test reveals a complete blood count with leukocytosis or leukopenia and urine catecholamines.

☐ Tumor markers show increase in vanillylmandelic acid.

☐ Child will need a biopsy and a computed tomography and or magnetic resonance imaging to look for metastasis.

☐ Treated with a surgical excision of the tumor, radiation, chemotherapy, and stem cell transplant.

☐ Monitor for side effects of chemotherapy and radiation treatments in infection, skin problems, and pancytopenia.

☐ Teach proper hand hygiene, infection prevention, and ways to monitor for infection.

Wilms Tumor

☐ Nephroblastoma, also known as Wilms tumor, is an embryonal cancer of the kidney.

☐ Wilms tumor can be caused by an inherited trait.

☐ Clinical manifestations of Wilms tumor include a firm, nontender mass located to one side of abdomen (which is often found by the parent during bath), hematuria, urinary frequency with urgency, and hypertension.

☐ A Wilms tumor is treated with surgical removal of the kidney, radiation, and chemotherapy for 6 to 15 months.

☐ Preoperatively, do not palpate abdomen and take care with activities of daily living to prevent the spread of cancerous cells.

☐ Monitor vital signs and respiratory status.

☐ The child may require treatment for hypertension.

☐ Post-op, monitor vital signs, renal status, I&O, daily weights, and pain levels.

Extracellular Fluid

☐ An infant has a much greater percentage of total body water in extracellular fluid (42% to 45%) than an adult does (20%).

☐ Because of the increased percentage of water in a child's extracellular fluid, a child's water turnover rate is two to three times greater than that of an adult.

☐ Every day, 50% of an infant's extracellular fluid is exchanged, compared with only 20% of an adult's; therefore, a child is more susceptible to dehydration than an adult.

☐ A neonate has a greater ratio of body surface area to body weight than an adult; this ratio results in greater fluid loss through the skin.

Pediatric Renal System

☐ A child's kidneys attain the adult number of nephrons (about a million in each kidney) shortly after birth.

☐ The nephrons, which form urine, continue to mature throughout early childhood.

- An infant's renal system can maintain a healthy fluid and electrolyte status; however, it doesn't function as efficiently as an adult's during periods of stress.
- An infant's kidneys don't concentrate urine at an adult level (average specific gravity is less than 1.010 for an infant, compared with 1.010 to 1.030 for an adult).
- An infant usually voids 5 to 10 mL/h, a 10-year-old child usually voids 10 to 25 mL/h, and an adult usually voids 35 mL/h.
- Children have short urethras; therefore, organisms can be easily transmitted into the bladder, increasing the risk of bladder infection.
- Enuresis is involuntary urination after age 5 years that generally occurs while the child is sleeping.
- Nephritis is a sudden inflammation that primarily affects the interstitial area and the renal pelvis or, less commonly, the renal tubules.

ENDOCRINE SYSTEM

Congenital Hypothyroidism

- A condition that affects infants from birth and results from a partial or complete loss of thyroid function and is associated with some gene mutations.
- In the first few months of life, the infant develops feeding difficulties, lethargy, and hoarse cry as well as cretinoid features such as a thick protuberate tongue, thick lips, and hypotonia.
- If not treated, congenital hypothyroidism will cause growth delay and intellectual disability.
- Congenital hypothyroidism is tested as part of the mandatory heel-stick neonatal testing program.
- Will require lifelong thyroid replacement and thyroid levels drawn periodically.
- Will need frequent measurement of height and bone age to assess growth patterns.
- Early recognition and treatment is essential to prevent delayed development of the central nervous system.
- Education about congenital hypothyroidism should occur as soon as the parents are ready so they'll understand the genetic implications for future children.

Hyperbilirubinemia

- A condition in the neonate in which there is an increase in the breakdown of red blood cells releasing bilirubin.
- There are two types: indirect (physiologic) and direct (obstruction).

- Clinical manifestations include jaundice, poor feeding, lethargy, encephalopathy, and elevated bilirubin levels (greater than 13 mg/dL [222.3 µmol/L]).
- Treated with light phototherapy and regular feedings.
- During phototherapy, protect neonate's eyes and monitor for dehydration.
- Monitor bilirubin levels.
- Teach parents about home phototherapy and to follow through with lab testing as ordered.
- Teach to report fever, poor feeding, worsening jaundice, or lethargy.

Diabetes Mellitus Type 1

- Thought to be an autoimmune process where there is destruction of beta cells, which leads to insulin deficiency.
- Heredity is a factor and onset typically in childhood.
- Clinical manifestations include polyuria, polydipsia, polyphagia, weight loss, and fatigue.
- Urinalysis reveals glucosuria and ketones.
- Medications include the administration of insulins such as rapid-acting Lispro, intermediate-acting NPH, and long-acting glargine.
- Child may need continuous insulin infusion until glucose stabilized.
- Treat dehydration and electrolyte imbalances.
- Monitor blood glucose and electrolytes.
- Assess neurologic status and monitor for diabetic ketoacidosis (DKA).
- DKA is determined by the presence of hyperglycemia (blood glucose level of 300 mg/dL [16.6 mmol/L] or higher), accompanied by acetone breath, dehydration, weak and rapid pulse, and a decreased level of consciousness.
- Educate the child and parents about diet, medication administration, signs and symptoms of hypoglycemia and hyperglycemia, foot care, and long-term complications.
- Food intake should be increased in children with diabetes when they are more physically active.
- A glycosylated hemoglobin (hemoglobin A1$_c$) level provides an overview of a person's blood glucose level over the previous 2 to 3 months.
- Teenagers with diabetes mellitus who drink alcohol may become hypoglycemic, but their symptoms of hypoglycemia may be misinterpreted as being intoxicated.

Growth Hormone Deficiency

- Idiopathic growth hormone deficiency is commonly associated with other pituitary hormone deficiencies, such as deficiencies of thyroid-stimulating hormone and corticotropin, and may be secondary to hypothalamic deficiency.

☐ During the school-age years, growth slows and doesn't accelerate again until adolescence.

☐ Familial short stature refers to otherwise healthy children who have ancestors with adult height in the lower percentiles and whose height during childhood is appropriate for genetic background.

☐ Children with delayed linear growth and skeletal and sexual maturation that is behind that of their peers are considered to have constitutional growth delay.

☐ The definitive treatment of growth hormone deficiency is replacement of the growth hormone; it is successful in 80% of affected children.

Hypopituitarism

☐ A rare disorder in which the pituitary gland either fails to produce growth hormone or does not produce enough hormones.

☐ Can be genetic or secondary to a tumor or absent or undeveloped pituitary gland.

☐ Generally, children with hypopituitarism are of average birth weight and grow at a normal pace for the first 2 or 3 years and then fall behind their peers in height, usually below the third percentile.

☐ Clinical manifestations include delayed growth pattern, short stature, absent or delayed puberty, and fatigue.

☐ Laboratory results reveal low insulin and growth factors levels.

☐ Child requires referral to an endocrinologist.

☐ Medications include grown hormone replacement for 3 weeks until height is achieved (around 14 to 16 years).

☐ Child may need surgery if caused by a tumor.

☐ Monitor height, weight, and growth over time.

☐ Promote normalcy.

☐ Teach the child how to do self-injections.

INTEGUMENTARY SYSTEM

Key Considerations

☐ Like most body systems, the integumentary system isn't mature at birth; therefore, it provides a less effective barrier to physical elements or microorganisms during birth and infancy than during childhood. This helps to explain why infants and young children are more prone to infection.

☐ Infants have poorly developed subcutaneous fat, predisposing them to hypothermia.

- Strawberry hemangiomas are rapidly growing vascular lesions that reach maximum growth by age 1 year, followed by an involution period of 6 to 12 months, and complete involution by age 2 or 3 years.
- When salmon patches appear on the nape of the neck, they're commonly called "stork bites."

Fifth Disease

- Fifth disease, also called erythema infectiosum, is a mild rash illness caused by parvovirus B19.
- Symptoms include 2 to 3 days with flulike symptoms (headache, chills, malaise, nausea), and 1 week later, a rash develops on the cheeks ("slapped cheek rash") that spreads to trunk and limbs (lacelike rash). The rash fades over 1 to 3 weeks.
- Laboratory results reveal increased IgM antibodies as body reacts to the parvovirus.
- Therapy is supportive encouraging rest, fluids, and antipyretics.
- Child should be placed on droplet precautions and isolated from pregnant women, immunocompromised children, and children with chronic anemia for up to 2 weeks.
- A child with fifth disease is contagious during the first stage, when symptoms of headache, body aches, fever, and chills are present, not after the rash appears.

Scarlet Fever

- Erythematous rash caused by a bacterial infection.
- Causative agent is group A beta-hemolytic streptococci.
- Clinical manifestations begin abruptly with fever, sore throat, headache, chills, and a red rash on the skin and mucous membranes.
- Give the child a soft or liquid diet.
- Medications include antipyretics and penicillin for streptococcal infection.
- Encourage rest and fluids.
- Monitor for complications such as pyelonephritis or rheumatic fever.
- Teach parent to make sure the child finishes the antibiotic prescription.

Varicella

- A highly contagious viral infection caused by varicella zoster virus.
- Varicella is spread via airborne and direct contact. The virus is communicable 1 to 2 days prior to rash until all lesions crusted.
- Clinical manifestations of varicella include a mild fever, malaise, and irritability.

☐ Varicella begins as macule on an erythematous base that is itchy and turns into a papule, and finally a blister-like vesicle.

☐ Vesicles can remain 1 to 3 weeks.

☐ Rash begins on the trunk before spreading to the scalp, face, and rest of the body.

☐ Management is supportive including rest, fluids, nonaspirin antipyretics, oral antihistamines, calamine lotion, and oatmeal baths.

☐ Child may need fingernails shortened and may need to wear mittens to prevent scratching, which can lead to localized infection.

☐ Place child on airborne and contact precautions.

☐ Monitor for complications such as pneumonia, meningitis, and cellulitis.

☐ Child may return to school after all lesions crusted.

☐ Encourage all parents to vaccinate their child for varicella to prevent infection.

Roseola

☐ A mild herpetic viral illness that causes an erythematous rash.

☐ It is generally mild and self-limiting infection.

☐ Clinical manifestations include a sudden high fever lasting 2 to 4 days before a pale pink maculopapular rash (fine pink) appears on the trunk. The rash spreads to the face, neck, and extremities and can last 1 to 2 days.

☐ Treatment is supportive including nonaspirin products, rest, and oral fluids.

☐ Maintain standard precautions.

☐ Monitor for seizures during fever.

☐ Teach the parents to treat temperature appropriately and explain that illness is self-limiting.

Rubeola

☐ Rubeola is a highly contagious measles virus spread through droplets and direct contact with respiratory droplets, blood, and urine.

☐ Clinical manifestations include high fever, cough, nasal congestion, malaise, buccal mucosa with bluish white Koplik spots, and macropapular rash that starts at the head and spreads to trunk then the extremities.

☐ Laboratory test reveals increased IgM antibodies.

☐ Treatment is supportive including humidified air, bulb syringe aspiration, rest, fluids, nonaspirin antipyretics, antipruritics, and antitussives.

- ☐ Place the child on airborne, droplet, and contact precautions for 4 to 5 days after onset of rash.
- ☐ Rubeola is a reportable disease.
- ☐ Complications include OM, bronchitis, and pneumonia.

Scabies

- ☐ Highly contagious skin infection caused by the female mite burrowing into epidermis to lay eggs.
- ☐ Clinical manifestations include intense pruritus (worse at night); lesions in web of fingers, palms, and waist; and irritability and restlessness.
- ☐ Medication includes 5% permethrin lotion over the entire body at bedtime. Leave on 8 to 12 hours and repeat the treatment in 1 week.
- ☐ Teach parent to treat all household members, wash all linen in hot water, and dry in a dryer for at least 20 minutes.
- ☐ Stress the importance of good hand hygiene.
- ☐ Pruritus may persist for 1 to 2 weeks after treatment and antihistamines may be prescribed to relieve the pruritus.

Child Abuse

- ☐ In cases of suspected child abuse, an accurate precise examination of all lesions must be properly and legally documented.
- ☐ Contusions that result from falls are typically confined to a single body area and are considered a reasonable finding in a child still learning to walk.
- ☐ Injuries from normal falls are usually not linear in nature.
- ☐ The bleeding from contusions can cause variations, but the color change is consistent.
- ☐ Burns that are bilateral as well as symmetrical are typical of child abuse.
- ☐ The shape of the burn may resemble the item used to create it, such as a cigarette.

Acne Vulgaris

- ☐ Chronic inflammatory disorder caused by the plugging of sebaceous glands.
- ☐ It is most common in 12- to 16-year-olds manifesting as blackheads, whiteheads, and pustules with inflammation.
- ☐ The goal of treatment is to prevent scarring using a stepwise approach.
- ☐ Benzoyl peroxide twice a day may cause dryness and scaling and redness.
- ☐ Topical retinoid tretinoin applied at sleep and wash off in the morning for 6 to 12 weeks.

☐ Ketolytic causes dryness and scaling and the child should avoid sunlight.

☐ Antibiotics including topical antibiotics (such as tetracycline or clindamycin [Clindagel]) and oral antibiotics for moderate to severe acne (such as doxycycline [Acticlate], tetracycline, or sulfamethoxazole and trimethoprim [Septra]).

☐ Oral retinoids such as isotretinoin (Absorica) for treatment for 16 to 20 weeks when other therapies fail.

☐ Other treatments include oral contraceptives for female children.

☐ Teach child about developing a good skin care routine.

Impetigo

☐ Highly contagious skin infection that is caused by staphylococcal or streptococcal organisms.

☐ Begins as red a macule that progresses to a vesicle usually on the face, hands, mouth, and extremities.

☐ The vesicles rupture and leave a honey colored crust and is spread by direct contact.

☐ Treated with topical antibiotics for 5 to 7 days.

☐ Teach parents that child is contagious for 48 hours after antibiotics initiated.

☐ Teach parents proper hand hygiene and surface cleaning.

☐ Teach parents to keep child's fingernails short to prevent breaks in skin integrity.

Port-Wine Stains

☐ Port-wine stains are associated with syndromes of the neonate, such as Sturge-Weber syndrome.

☐ Port-wine stains found on the face or extremities may be associated with soft tissue and bone hypertrophy.

Warts

☐ Plantar warts found on the soles of feet and common warts occur anywhere.

☐ Common cause of health care visits in children.

☐ Visual inspection shows rough scaly papules or plaques.

☐ May need no intervention because warts can resolve spontaneously.

☐ Treated with caustic agents like salicylic acid or cryotherapy.

☐ Teach the child not to bite or pick at wart to prevent spreading warts to surrounding tissues, wear shoes in public showers, and frequently hand wash.

Tinea Fungal Infections

☐ Tinea is a fungal infection of the skin, hair, and nails. (See Table 3.4 for more information on tinea infections.)

Candidiasis (Thrush)

☐ Most cases, the cause is the host's normal flora that has over grown due to immunosuppression or antibiotic use.

☐ Clinical manifestations include creamy white plagues on buccal mucosa and tongue (thrush).

☐ May be mistaken for milk residue.

☐ Treated with a nystatin suspension.

☐ Encourage soft and nonacidic foods.

TABLE 3.4 Tinea Infections		
Type	Clinical Manifestations	Treatment
Tinea capitis	■ Scaly, erythematous patches on scalp	■ Selenium sulfide shampoo for 2 wk ■ If resistant, griseofulvin, terbinafine (Lamisil), or fluconazole (Diflucan) for 6–8 wk
Tinea corporis	■ Annular lesion on the body with a raised erythematous border ■ Itchy and scaly	■ Wash body with selenium sulfide shampoo. ■ Apply miconazole topical cream bid 2–4 wk.
Tinea cruris	■ Erythematous patches of the groin ■ Also known as jock itch	■ Wash body with selenium sulfide shampoo. ■ Apply miconazole cream 2–4 wk.
Tinea pedis	■ Itchy and scaly erythematous patches on the feet ■ Also known as athlete's foot	■ Topical antifungal cream ■ Apply absorbent talc. ■ Keep feet dry. ■ Wear cotton socks.

REVIEW QUESTIONS ||||||||||

1. For an infant who's about to undergo a lumbar puncture, the nurse should place the infant in which position?

1. An arched, sidelying position, with the neck flexed onto the chest
2. An arched, sidelying position, avoiding flexion of the neck onto the chest
3. A mummy restraint
4. A prone position, with the head over the edge of the bed

2. A nurse teaches a parent about frequent assessment tests necessary to assess and treat congenital hypothyroidism. Which of the following test if identified by the parent would show the teaching was effective?

1. Blood electrolyte levels
2. Metabolic rate
3. Muscular coordination
4. Bone age

3. A toddler is brought to the emergency room after ingesting an undetermined amount of drain cleaner. The nurse should expect to assist with which of the following **first**?

1. Administering an emetic
2. Performing a tracheostomy
3. Performing gastric lavage
4. Inserting an indwelling urinary (Foley) catheter

4. A nurse is teaching the parents of a child diagnosed with a urinary tract infection secondary to vesicoureteral reflux. How can the nurse **best** explain the way reflux contributes to the infection?

1. "It prevents complete emptying of the bladder."
2. "It causes urine backflow into the kidney."
3. "It results in painful bladder spasms."
4. "It causes painful urination."

5. A nurse is making an initial visit to a family with a 3-year-old child with early Duchenne muscular dystrophy. Which of the following findings is expected when assessing this child?

1. Contractures of the large joints
2. Enlarged calf muscles
3. Difficulty riding a tricycle
4. Small, weak muscles

Chapter References

Ateah, C. A., Scott, S. D., & Kyle, T. (2012). *Canadian essentials of pediatric nursing.* Philadelphia, PA: Lippincott Williams & Wilkins.

Hatfield, N. T. (2013). *Introductory maternity and pediatric nursing.* Philadelphia, PA: Lippincott Williams & Wilkins.

Kyle, T., & Carmen, S. (2016). *Essentials of pediatric nursing* (3rd ed.). Philadelphia, PA: Wolters Kluwer.

Ricci, S. S., Kyle, T., & Carman, S. (2012). *Maternity and pediatric nursing.* Philadelphia, PA: Lippincott Williams & Wilkins.

4

Psychiatric Care

ESSENTIALS OF PSYCHIATRIC CARE

KEY TERMS

- ☐ **Maslow's hierarchy of needs** is a theory developed by Abraham Maslow that directly applies to prioritizing safety when caring for a psychiatric patient.

- ☐ **Unconditional positive regard** is a phrase from Carl Rogers's client-centered therapy that describes a supportive, nonjudgmental, neutral approach by a therapist.

- ☐ **Transference** is the unconscious assignment of negative or positive feelings evoked by a significant person in the client's past to another person.

- ☐ **Countertransference** is the unconscious assignment of negative or positive feelings evoked by a significant person in the practitioner's past to the patient.

- ☐ **Interpretation** is a technique in which the nurse attempts to describe the client's feelings.

- ☐ **Validation** is a technique in which the nurse seeks to clarify what the client is describing.

- ☐ **Open-ended statements** introduce a topic in order to get the client's feedback past a "yes" or "no" reply.

- ☐ **Doubt** is a technique used by the nurse to prompt the client to assess if his or her feelings are based on truth.

- ☐ **Confrontation** is similar to doubt; however, confrontation is when the nurse provides directly contradicting evidence to the client's statement to immediately demonstrate reality.

- ☐ **Observation** is a technique in which the nurse shares with the client objective information about the client or the situation to initiate discussion.

- ☐ **Restatement** is a technique in which the nurse rephrases the client's statements in order to demonstrate that the nurse is listening.

- ☐ **Therapeutic silence** is a technique that demonstrates active listening skills through the use of nonverbal communication. It allows the client to know that they are being heard and prompts the client to continue sharing at their own pace.

☐ **Triangulation** refers to conflicts involving three family members.

Overview

☐ Therapeutic communication is the foundation for developing a nurse–client relationship.

☐ Suicide and homicide risk should be assessed directly. For instance, a nurse could ask, "Are you currently thinking about killing yourself?" to assess suicidal ideation. Additionally, intent, plan, and means to accomplish the plan should be assessed for both suicidal and homicidal clients.

☐ Impulsive behavior, overwhelming guilt, and chronic illness are factors that contribute to suicide potential.

☐ In an examination of the psychiatric client, the nurse should assess the client's general appearance, behavior, mood, affect, thought processes and cognitive function, coping mechanisms, and potential for self-destructive behavior. Mood is a subjective assessment, whereas affect is objective.

☐ The *Diagnostic and Statistical Manual of Mental Disorders, 5th ed.* (*DSM-5*) includes a complete description and diagnostic criteria of psychiatric disorders.

☐ See Table 4.1 for a list and description of defense mechanisms.

Therapies

☐ Biologic therapy includes psychoactive drugs, electroconvulsive therapy (ECT), and nonconvulsive electrical stimulation.

☐ Analysis of free association is characteristic of the Freudian therapy psychoanalysis.

☐ Cognitive therapy uses strategies such as role-playing and thought substitution to modify the beliefs and attitudes that influence a client's feelings and behaviors.

☐ Cognitive-behavioral therapy identifies negative automatic thought patterns in order to examine and replace them with positive thought patterns.

☐ Classical conditioning is characteristic of a pure behavioral intervention.

☐ Family therapy involves the entire family to improve family function.

☐ Group therapy aims to increase self-awareness, change maladaptive behaviors, and improve interpersonal relationships.

☐ Yalom's curative, or therapeutic, factors of group therapy represent different mechanisms that evoke change within a group.

TABLE 4.1 Defense Mechanisms	
Mechanism	Description
Denial	Avoiding the awareness of truth or reality
Devaluation	Assigning excessive negative qualities to oneself or another person
Displacement	Shifting of an emotion from its original object to a substitute
Fantasy	Creation of unrealistic or improbable images to escape from daily pressures and responsibilities
Identification	Unconscious adoption of the personality characteristics, attitudes, values, and behavior of another person
Idealization	Assigning excessive positive qualities to oneself or another person
Intellectualization	Implementing inappropriate generalizations or abstract thinking to compensate for negative feelings
Passive aggression	Indirectly expressing aggression, resistance, resentment, or hostility toward others while appearing compliant
Projection	Displacement of negative feelings onto another person
Rationalization	Substitution of acceptable reasons for the real or actual reasons behind behavior
Reaction formation	Conduct in a manner opposite from the way the person feels
Regression	Returning to the behavior of an earlier, less worrisome time in life
Repression	Exclusion of distressing thoughts and feelings from the conscious mind
Sublimation	Channeling maladaptive urges into socially acceptable activities
Undoing	Verbalizations or actions intending to compensate for unacceptable thoughts or behavior

TABLE 4.2 Yalom's Curative Factors of Group Therapy

Factor	Description
Altruism	Giving to another group member in order to increase self-esteem
Catharsis	Open expression of a deep feeling
Corrective recapitulation	Reliving and correcting past family conflicts
Development of socializing techniques	Learning social skills
Existential factors	Realization that concerns about existence and death are universal and limitedly controllable
Group cohesiveness	Connectivity among group members and the group leader
Imitative behavior	Demonstrating growth by copying healthy behaviors of another group member or group leader
Imparting of information	Information is shared among group members or by the group leader to the group
Instillation of hope	Belief among the group that improvement is possible
Interpersonal learning	Learning about oneself via feedback from group members
Universality	Multiple group members experience the same feeling or thought, demonstrating that one member is not alone

See Table 4.2 for more information on Yalom's curative factors of group therapy.

Therapeutic Milieu

☐ A therapeutic milieu implies that the nurse utilizes all aspects of the hospital environment in a therapeutic manner to encourage communication and decision making.

☐ A therapeutic milieu provides opportunities for enhancing self-esteem as well as learning new skills and behaviors.

☐ See Table 4.3 for a list of clinical assessment tools.

TABLE 4.3	Clinical Assessment Tools
Tool	**What It Assesses or Measures?**
Mini-Mental State Examination	▪ Orientation ▪ Registration ▪ Recall ▪ Calculation ▪ Language ▪ Motor skills
Beck Depression Inventory	▪ Depressive symptoms ▪ Severity of depression ▪ Client's response to treatment
Hamilton Rating Scale for Depression	▪ Depressive symptoms ▪ Severity of depression ▪ Client's response to treatment
Patient Health Questionnaire (PHQ-9)	▪ Depressive symptoms ▪ Severity of depression ▪ Client's response to treatment
Beck Anxiety Inventory	▪ Anxiety ▪ Severity of anxiety ▪ Client's response to treatment
Eating Attitudes Test	▪ Patterns that suggest an eating disorder
Yale-Brown Obsessive-Compulsive Scale (Y-BOCS)	▪ Severity of obsessions and compulsions
The CAGE Questionnaire	▪ Client's alcohol consumption
Positive and Negative Syndrome Scale (PAN SS)	▪ Positive and negative psychotic symptoms
Abnormal Involuntary Movement Scale (AIMS)	▪ Extrapyramidal symptoms commonly associated with antipsychotics

NEURODEVELOPMENTAL DISORDERS

KEY TERMS

☐ **Inattention** is the inability or difficulty to focus on a topic or object for a sustained period of time.

☐ **Impulsivity** is the pattern of acting abruptly without sufficiently weighing the consequences of the action.

- **Hyperactivity** is restless behavior and/or excessive speech.
- **Motor tics** are repetitive and stereotyped movements such as shrugging or blinking.
- **Phonic tics** are repetitive, audible sounds such as grunting or spoken words.

Overview

- The *DSM-5* lists neurodevelopmental disorders including autism spectrum disorder, attention deficit hyperactivity disorder (ADHD), and tic disorders.

Autism Spectrum Disorder

- Hallmarks of this spectrum disorder include repetitive or stereotypic behaviors, inflexibility in routines or rules, fixation with specific stimuli, and impaired social skills.
- Delayed or loss of milestone progression may indicate autism spectrum disorder. Loss of language skills is particularly a "red flag" in autism spectrum disorder, typically noted between 12 and 24 months of age.
- Clients with autism spectrum disorder may or may not have decreased intellectual functioning.
- Males more commonly present with autism spectrum disorder than females.
- Commonly, clients with autism spectrum disorder struggle to tolerate stress and will express outbursts of emotions in response to distress or overstimulation.
- Medication is only indicated for symptom management such as atypical antipsychotics for agitation.
- Involvement of clients' family members in the nursing care process is highly encouraged in order for behavioral interventions to be most effective.

Attention Deficit Hyperactivity Disorder (ADHD)

- Clients with ADHD may struggle to shift their focus, maintain attention, filter out extraneous stimuli in their environment, organize, wait for their turn, consider consequences before acting, remain seated calmly, or endure lengthy or complex tasks.
- Most commonly, females present with predominantly inattentive features.
- ADHD is more common in children exposed to tobacco in utero.
- Depression, mood lability, and anxiety should be assessed in these clients due to increased rates of comorbidity.
- Due to impulsivity, these clients are particularly a safety concern; suicide, self-harm, and substance use should be directly assessed.

☐ Standardized tools used to help identify ADHD include the Conners Parent Questionnaire, the ADHD Rating Scale, and the Child Behavior Checklist.

☐ First-line medications for treatment of ADHD include stimulants (either methylphenidate or amphetamine classes).

☐ When taking stimulant medication, the client and their family should be educated that stimulants may suppress appetite and accordingly inhibit growth in children.

☐ Additionally, stimulants should not be taken before bed due to increased wakefulness and should be stored in a secure area due to their abuse potential as controlled substances.

☐ Stimulants may also cause cardiac complications; therefore, client's personal and family cardiac history should be assessed prior to taking this type of medication.

☐ Sleep hygiene should be encouraged in this population as well as behavior modification to promote symptom management.

☐ Encourage clients to complete homework and expected tasks in low-stimulus environment with clear limits and consequences established.

Tic Disorders

☐ Tourette syndrome is defined by the presence of multiple tics for at least 1 year.

☐ Tics typically present in childhood around age 7 and decrease in severity in adulthood.

☐ Tics may be transient or chronic. Transient tics are more common.

☐ Tics typically subside with a relief of stress.

SCHIZOPHRENIA SPECTRUM AND OTHER PSYCHOTIC DISORDERS

KEY TERMS

☐ **Negative symptoms** focus on a *loss* of normal functions.

☐ **Positive symptoms** focus on a *distortion* of normal functions.

☐ **Hallucinations** are the phenomenon of seeing, hearing, feeling, smelling, or tasting something that is not actually present.

☐ **Illusions** are a visual distortion of something that is actually present.

☐ **Delusions** are false, fixed beliefs that aren't shared by other members of the client's social, cultural, or religious background.

☐ **Clang associations** are nonsensical verbalizations of rhyming words.

☐ **Neologism** involves the use of invented words.

☐ **Echolalia** is the repetition of words heard.

- **Perseveration** is the repetitive use of words or phrases.
- **Waxy flexibility** is a posture held in odd or unusual fixed positions for an extended period.
- **Catatonia** is the formation of bizarre postures, waxy flexibility, and resistance to being moved.
- **Flat affect** is a loss of emotional expression.
- **Alogia** is poverty of speech.
- **Avolition** is a lack of self-initiated behaviors.
- **Anhedonia** is a loss of enjoyment in activities or hobbies.

Overview

- The *DSM-5* lists psychotic disorders including brief psychotic disorder, schizophreniform disorder, schizophrenia, schizoaffective disorder, and delusional disorder.
- A psychotic illness is a brain disorder characterized by an impaired perception of reality.
- Psychosis can be either progressive or episodic.
- Pharmacologic treatment options for psychosis include typical antipsychotics and atypical antipsychotics, both of which block dopamine. The difference between these two drug classes' mechanisms of action is that atypical antipsychotics also block serotonin and actually more potently than dopamine.
- The Abnormal Involuntary Movement Scale (AIMS) is used to assess and monitor extrapyramidal symptoms (EPS) most commonly associated with typical antipsychotics. EPS include symptoms such as tremors as well as perioral and tongue movements.
- Atypical antipsychotics can cause metabolic syndrome, a combination of hypertension, hypercholesterolemia, hyperglycemia, and weight gain. Patients taking atypical antipsychotics should be monitored accordingly.
- Clozapine is an atypical antipsychotic that is known to cause agranulocytosis; therefore, absolute neutrophil count and signs of infection should be monitored closely when receiving this medication.

Neuroleptic Malignant Syndrome (NMS)

- NMS is a life-threatening adverse effect of antipsychotic medications.
- Symptoms of NMS include hyperthermia, hypertension, tachycardia, tachypnea, diaphoresis, muscle rigidity, hyporeflexia, and elevated creatine phosphokinase (CPK).
- If these symptoms present, the client should be prepared to go to the hospital or transferred to an intensive care unit.

Hallucinations

☐ If a client experiences hallucinations, don't attempt to reason with the client or challenge their perception of the hallucinations; instead, ensure the client's safety and provide comfort and support.

☐ Attempts to reason with the client experiencing hallucinations will increase the client's anxiety and possibly make the hallucinations worse.

☐ Encourage the client with auditory hallucinations to reveal the content of the hallucinations to help prevent harm to the client and others.

Delusions

☐ Delusions may occur in the form of thought broadcasting, in which the client believes that their personal thoughts are available to the external world.

☐ The client with delusions may or may not believe that their feelings, thoughts, or actions are his or her own.

☐ Delusional themes are described as persecutory, erotomanic, somatic, jealous, or grandiose.

☐ An example of a persecutory delusion is the idea that one is being followed, tricked, tormented, or made the subject of ridicule.

☐ The client with erotomanic delusions falsely believes he or she shares an idealized relationship with another person, usually someone of higher status such as a celebrity.

☐ An example of a somatic delusion is a client who believes his or her body is deteriorating from within.

☐ An example of a jealous delusion is a client who feels that his or her spouse or partner is unfaithful with no evidence of unfaithfulness.

☐ The client with grandiose delusions has an exaggerated sense of self-importance.

Disorganized Thinking

☐ In disorganized thinking, the client's speech shifts randomly from one topic to another with only a vague connection between topics.

☐ The client with disorganized thinking may have neologisms, perseveration, clang association, or echolalia.

Brief Psychotic Disorder

☐ This condition is identified when positive symptoms are present for 1 day to 1 month.

☐ Suicide risk is important to consider in this population due to confusion and unpredictability.

Schizophreniform Disorder

☐ This condition is identified when positive symptoms are present for 1 to 6 months.

☐ Clients with brief psychotic disorder often develop schizophrenia; however, about 1/3 of clients with brief psychotic disorder resume baseline level of functioning.

Schizophrenia

☐ Schizophrenia is characterized by disturbances (for at least 6 months) in thought content and form, perception, affect, sense of self, volition, interpersonal relationships, work, and self-care.

☐ Schizophrenia is usually a chronic disorder that begins in late adolescence or early adulthood. Men typically are diagnosed between ages 18 and 25; women experience a slightly later onset ranging from ages 25 to 35.

☐ Earlier onset of schizophrenia is associated with poorer prognosis.

☐ Risk factors for developing schizophrenia include genetic predisposition, prenatal malnutrition, obstetrical complications, stressful life events, and lifetime cannabis use.

☐ The client with schizophrenia may demonstrate negative symptoms such as a blunted, flat, or inappropriate affect manifested by poor eye contact; a distant, unresponsive facial expression; and very limited body language.

☐ Clients with schizophrenia experience positive symptoms, most commonly auditory hallucinations and delusions of persecution or paranoia. (See Table 4.4 for positive and negative symptoms of schizophrenia.)

☐ When the client with schizophrenia hears voices, the client perceives these voices as being separate from their own thoughts.

☐ The content of the voices a client with schizophrenia hears is often threatening and derogatory; many times, the voices tell the client to commit an act of violence against themselves or others. The nurse should consistently assess for the presence and content of hallucinations.

☐ Clients with schizophrenia commonly will present with comorbid psychiatric conditions such as substance abuse and depression. Both of these comorbidities increase the already elevated suicide risk for clients with schizophrenia.

TABLE 4.4 Positive and Negative Symptoms of Schizophrenia	
Positive Symptoms	**Negative Symptoms**
■ Delusions	■ Flat affect (loss of emotional expression)
■ Hallucinations	■ Alogia (poverty of speech)
■ Disorganized speech	■ Avolition (lack of self-initiated behaviors)
■ Grossly disorganized or catatonic behavior	■ Anhedonia (loss of enjoyment in activities or hobbies)

Schizoaffective Disorder

☐ This condition combines features of both schizophrenia and mood disorders.

☐ Clients with schizoaffective disorder have mood episodes with persistent psychotic features independent of their presenting mood severity. This differs from mood disorders with psychotic features, which only present in those individuals with severe mania or severe depression.

☐ Due to the complexity of mood and psychotic features, clients with schizoaffective disorder are highly susceptible to suicide. Nurses should assess these clients accordingly with direct questions.

☐ Medication compliance is a key concept for nurses educating clients with schizoaffective disorder.

☐ Common medications used for this client population include antipsychotics, antidepressants, and mood stabilizers.

Delusional Disorder

☐ Clients with delusional disorder hold firmly to false belief despite contradictory information.

☐ The presence of delusions does not indicate a lack of competence.

☐ Clients with delusional disorder exhibit impaired social and personal relationships.

☐ One indication of delusional disorder is an absence of hallucinations.

☐ Explore events that trigger delusions with the client with delusional disorder; also, discuss anxiety associated with triggering events, which can help you understand the dynamics of the client's delusional system.

☐ Do not directly attack the client's delusion because doing so will increase the client's anxiety.

☐ When the dynamics of the delusions are understood, discourage repetitive talk about delusions and refocus the conversation on the client's underlying feelings.

MOOD DISORDERS

KEY TERMS

☐ **Grandiosity** is a symptom of mania or hypomania when a client experiences an inflated self-esteem.

☐ **Flight of ideas** is a speech pattern characterized by rapid transition from topic to topic, typically without finishing one idea due to racing thoughts, and is common in mania.

Overview

- ☐ The *DSM-5* lists mood disorders including bipolar disorders, major depressive disorder, dysthymia, and seasonal affective disorder.
- ☐ During episodes of hypomania, the client may demonstrate an elevated and irritable mood, along with mild symptoms of mania that do not impair functioning.
- ☐ Psychotic symptoms may sometimes present in mood disorders, but only when mood states are severely high or severely low.
- ☐ Suicidal risk is elevated in mood disorders.
- ☐ Nonverbal clues to suicidal ideation include giving away personal possessions, a sudden calmness, and risk-taking behaviors.

Bipolar Disorders

- ☐ There are two main types of bipolar disorders. Bipolar type I can be diagnosed whenever a client has experienced a manic episode at any point in their lifetime. Bipolar type II can be diagnosed whenever a client has experienced oscillation of mood states without ever having experienced a manic episode.
- ☐ Thoughtless or reckless spending is a common indication of a manic episode.
- ◎ ☐ Symptoms of a manic episode include grandiosity, decreased need for sleep, increased rate of speech, racing thoughts, distractibility, increased productivity or psychomotor agitation, and increased risk taking. Symptoms persist for at least 1 week.
- ☐ The client must present with an elevated or irritable mood as well as increased energy or productivity level.
- ☐ During episodes of mania, a client may in fact interact with many people and participate in unsafe sexual behavior.
- ☐ To decrease stimulation in the client with mania, the nurse should attempt to redirect and focus the client's communication in a calm environment.
- ☐ For a manic client, it may be more effective to ask closed-ended questions, because open-ended questions may enable the client to talk endlessly, possibly contributing to the client feeling out of control.
- ☐ A manic client is often highly active and struggles to manage to eat and drink sufficiently as a result. The nurse should encourage hydration and foods that can be consumed without needing a structured sit-down meal.
- ☐ Pharmacologic treatment for bipolar disorder commonly includes a mood stabilizer.
- ☐ Lithium is often used as a mood stabilizer for bipolar patients; however, when it is used, trough serum concentration levels for this

medication must be strictly monitored in order to prevent toxicity, which can occur at blood levels at or above 1.5 mEq/L (1.5 mmol/L).

- Common mild side effects of lithium include nausea, thirst, and a metallic taste in the client's mouth.
- Signs of lithium toxicity include nausea and vomiting, diarrhea, muscle weakness, tremors, blurred vision, confusion, seizures, coma, and death.
- Mood-stabilizing agent lamotrigine has a high risk of a life-threatening condition called Stevens-Johnson syndrome. Therefore, when this medication is used, it is important to promote strict medication adherence and to teach clients to monitor for a rash. If a rash presents, clients taking lamotrigine should be taught to seek care immediately.

Major Depressive Disorder

- Major depressive disorder can be diagnosed when a client has experienced at least one major depressive episode without any episodes of mania or hypomania in their lifetime.
- Symptoms of a major depressive episode include persistently low mood, anhedonia, insomnia or hypersomnia, decreased or increased appetite, weight loss or gain, psychomotor agitation or retardation, excessive feelings of guilt or worthlessness, fatigue, decreased concentration or decisiveness, and thoughts about death or suicide.
- Symptoms persist for at least 2 weeks. Either low mood or anhedonia must be present.
- First-line pharmacologic treatment for major depressive disorder includes antidepressants such as selective serotonin reuptake inhibitors (SSRIs). Other antidepressants include selective norepinephrine reuptake inhibitors (SNRIs), tricyclic antidepressants (TCAs), and monoamine oxidase inhibitors (MAOIs).
- TCAs are not as commonly used because of their high risk for lethal overdose.
- MAOIs are not as commonly used because of their strict dietary restriction for foods that contain tyramine, such as cured meats and aged cheeses.
- ECT is most commonly used to treat major depression in clients who haven't responded to antidepressants or who have medical problems that contraindicate the use of antidepressants.
- The nurse must assess for difficulty swallowing before allowing the client to eat or drink after an ECT procedure. The nurse must also assess for altered orientation after an ECT procedure.

☐ Serotonin syndrome is a life-threatening adverse effect of serotonergic medications such as SSRIs and SNRIs. It is associated with hyperthermia, hypertension, tachycardia, tachypnea, diaphoresis, and increased muscle tone. If these symptoms are detected, the client should be prepared to go to the hospital or transferred to an intensive care unit.

Dysthymia

☐ Dysthymia is a mood disorder similar to major depression, but it remains mild to moderate in severity.

☐ The depressive mood present in dysthymia is present for at least 2 years, rather than 2 weeks in a major depressive episode.

Seasonal Affective Disorder

☐ Seasonal affective disorder is a form of depression occurring in the fall and winter due to changes in exposure to light.

☐ Phototherapy is an evidenced treatment option for clients with seasonal affective disorder.

ANXIETY DISORDERS

KEY TERMS

☐ **Derealization** is when a situation does not feel real to a client.

☐ **Depersonalization** is when clients feel outside of their own body or no longer associated with their own body or identity.

Overview

☐ The *DSM-5* lists anxiety disorders including generalized anxiety, panic disorder, and phobias.

☐ Clients with anxiety disorders commonly experience somatic symptoms, such as a headache or upset stomach. This is especially common in children with anxiety.

☐ The use of substances is a way for the client to deny problems and self-medicate distress.

☐ Clients with anxiety tend to cling to maladaptive behaviors in an attempt to alleviate their own distress.

☐ Avoiding, rationalizing, and hiding behaviors demonstrate maladaptive methods for managing stress and anxiety.

☐ Verbalizing the relationship between anxiety-provoking stressor and maladaptive behaviors indicates that the client understands the disease process.

☐ Benzodiazepines can be used for short-term pharmacologic treatment of acute anxiety.

☐ SSRIs (such as fluoxetine) and SNRIs (such as venlafaxine) are treatment options for long-term management of anxiety disorders.

Generalized Anxiety Disorder

☐ Generalized anxiety disorder is characterized by a client consistently worrying about multiple things.

☐ Generalized anxiety disorder is also associated with symptoms such as muscle tension, irritability, difficulty concentrating, and insomnia.

☐ Clients with generalized anxiety disorder also may have a diagnosis of major depressive disorder, dysthymia, phobias, panic disorder, or substance abuse.

☐ A client with generalized anxiety disorder may be too worried to take medication; therefore, medication education and reinforcement of medication compliance are especially important.

Panic Attacks

☐ Panic attack symptoms include elevated heart rate, elevated blood pressure, chest pain, shortness of breath, tingling, numbness, diaphoresis, shaking, depersonalization or derealization, GI disturbances, dizziness, feeling of choking, temperature intolerance, and fear of dying, losing control, or going crazy.

☐ People who fear loss of control during a panic attack commonly make statements about feeling trapped, getting hurt, or having little or no personal control over their situations.

☐ During a panic attack, the nurse should remain with the client and direct what's said toward changing the physiologic response, such as having the client take deep breaths. Communication directed toward the panicking client should be short and direct.

☐ A therapy intervention that is of primary importance to a client with panic disorder is discussing new ways of thinking to counter feelings of panic, called restructuring.

☐ Restructuring an anxiety-producing event allows the client with panic disorder to gain control over the situation during therapy.

Phobias

☐ Agoraphobia is characterized by fear of open or confined places from which escape may be difficult.

☐ The client with agoraphobia typically stays at home and cannot carry out normal socializing and life-sustaining activities.

☐ People who have a social phobia fear social gatherings and dislike being the center of attention; they are very critical of themselves and believe that others will also be critical.

☐ Clients with blood injection injury phobia may avoid all medical care, endangering their health.

☐ Systematic desensitization is a common behavior modification technique successfully used to help treat phobias by gradual exposure to the feared object or situation.

OBSESSIVE-COMPULSIVE AND RELATED DISORDERS

KEY TERMS

☐ **Obsessions** are thoughts that are excessive, unwanted, and intrude on daily functioning.

☐ **Compulsions** are repeated actions that are directed at diminishing anxiety and distress from obsessions.

Overview

☐ The *DSM-5* lists obsessive-compulsive and related disorders including obsessive-compulsive disorder (OCD), excoriation disorder, trichotillomania, and body dysmorphic disorder.

Obsessive-Compulsive Disorder

☐ OCD combines both obsessions and compulsions.

☐ Dissociation is a common defense mechanism found in clients with OCD.

☐ The nurse must consider cultural and religious norms when assessing for the presence of obsessions or compulsions.

☐ The Yale-Brown Obsessive-Compulsive Scale (Y-BOCS) is a standardized tool to assess the severity of obsessions and compulsions.

☐ Common obsessions include fear of harm, fear of contamination, and need for symmetry or order.

☐ Common compulsions include counting, checking, washing, sorting, or hoarding.

☐ One therapeutic goal for OCD is to decrease the amount of time spent on obsessions/compulsions, thereby improving ability to function in daily role.

☐ OCD must be carefully diagnosed, as these symptoms can be induced by both cocaine and amphetamine class stimulants.

☐ Additionally, obsessive-compulsive symptoms can develop from medical conditions such as pediatric autoimmune neuropsychiatric disorders associated with streptococcal infections (PANDAS).

☐ Behavioral therapy focuses on breaking the cycle of using compulsions to achieve a decrease in anxiety.

☐ Cognitive-behavioral therapy aids in restructuring thought distortions found in OCD.

☐ Medications commonly used to effectively treat OCD include SSRIs and TCAs.

Excoriation (Skin-Picking) Disorder

☐ This condition is indicated by a client repeatedly picking at their skin as a means of relieving stress.

☐ The therapeutic goal for this client is to substitute this harmful coping skill with positive coping skills.

Trichotillomania
☐ This condition is indicated by a client repeatedly pulling out their hair as a means of relieving stress.
☐ Clients may also exhibit hair-eating behaviors, which can put them at risk for gastrointestinal complications.
☐ The therapeutic goal for this client is to substitute this harmful coping skill with positive coping skills.

Body Dysmorphic Disorder
☐ Clients with body dysmorphic disorder have a distorted perception of their physical appearance.
☐ As a result of their dysmorphia, these clients will often isolate socially and avoid work or school due to the anxiety caused by their appearance.
☐ Comorbidity with depression is increased in this population, and suicide risk is high. Direct mood and suicide assessment is imperative for care of these clients.

TRAUMA- AND STRESSOR-RELATED DISORDERS

KEY TERMS
☐ **Intrusion** is when thoughts or dreams, sometimes triggered by an external cue, occur involuntarily and distress the client. Flashbacks and nightmares are examples of intrusion.
☐ **Derealization** is when a situation does not feel real to a client.
☐ **Depersonalization** is when clients feel outside of their own body or no longer associated with their own body or identity.
☐ **Hyperarousal** is when a client is excessively on edge and alert for signs of danger, startles easily, and reacts markedly to stimuli.
☐ **Kindling** may result after a trauma and be demonstrated by a heightened response to a mild stressor.

Overview
☐ The *DSM-5* lists trauma- and stressor-related disorders including posttraumatic stress disorder (PTSD) and reactive attachment disorder.
☐ Improving stress management skills, verbalizing feelings, and anticipating and planning for stressful situations are adaptive responses to stress.
☐ Clients who have had a severe trauma commonly experience an inability to trust others.

Posttraumatic Stress Disorder (PTSD)

☐ Examples of traumas include near-death experiences, exposure to dead bodies, or exposure to extreme details of a traumatic event.

☐ After experiencing a trauma, the client with PTSD may have strong reactions to stimuli similar to those that occurred during the traumatic event.

☐ Symptoms of PTSD include intrusion, dissociative symptoms (depersonalization/derealization), hyperarousal, avoidance, and altered mood.

☐ Sleep disturbance often results from hypervigilance.

☐ Clients who experience PTSD are at high risk for suicide and other forms of violent behaviors. Nurses should be diligent about directly assessing for suicidal and homicidal ideation, intent, plan, and means.

☐ Listening attentively and staying with the client are effective communication strategies for a nurse to use with a client with PTSD.

☐ Pharmacologic treatment for PTSD is aimed at symptom management, including use of antidepressants, antipsychotics, and anxiolytics.

☐ Cognitive-behavioral therapy and eye movement desensitization and reprocessing (EMDR) are both nonpharmacologic treatment modalities used for PTSD.

Reactive Attachment Disorder

☐ Clients with reactive attachment disorder will exhibit withdrawn behavior, especially noted when affection is attempted to be shown toward the client by an adult caregiver.

☐ Clients with reactive attachment disorder avoid seeking or receiving comfort when in distress.

☐ This disorder is common among children in foster care due to repeated change in caregivers.

DISSOCIATIVE DISORDERS

KEY TERMS

☐ **Reality testing** is the ability to distinguish fact from fantasy.

☐ **Dissociation** is a mechanism used to protect the self and gain relief from overwhelming anxiety.

Overview

☐ The *DSM-5* lists dissociative disorders including dissociative amnesia and dissociative identity disorder.

☐ A client with a dissociative disorder experiences a disruption in the usual relationship among memory, identity, consciousness, and perceptions. The disturbance may occur suddenly or appear gradually.

- ☐ Dissociative disorders are characterized by lost periods of time.
- ☐ Dissociative disorders are more common in women than in men.
- ☐ Hypnosis is one of the main therapies for clients who dissociate as well as psychoanalytic and cognitive-behavioral therapies.
- ☐ Pharmacologic treatment is focused on symptom relief of co-occurring mood, anxiety, and trauma-related or personality disorders.

Dissociative Amnesia
- ☐ In dissociative amnesia, the client may not recall important life events in an attempt to avoid traumatic memories.
- ☐ Contributing factors to dissociative amnesia are emotional abuse, low self-esteem, past trauma, physical abuse, or sexual abuse.
- ☐ Recovery from dissociative amnesia is common; recurrences are rare.

Dissociative Identity Disorder
- ☐ In dissociative identity disorder, formerly known as multiple personality disorder, the client has at least two unique identities. Each identity can have unique behavior patterns and unique memories, although usually, one primary identity is associated with the client's name.
- ☐ In dissociative identity disorder, the client may also have traumatic memories that intrude into their awareness.
- ☐ Dissociative identity disorder tends to be chronic and recurrent.
- ☐ Contributing factors in dissociative identity disorder include emotional, physical, or sexual abuse; genetic predisposition; lack of nurturing experiences to assist in recovery from abuse; low self-esteem; and a traumatic experience before age 15.

SOMATIC SYMPTOM AND RELATED DISORDERS

KEY TERMS
- ☐ **Psychosomatic** is a term used to describe conditions in which a psychological state contributes to the development of a physical illness.
- ☐ **Somatization** is the manifestation of physical symptoms that result from psychological distress.
- ☐ **Internalization** is when a client's anxiety, stress, and frustration are expressed through physical symptoms rather than confronted directly.

Overview
- ☐ The *DSM-5* lists somatic symptom and related disorders including somatic symptom disorder, illness anxiety disorder, and conversion disorder.

Somatic Symptom Disorder

☐ The client with a somatic symptom disorder commonly suffers physical symptoms related to an inability to handle stress; the physical symptoms have no physiologic cause but are overwhelming to the client.

☐ Because the client with a somatic symptom disorder doesn't produce the symptoms intentionally or feel a sense of control over them, he or she is usually unable to accept that his or her illness has a psychological cause.

Illness Anxiety Disorder

☐ In illness anxiety disorder, the client is preoccupied by fear of a serious illness, despite medical assurance of good health.

☐ The client with illness anxiety disorder interprets all physical sensations as indications of illness, impairing his or her ability to function normally.

☐ The pain with illness anxiety disorder is not intentionally produced or feigned by the client. The pain becomes a major focus of life, and the client is often unable to function socially or at work.

☐ The client with illness anxiety disorder may have a physical ailment but should not be experiencing such intense pain. When a physical condition is diagnosable, the client's preoccupation and concept of severity are excessive.

Conversion Disorder

☐ The onset of symptoms in a client with conversion disorder is preceded by psychological trauma or conflict.

☐ The physical symptoms associated with conversion disorder are a manifestation of the conflict, and resolution of the symptoms usually occurs spontaneously.

FEEDING AND EATING DISORDERS

KEY TERMS

☐ **Binging** is the act of consuming an excessive amount of food without control during one period of time.

☐ **Purging** is the compensatory act of preventing weight gain that can be self-induced vomiting, laxative abuse, diuretic abuse, excessive exercise, or fasting after a binge episode.

☐ **Rumination** is a condition when food is regurgitated and masticated in a repeated cycle, possibly eventually being spit out.

Overview

- The *DSM-5* lists feeding and eating disorders including anorexia nervosa, bulimia nervosa, and binge-eating disorder.
- Eating disorders are characterized by severe disturbances in eating behaviors typically related to a need for control.
- Clients with eating disorders commonly use manipulation to resist weight gain (if they restrict food intake) or to maintain purging practices (if they have bulimia nervosa).
- The two most common eating disorders, anorexia nervosa and bulimia nervosa, put the client at risk for severe cardiovascular and GI complications and can ultimately result in death.
- Constant binging and purging behaviors can result in severe electrolyte imbalances, erosion of tooth enamel from constant exposure to gastric acids, menstrual irregularities, esophageal tears, and, in severe cases, gastric rupture.
- Psychotherapy modalities commonly used with anorexia nervosa and bulimia nervosa include behavioral therapy and interpersonal therapy.
- Nutritional supplements are commonly prescribed for clients with a low nutritional status.

Anorexia Nervosa

- A client with anorexia nervosa wants to become as thin as possible and refuses to maintain an appropriate weight.
- A key clinical finding in anorexia nervosa is a refusal to sustain weight at or above minimum requirements for the client's age and height and an intense fear of gaining weight or becoming fat.
- Physical manifestations of anorexia nervosa include low body mass index, amenorrhea, and lanugo.
- Perfectionism is more commonly seen in clients with anorexia nervosa.
- If left untreated, anorexia nervosa can be fatal.
- Anxiolytics can be prescribed prior to meal times in order to help diminish anxiety surrounding food consumption.

Bulimia Nervosa

- Bulimia nervosa is characterized by episodic binge eating followed by purging.
- Contributing factors to bulimia nervosa are thought to include a distorted body image, history of sexual abuse, low self-esteem, neurochemical changes, and poor family relations.
- Bruised or scarred knuckles due to repeated self-induced vomiting may be observed in bulimia nervosa.

☐ In bulimia nervosa, metabolic acidosis may occur from diarrhea caused by enemas and excessive laxative use.

☐ In bulimia nervosa, metabolic alkalosis may occur from frequent vomiting and is the most common metabolic complication found in clients with this disorder.

☐ Prevent the client with bulimia nervosa from using the bathroom directly after eating to help the client avoid purging behavior.

Binge-Eating Disorder

☐ Binge-eating disorder is a condition marked by binge eating without the presence of purging behaviors.

☐ The body mass index (BMI) of clients with binge-eating disorder often indicates obesity.

ELIMINATION DISORDER

KEY TERMS

☐ **Enuresis** is repeated, inappropriate urination after the developmental age of bladder control.

☐ **Encopresis** is repeated, inappropriate defecation after the developmental age of bowel control.

Overview

☐ Bladder control is typically achieved by developmental age 5.

☐ Bowel control is typically achieved by developmental age 4.

☐ Both enuresis and encopresis may be involuntary or intentional.

☐ Behavioral treatment approaches are common to stimulate elimination control.

SLEEP-WAKE DISORDERS

KEY TERMS

☐ **Insomnia** is difficulty falling or staying asleep.

☐ **Hypersomnia** is sleeping for excessive periods of time.

☐ **Dyssomnias** involve excessive sleep or difficulty initiating and maintaining sleep.

☐ **Parasomnias** are physiologic or behavioral reactions during sleep that are characterized by abnormal, unpleasant motor or verbal arousals and behaviors that occur during sleep.

Overview

☐ The *DSM-5* lists sleep-wake disorders including breathing-related disorders, circadian rhythm sleep-wake disorders, narcolepsy, and restless leg syndrome.

☐ The client with a sleep disorder commonly suffers from excessive daytime sleepiness and impaired ability to perform daily tasks safely or properly.

☐ Primary insomnia is characterized by subjective complaint of difficulty initiating or maintaining sleep that lasts for at least 1 month; alternatively, the client may report that sleep isn't refreshing.

☐ A key symptom of primary insomnia is the client's intense focus and anxiety about not getting sleep, resulting in significant distress or impairment; commonly, the client reports being a "light sleeper."

☐ Polysomnography includes measurement of electroencephalogram (EEG) activity.

Breathing-Related Disorders

☐ Obstructive sleep apnea syndrome is the most commonly diagnosed breathing-related sleep disorder.

☐ In breathing-related sleep disorders, a disturbance in breathing leads to a disruption in sleep that leads to excessive sleepiness or insomnia.

☐ Excessive sleepiness is the most common complaint of clients with breathing-related sleep disorder.

☐ In breathing-related sleep disorders, naps usually aren't refreshing and may be accompanied by a dull headache.

☐ The apnea in breathing-related disorders is concerning due to compromised oxygenation.

Narcolepsy

☐ In narcolepsy, the client falls asleep regardless of the amount of previous sleep.

☐ In narcolepsy, the client may fall asleep two to six times a day during inappropriate times, such as while driving a car or attending class.

☐ In narcolepsy, the client's sleepiness typically decreases after a sleep attack, only to return several hours later. The sleep attacks in narcolepsy must occur daily over a period of 3 months to confirm the diagnosis.

Circadian Rhythm Sleep-Wake Disorders

☐ In circadian rhythm sleep disorder, there is a mismatch between the internal sleep-wake circadian rhythm and the timing and duration of sleep.

☐ In circadian rhythm sleep disorder, the client may report insomnia at particular times during the day and excessive sleepiness at other times.

☐ Causes of circadian rhythm sleep disorder can be intrinsic, such as delays in the sleep phases, or extrinsic, as in jet lag or shift work.

- In circadian rhythm sleep disorder, polysomnography shows short sleep latency (length of time it takes to fall asleep), reduced sleep duration, and sleep continuity disturbances.

Restless Leg Syndrome

- Restless leg syndrome is a condition marked by an urge to move one's legs; resisting to do so results in extreme discomfort.
- Clients with restless leg syndrome may report symptoms such as tingling, burning, or crawling sensations in their legs with worsened symptoms during periods of inactivity such as sleep.
- Treatment involves promotion of good sleep hygiene such as limiting caffeine, alcohol, and food consumption in the hours prior to bedtime.

SEXUAL DYSFUNCTIONS

KEY TERMS

- **Dyspareunia** is genital pain associated with sexual intercourse.
- **Vaginismus** is recurrent or persistent involuntary tightening when penetration is anticipated or attempted.

Overview

- The *DSM-5* lists sexual dysfunctions including orgasmic disorders, sexual arousal disorders, sexual desire disorders, sexual pain disorders, and substance-induced sexual dysfunction.
- Sexual dysfunctions are characterized by a deficiency or loss of desire for sexual activity or by a disturbance in the sexual response cycle.
- Male and female orgasmic disorders are characterized by a persistent or recurrent delay in or absence of orgasm following a normal sexual excitement phase.
- With female sexual arousal disorder, the client has a persistent or recurrent inability to attain or maintain adequate lubrication, swelling, and response of sexual excitement until the completion of sexual activity.
- In male erectile disorder, the client has a persistent or recurrent inability to attain or maintain an adequate erection until completion of sexual activity.
- The key feature of hypoactive sexual desire disorder is a deficiency or absence of sexual fantasies and the desire for sexual activity. The client usually doesn't initiate sexual activity and may only engage in it reluctantly when it's initiated by the partner.
- With sexual aversion disorder, the client has an aversion to and active avoidance of genital sexual contact with a sexual partner.

- ☐ Sexual pain disorders include dyspareunia (genital pain associated with sexual intercourse) and vaginismus (recurrent or persistent involuntary tightening when penetration is anticipated or attempted).
- ☐ In sexual dysfunction due to a medical condition, the sexual dysfunction may occur as a result of a physiologic problem.
- ☐ Substance-induced sexual dysfunction refers to sexual dysfunction resulting from direct physiologic effects associated with drug abuse, medication use, or toxin exposure.

GENDER DYSPHORIA

KEY TERMS

- ☐ **Sex** refers to biologic indicators of males and females.
- ☐ **Gender** refers to the public role identity of males and females.

Overview

- ☐ Gender dysphoria is characterized by intense and ongoing cross-gender identification.
- ☐ Clients with gender dysphoria may experience dislike of their sex-specific body parts.

DISRUPTIVE, IMPULSE CONTROL, AND CONDUCT DISORDERS

Overview

- ☐ The *DSM-5* lists disruptive, impulse control and conduct disorders including oppositional defiant disorder, conduct disorder, and intermittent explosive disorder.

Oppositional Defiant Disorder

- ☐ Oppositional defiant disorder is characterized by disobedience, argumentativeness, irritability, and negative outbursts.
- ☐ Clients with oppositional defiant disorder are often notably impaired in the ability to make friends and avoid conflict with adults and/or authority figures.
- ☐ Goals for this client population include increasing responsibility for behavior and increasing problem-solving skills during times of interpersonal conflict.
- ☐ Parent management helps to improve interactions between parents and their child with oppositional defiant disorder.
- ☐ Common techniques encouraged in parent management are increased positive reinforcement for desired behavior, limit setting, and teaching the use of appropriate punishment.

Conduct Disorder

□ Compared to oppositional defiant disorder, clients with conduct disorder exhibit more serious behavior such as aggression, destroying property, behaving cruelly toward animals, truancy from school, and illegal activity.

□ Conduct disorder increases the risk of developing mood disorders, anxiety disorders, and substance use disorders.

□ Goals and parent management techniques are the same as those used for oppositional defiant disorder.

□ Setting limits and removing the client from the situation are the best ways to handle aggression.

Intermittent Explosive Disorder

□ Clients with intermittent explosive disorder present with aggressive or destructive reactions to disproportionally milder provocation.

□ Intermittent explosive disorder most commonly presents in childhood.

□ While symptom management with medication can be utilized, anger management is an important treatment for this client population.

SUBSTANCE-RELATED AND ADDICTIVE DISORDERS

KEY TERMS

□ **Substance intoxication** is the development of a reversible substance-specific syndrome due to ingestion of or exposure to a substance.

□ **Substance abuse** is the consumption of a substance in an illegal manner or other than its indicated purpose.

□ **Substance dependence** is characterized by physical, behavioral, and cognitive changes resulting from persistent substance use.

□ **Tolerance** is defined as an increased need for a substance or a need for an increased amount of the substance to achieve an effect.

□ **Withdrawal** occurs when the tissue and blood levels of a substance decrease in a person who has engaged in prolonged, heavy use of the substance.

□ **Relapse** is when use of a substance has resumed after abstinence had been achieved.

Overview

□ The clinically significant maladaptive behavior or psychological changes in substance abuse disorders vary depending on the substance.

□ Likewise, withdrawal symptoms vary depending on the substance. For example, life-threatening seizures known as delirium tremens are the specific and primary concern for alcohol withdrawal.

- Features of substance use disorders include a maladaptive pattern of substance use coupled with recurrent and significant adverse consequences.
- Persistent drug use can result in tolerance and withdrawal.
- When uncomfortable withdrawal symptoms persist, the person usually takes the drug to relieve the symptoms.
- Respiratory depression is of particular concern with abuse of CNS depressants such as alcohol, opioids, and benzodiazepines.
- Benzodiazepine tapers can be used to manage withdrawal from alcohol.
- In treating alcohol use disorder, vitamin supplements are used due to the nutritional deficiencies associated with excessive alcohol consumption.
- Naloxone, an opioid antagonist, is used as a pharmacologic intervention for opioid intoxication.
- Individuals exposed to cocaine develop dependence after a very short period followed by maladaptive behavior resulting in social dysfunction.
- Cocaine use can cause serious physical complications, such as cardiac arrhythmias, myocardial infarction, seizures, and stroke.
- See Table 4.5 for more information on symptoms of intoxication/overdose and withdrawal.

TABLE 4.5	Symptoms of Intoxication/Overdose and Withdrawal	
Substance	**Intoxication/Overdose**	**Withdrawal**
Alcohol	■ Sedation ■ Disinhibition ■ Uncoordinated movement ■ Slurred speech ■ Respiratory depression	■ Tremors ■ Tachycardia ■ Hypertension ■ Headache ■ Nausea and vomiting ■ Anxiety ■ Hallucinations ■ Delirium tremens
Stimulants (cocaine, amphetamines)	■ Euphoria ■ CNS stimulation followed by depression ■ Increased wakefulness ■ Appetite suppression ■ Aggression ■ Paranoia ■ Respiratory depression ■ Cardiac arrhythmias ■ Cardiac arrest ■ Seizures ■ Coma	■ Depression ■ Anxiety ■ Cravings ■ Vivid dreams

(Continued)

TABLE 4.5	Symptoms of Intoxication/Overdose and Withdrawal (*Continued*)	
Substance	Intoxication/Overdose	Withdrawal
Opioids	■ Euphoria ■ Sedation ■ Decreased concentration ■ Memory lapses ■ Pain relief ■ Constipation ■ Decreased libido ■ Constricted pupils ■ Respiratory depression ■ Coma	■ Abdominal cramps ■ Nausea ■ Diarrhea ■ Rhinorrhea ■ Watery eyes ■ Dilated pupils ■ Yawning ■ Piloerection ■ Diaphoresis ■ Insomnia ■ Hyperthermia
Sedatives, hypnotics, and anxiolytics	■ Euphoria ■ Sedation ■ Impaired judgment ■ Respiratory depression ■ Cardiac arrest	■ Anxiety ■ Agitation ■ Tachycardia ■ Hypertension ■ Diaphoresis ■ Hyperthermia ■ Seizures

NEUROCOGNITIVE DISORDERS

KEY TERMS

☐ **Sundowning** is an increase in agitation that occurs in the evening accompanied by confusion and is commonly seen in clients with dementia.

☐ **Confabulation** is unintentional inaccurate memory recall due to lapses in memory often seen in clients with dementia.

Overview

☐ The *DSM-5* lists neurocognitive disorders including delirium and dementia.

☐ Symptoms of neurocognitive disorders include neurocognitive impairment, behavioral dysfunction, and personality changes.

☐ Neurocognitive disorders result from any condition that alters or destroys brain tissue and, in turn, impairs neurologic functioning.

☐ Neurocognitive disorders may result from a primary brain disease, a medical condition, or exposure to a drug.

☐ Delirium can easily be mistaken for dementia, so the cause needs to be thoroughly investigated.

☐ Unlike delirium, dementia is caused by primary brain pathology; therefore, reversal of cognitive defects is less likely.

☐ The Mini-Mental State Examination measures orientation, registration, recall, calculation, language, and motor skills. It is used to assess the severity of cognitive impairment.

Delirium

☐ Delirium is characterized by an acute onset and may last from several hours to several days.

☐ Delirium is commonly caused by the disruption of brain homeostasis; when the source of the disturbance is eliminated, cognitive deficits generally resolve.

☐ Common causes of delirium include postoperative conditions or metabolic disorders, withdrawal from alcohol and drugs, and exposure to toxic substances.

☐ Delirium is potentially reversible but can be life-threatening if not treated.

Vascular Dementia

☐ Vascular dementia is temporally related to one or more cerebrovascular events.

☐ Vascular dementia is caused by an irreversible alteration in brain function that damages or destroys brain tissue.

☐ Vascular dementia impairs the client's cognitive functioning, memory, and personality but does not affect the client's level of consciousness.

Alzheimer-Type Dementia

☐ A client with Alzheimer-type dementia suffers from a global impairment of neurocognitive functioning, memory, and personality.

☐ The dementia with Alzheimer-type dementia occurs gradually but with continuous decline.

☐ Damage from Alzheimer-type dementia is irreversible.

☐ Because of the difficulty in obtaining direct pathologic evidence of Alzheimer disease, the diagnosis is given only when other etiologies for the dementia have been eliminated.

☐ Causes of Alzheimer-type dementia include alterations in acetylcholine levels (a neurotransmitter); altered immune function, with autoantibody production in the brain; familial history; increased brain atrophy with wider sulci and cerebral ventricles than seen in normal aging; and presence of neurofibrillary tangles and beta amyloid neuritic plaques, mainly in the cerebral cortex and hippocampus (early) and later in the frontal, parietal, and temporal lobes.

- ☐ Most health care providers categorize three stages of Alzheimer-type dementia: mild, moderate, and severe.
- ☐ A client with stage 1 (mild) Alzheimer-type dementia demonstrates memory loss, language difficulties, mood fluctuation, and impaired judgment.
- ☐ A client with stage 2 (moderate) Alzheimer-type dementia demonstrates confusion, agitation, personality changes, increasingly worse memory loss, anxiety, and difficulty performing activities of daily living such as feeding and bathing.
- ☐ A client with stage 3 (severe) Alzheimer-type dementia demonstrates loss of bowel and bladder control, motor disturbances, inability to perform activities of daily living, and immense dependence on caregiver.

PERSONALITY DISORDERS

KEY TERMS

- ☐ **Lability** is used to describe highly fluctuating moods.
- ☐ **Dichotomous thinking** is exhibited when a client thinks about things in a mutually exclusive manner. This type of thinking fosters thinking in extremes, such as good or bad, right or wrong, etc.
- ☐ **Splitting** is a defense mechanism commonly seen in clients with personality disorders in which the world is perceived as all good or all bad.

Overview

- ☐ According to the *DSM-5*, personality disorders can be broken down into clusters.
- ☐ Cluster A disorders tend to show odd, eccentric mannerisms and include paranoid personality disorder, schizoid personality disorder, and schizotypal personality disorder.
- ☐ Cluster B disorders tend to show highly dramatic, emotionally erratic behavior and include borderline personality disorder, antisocial personality disorder, narcissistic personality disorder, and histrionic personality disorder.
- ☐ Cluster C disorders tend to focus on fear or anxiety; this cluster includes dependent personality disorder, avoidant personality disorder, and obsessive-compulsive personality disorder.
- ☐ Personality traits are patterns of behavior that reflect how people perceive and relate to others and themselves. Personality disorders occur when these traits become rigid and maladaptive.
- ☐ A client with a personality disorder uses maladaptive behavior to relate to others and fulfill basic emotional needs.

□ Psychotherapy is a mainstay of treating personality disorders due to the rigidity and chronicity of the maladaptive behaviors.

Paranoid Personality Disorder

□ Paranoid personality disorder is characterized by extreme distrust of others.

□ Clients with paranoid personality disorder appear guarded, unfriendly, and often jealous.

□ Clients with paranoid personality disorder do not report feeling isolated or endorse a desire for social contact.

□ Clients with paranoid personality disorder avoid relationships in which they are not in control or have the potential of losing control.

□ Achieving a nurse–patient rapport is particularly difficult with this client population.

Schizoid Personality Disorder

□ Schizoid personality disorder is characterized by a disinterest in social engagement and a preferable focus on objects or abstract concepts.

□ A primary nursing diagnosis for this client population is impaired social interaction.

□ A goal for treatment would be increasing emotional responsiveness to others. This goal is achieved by increasing social interactions while managing the client's associated anxiety with such situations.

Schizotypal Personality Disorder

□ Schizotypal personality disorder is characterized by positive psychotic symptoms that present as maladaptive behaviors.

□ Due to eccentricity, clients with schizotypal personality disorder often have impaired social skills. Understandably, social skill development consistent with cultural norms is a focus of treatment.

□ Medications are rarely used to control the symptoms of this condition.

Borderline Personality Disorder

□ Borderline personality disorder is characterized by a pattern of mood lability, unstable interpersonal relationships, self-injurious behavior, low self-esteem, and poor self-identity.

□ Clients with borderline personality disorder commonly exhibit an intense fear of abandonment.

□ Borderline personality disorder appears to be related to sexual abuse in childhood.

Antisocial Personality Disorder

☐ Antisocial personality disorder is characterized by a total disregard for the rights of others.

☐ Clients with antisocial personality disorder commonly will rationalize why their aggressive behavior was warranted and deny responsibility for their actions.

☐ Aggressive behavior makes caring for clients with antisocial personality disorder a challenge, because these clients are typically impulsive and tend to lash out at those who interfere with their need for immediate gratification.

☐ Setting limits and removing the client from the situation are the best ways to handle aggression.

Narcissistic Personality Disorder

☐ Clients with narcissistic personality disorder exhibit a sense of superiority and grandiosity. These characteristics are developed early on in life and foster an inability to show empathy or sensitivity toward others, unless there is a direct personal gain.

☐ Clients with narcissistic personality disorder appear overly confident, self-centered, unrealistically knowledgeable, and above social conventions.

☐ Clients with narcissistic personality disorder often are ambitious and strive for success in careers associated with high respect or status including doctors, lawyers, athletes, or celebrities. However, their success often comes at the expense of distancing others.

☐ Clients with narcissistic personality disorder have difficulty managing criticism and either become enraged by it or act indifferently.

Histrionic Personality Disorder

☐ Clients with histrionic personality disorder exhibit dramatic and often seductive behavior that calls attention to them.

☐ While clients with histrionic personality disorder may be quick to make friends, their relentless need to talk about and call attention to themselves often impairs their ability to truly achieve intimacy with others.

☐ Difficulty with intimacy may lead to a lack of fidelity in romantic relationships.

☐ Reinforcing positive qualities of the client with histrionic personality disorder while examining their own personal negative perceptions is important in the treatment process.

Dependent Personality Disorder

☐ Clients with dependent personality disorder exhibit the need to be taken care of, which leads to submissive, clinging behavior, fear of separation, and difficulty or inability to make decisions.

- ☐ These characteristics develop by early adulthood, when behaviors designed to elicit caring from others become predominant and arise from the client's perception that they are unable to function adequately without others.
- ☐ Basic personal management, including cleaning and paying bills, may be problematic for this client population.
- ☐ Clients with dependent personality disorder are eager to form a relationship with the nurse.
- ☐ To promote therapeutic outcomes, the nurse must encourage the client to make decisions independently.

Avoidant Personality Disorder

- ☐ Clients with avoidant personality disorder exhibit an extreme fear of rejection and criticism.
- ☐ These characteristics cause avoidance of social situations and career endeavors, impairing their level of functioning and ability for personal achievement.

PARAPHILIC DISORDERS

KEY TERMS

- ☐ **Exhibitionism** is exposing one's genitals in public to become intensely sexually aroused.
- ☐ **Fetishism** includes the use of an object to become intensely sexually aroused.
- ☐ **Frotteurism** is rubbing one's genitals on another nonconsenting person to become intensely sexually aroused.
- ☐ **Voyeurism** is deriving intense sexual arousal from observing the naked body or sexual acts of an unaware individual.
- ☐ **Masochism** is deriving sexual arousal from being submissive or humiliated.
- ☐ **Sadism** is deriving sexual arousal from the suffering of another person.
- ☐ **Pedophilia** is deriving sexual arousal from sexual activity with prepubescent individuals.

Paraphilias

- ☐ Paraphilias are characterized by an intense, recurring sexual urge.
- ☐ A paraphilic disorder is defined as a recurrent, intense sexual urge or fantasy that is distressful, impairing, or harmful.
- ☐ Paraphilic disorders generally involve nonhuman subjects; corpses; children; nonconsenting partners; or the degradation, suffering, and humiliation of the client or their partners.

☐ The client with a paraphilic disorder may report that the fantasy is always present but that the frequency of the fantasy and intensity of the urge may vary.

☐ Inappropriate sexual behavior may increase in response to psychological stressors, in relation to other mental disorders, or when opportunity to engage in the paraphilia becomes more available.

☐ Paraphilia tends to be lifelong, but in adults, both the fantasy and behavior commonly diminish with advancing age.

REVIEW QUESTIONS

1. A client is admitted to the psychiatric emergency department. The client's significant other reports that the client has a decreased need for sleep, has poor judgment, and is distractible at times. The client's speech is rapid and loose. The client reports being a special messenger from the Messiah. The client has a history of depressed mood and has been taking an antidepressant. Which diagnosis should the nurse suspect?
   1. Schizophrenia
   2. Paranoid personality disorder
   3. Bipolar disorder
   4. Obsessive-compulsive disorder (OCD)

2. A client who is taking lithium has nausea, thirst, and complains of a metallic taste in his mouth. The nurse should tell the client:
   1. "We need to check the level of lithium in your blood."
   2. "These common mild side effects of lithium will go away after 6 weeks."
   3. "Your symptoms really are no cause for concern."
   4. "I'll hold off on giving you your lithium until you feel better."

3. A client is experiencing an acute exacerbation of schizophrenia. The client's vivid auditory hallucinations are making the client agitated. The nurse's **best** response at this time is to:
   1. take the client's vital signs.
   2. explore the content of the client's hallucinations.
   3. tell the client that their fear is unrealistic.
   4. engage the client in reality-oriented activities.

4. A client has just been diagnosed with panic disorder. Which medication does the nurse anticipate administering long-term for this diagnosis?
   1. Fluoxetine
   2. Propranolol
   3. Diazepam
   4. Clozapine

5. A client diagnosed with depression tells a nurse that "I will not allow myself to cry because my crying upsets the whole family." This is an example of:

1. manipulation.
2. insight.
3. rationalization.
4. repression.

Chapter References

American Psychiatric Association. (2013). *Diagnostic and statistical manual of mental disorders* (5th ed.). Arlington, VA: American Psychiatric Publishing.

Austin, W., & Boyd, M. A. (2014). *Psychiatric & mental health nursing for Canadian practice* (3rd ed.). Philadelphia, PA: Lippincott Williams & Wilkins.

Boyd, M. A. (2015). *Psychiatric nursing contemporary practice* (5th ed.). Philadelphia, PA: Wolters Kluwer.

Mohr, W. (2012). *Psychiatric-mental health nursing: Evidence-based concepts, skills, and practices* (8th ed.). Philadelphia, PA: Lippincott Williams & Wilkins.

Videbeck, S. (2013). *Psychiatric-mental health nursing* (6th ed.). Philadelphia, PA: Lippincott Williams & Wilkins.

5

Pharmacology

MEDICATION ADMINISTRATION ROUTES

General Guidelines for Medication Administration

☐ The three checks when preparing medications include the label with the MAR when removing the med, the label immediately before opening or pouring, and the label again before returning or throwing away.

☐ The six rights include "right medication," "right patient," "right dosage," "right route," "right time," and "right documentation."

☐ Other rights include "right education," "right to refuse," "right preparation," "right assessment," and "right evaluation."

⊚ ☐ Always check your client's name against their ID band before administering medications. If the client does not have an ID band and cannot identify their name and birthdate, a responsible party must identify the client and the ID band replaced.

⊚ ☐ A stated name is not sufficient to identify a client for medication administration.

☐ Don't open a unit dose medication until you're at the client's bedside.

☐ To assess the client's response to medication, be aware of the client's medical condition and what the drug's desired or expected effect should be.

☐ After administering a drug, document on the client's medication administration record. Be sure to include the following: the drug name, dosage, route and time of administration, and your signature and title.

☐ In the nurse's notes, include any assessment data that refer to the client's response to the medication and any adverse effects of the medication.

☐ Enteric-coated, buccal, and sublingual tablets should never be crushed or chewed.

☐ Children absorb topical medications at a higher rate than adults.

⊚ ☐ Body surface area in relation to weight is the most reliable method for estimating proper medication dosage for a child.

☐ Drug toxicities occur when a drug level rises as a result of impaired metabolism or excretion. Most drug toxicities are dosage-related and usually reversible upon dosage adjustment.

☐ The Food and Drug Administration (FDA) has assigned a pregnancy risk category to each drug based on available information reflecting a drug's potential to cause birth defects. (See Table 5.1 for more information on FDA Pregnancy Risk Categories.)

☐ Although drugs should ideally be avoided during pregnancy, sometimes, they're needed; the pregnancy risk category rating system permits rapid assessment of the risk-benefit ratio.

☐ Pregnant women should avoid oral antidiabetic agents and use insulin therapy to maintain glucose levels as close to normal as possible.

TABLE 5.1	FDA Pregnancy Risk Categories
Category	Pregnancy Risk
A	■ Adequate studies in pregnant women have failed to show a risk to the fetus.
B	■ Animal studies haven't shown a risk to the fetus, but controlled studies haven't been conducted in pregnant women. ■ Also includes those drugs in which animal studies have shown an adverse effect on the fetus, but no adequate studies have been performed in pregnant women to show a risk to the fetus.
C	■ Animal studies have shown an adverse effect on the fetus, but adequate studies haven't been conducted in humans. ■ The benefits from use in pregnant women may be acceptable despite potential risks.
D	■ There is positive evidence of human fetal risk, but the potential benefits of use in pregnant women may be acceptable despite the risks (such as in a life-threatening situation or a serious disease for which safer drugs can't be used or are ineffective).
X	■ Studies in animals or humans show fetal abnormalities or adverse reaction reports indicate evidence of fetal risk, and the risks involved clearly outweigh potential benefits.
NR	■ Not rated

Oral Route

- ☐ The rate of enteral absorption is dependent on food in stomach, gastric motility, and gastric pH.
- ☐ Oral or PO medications are sometimes prescribed in higher dosages than their parenteral equivalents because, after absorption through the GI system, the liver breaks them down before they reach the systemic circulation.

Buccal, Sublingual, and Translingual Administration

- ☐ Drugs that are given buccally include nitroglycerin and methyltestosterone.
- ☐ Drugs that are given sublingually include ergotamine tartrate, isosorbide, and nitroglycerin.
- ☐ Translingual drugs, which are sprayed onto the tongue, include nitrate preparations for clients with chronic angina.

Otic Route

- ☐ To administer eardrops to an infant or a child younger than age 3, gently pull the auricle down and back; the ear canal is straighter at this age.
- ☐ To administer eardrops to a child older than 3 or an adult, gently pull the auricle up and back.

Optic Route

- ☐ When teaching an elderly client how to instill eye drops, keep in mind that the client may have difficulty sensing drops in the eye; suggest chilling the medication slightly to enhance the sensation.
- ☐ To apply eye ointment, squeeze a small ribbon of medication on the edge of the conjunctival sac, from the inner to the outer canthus.
- ☐ To maintain the sterility of the drug container, never touch the tip of the dropper or bottle to the eye area.

Nasal Route

- ☐ To instill nose drops into the ethmoidal and sphenoidal sinuses, have the client lie supine with their neck hyperextended and the client's head tilted back over the edge of the bed, while supporting the client's head with one hand to prevent neck strain.
- ☐ To instill nose drops into the maxillary and frontal sinuses, have the client lie supine with the head toward the affected side and hanging slightly over the edge of the bed, and then, ask the client to rotate the head laterally after hyperextension.
- ☐ Calcitonin, a hormone used for osteoporosis, should be given in only one nostril daily, with the nostrils alternated each day.

Rectal Route

- ☐ Because the intake of food and fluid stimulates peristalsis, a suppository for relieving constipation should be inserted about 30 minutes before mealtime to help soften the stool and facilitate defecation.

- ☐ Suppositories are inserted, lubricated, with the "pointed" end first, 1 inch into the rectum.

- ☐ Clients should be instructed to lie down for about 5 minutes after insertion to help hold the suppository in place.

Transdermal

- ☐ Apply daily transdermal medications at the same time every day to ensure a continuous effect, but alternate the application sites to avoid skin irritation.

- ☐ Transdermal sites should be rotated.

- ☐ All transdermal medication should be removed before a new patch or paste is applied.

- ☐ Transdermal patches administer drugs by passive diffusion at a constant rate.

Enteral

- ☐ To confirm the placement of a nasogastric tube, place a small amount of gastric contents from the tube on a pH test strip; the appearance of gastric contents and pH (equal to or less than 5) implies that the tube is patent and in the stomach. If the client is receiving a proton pump inhibitor or antacid, the pH may not be less or equal to 5.

- ☐ When giving medication through a nasogastric tube by gravity, as the last of the medication flows out of the syringe, start to irrigate the tube by adding 30 to 50 mL of water (15 to 30 mL for a child). Check for fluid restrictions prior to irrigation.

- ☐ Administer medication before tube feeding and never mix.

- ☐ Tube feedings must be withheld 2 hours before and 2 hours after phenytoin or warfarin administration.

- ☐ Residual (stomach content) is assessed by pulling back on syringe and is placed back into the stomach after measurement.

- ☐ If residual stomach contents exceed 100 mL, standard procedure is to wait to administer the feeding or medication and recheck within an hour.

- ☐ Excess residual may indicate delayed gastric emptying, intestinal obstruction, or paralytic ileus.

Z-Track

- ☐ The Z-track IM injection method prevents leakage, or tracking, into the subcutaneous tissue and is typically used to administer drugs that irritate and discolor subcutaneous tissue, primarily iron preparations such as iron dextran.

☐ The Z-track method for injection may be used in elderly clients who have decreased muscle mass.

Epidural Route

☐ When giving an epidural analgesic, the health care provider injects or infuses the drug into the epidural space and thus into the cerebrospinal fluid, so that the medication can bypass the blood-brain barrier.

☐ Clients receiving epidural anesthesia should be assessed frequently, including respiratory rate and blood pressure. Institutional policy should be reviewed for frequency guidelines.

Central Venous Access Catheter Medication Administration

☐ The central venous access catheter is inserted through a large vein, such as the subclavian vein, the jugular vein, or peripheral veins.

☐ The tip of the central venous access catheter must be placed in the superior vena cava for the catheter to be considered a central venous access catheter.

☐ Allow the administration of intravenous fluids in large amounts and can remain in place for long-term therapy.

☐ Can be utilized for fluids that put the vein at risk including chemotherapy, potassium, and hypertonic solutions like total parenteral nutrition.

☐ In addition to administration, the central venous access catheter can be utilized to draw blood samples.

☐ Pneumothorax can occur during central venous access catheter insertion.

☐ Sepsis can occur anytime during therapy with a central venous access catheter.

☐ Thrombus formation and air embolism can occur with a central venous access catheter. The nurse assesses for changes in respiratory rate, heart rate, and chest pain.

Peripherally Inserted Central Catheters (PICC)

☐ Usually enters at the arm's basilic vein and terminates in the superior vena cava.

☐ Can be used for long-term medication therapy and can be safely used at home.

☐ May be used in a client who has a chest injury; neck, chest, or shoulder burns; compromised respiratory function; or a surgical site that's close to a central venous line placement site.

Central Venous Access Catheter Maintenance

☐ All lumens of the central venous access catheter must be flushed regularly. Institutional policy should be followed.

☐ The central venous access catheter is flushed vigorously, using only low-pressure 10-mL syringes.

☐ Blood return should be assessed prior to flushing a central venous access catheter lumen.

☐ After flushing the central venous access catheter, pressure is kept on the plunger of the syringe to prevent backflow of blood.

☐ Clamps are closed before the last of the flush is pushed in.

☐ Caps are changed on lumens of the central venous access catheter according to policy, using aseptic technique.

☐ The client performs a Valsalva maneuver when the old cap is removed.

☐ If the client cannot perform the Valsalva, a padded clamp is used to prevent air from entering the catheter.

Central Venous Access Catheter Removal

☐ Central venous access catheter removal is a sterile procedure.

☐ Only a nurse trained in the care of peripherally inserted central catheter (PICC) lines may remove a PICC line.

☐ If the client has an infection, the removal procedure includes sending the tip to the laboratory for culture.

Parenteral Therapy

☐ Parenteral means outside the intestine and miss first-pass metabolism by the liver.

☐ Parenteral drugs are administered through the skin, subcutaneous tissue, muscle, or veins.

☐ Intradermal medications are injected into the dermis, or outer layer of the skin.

☐ Common uses for intradermal injections include anesthetizing skin for invasive procedures and testing for allergies, tuberculosis, and other diseases.

☐ When giving an intradermal injection, stretch the skin taut with one hand and insert the needle with your other hand at a 10- to 15-degree angle.

☐ A subcutaneous injection is given typically into the lateral upper arm, thigh, abdomen, and upper back.

☐ Administer a subcutaneous injection by pinching the skin if the client is thin and inserting the needle at a 45-degree angle; if the client is obese, do not pinch the skin but insert the needle into the fatty tissue at a 90-degree angle.

☐ Do not massage the skin after giving an injection of heparin or insulin.

☐ After administering an intramuscular injection, pressure should be applied to the site; it should not be rubbed.

☐ The IM route is used to administer drugs that need to be absorbed quickly.

☐ A volume for IM injections to a child should only receive no more than 1 mL.

☐ The ventrogluteal site is the safest site for intramuscular injections.

☐ When administering intramuscular injections to a child, use the vastus lateralis muscle.

☐ When giving an injection, avoid any site that's inflamed, edematous, or irritated or that contains moles, birthmarks, scar tissue, or other lesions.

☐ See Table 5.2 for facts on selecting needle size.

Intravenous (IV) Therapy

☐ Intravenous drug administration involves venipuncture.

☐ Selection of a venipuncture device and site for peripheral IV catheter insertion depends on the type of solution to be used; the frequency and duration of infusion; the patency and location of accessible veins; the client's age, size, and condition; and, when possible, the client's preference.

☐ The nondominate side is preferred for IV therapy as decreased movement decreases the risk of dislodging of the catheter.

☐ A paralyzed limb is never used for IV therapy, as the client would not be able to sense infiltration or any other complication.

Route	Total to be Administered	Needle Gauge	Needle Length	Angle for Administration
Intradermal injection	Small volumes (about 0.1 ml)	25–27 gauge	⅜–⅝ inches long (9–16 mm)	15 degrees
Subcutaneous injection (Subcut)	1 mL	25–28 gauge	½–⅝ inches long (12–16 mm)	45–90 degrees
Intramuscular injection (IM)	Up to 3 mL (depending on site)	18–23 gauge	1–3 inches long (25–75 mm)	90 degrees

TABLE 5.2 Selecting Needle Size

- Clients who have had a mastectomy or lymph node removal should not have an IV catheter inserted on the affected side. If an infection develops, this could result in unresolvable lymphedema.
- An arm with an arteriovenous fistula for dialysis cannot be utilized for IV therapy due to the risk of damaging the fistula.
- Leg and feet are not typically used for venipuncture due to the increased risk of thrombophlebitis.
- Attempts at venipuncture should begin at the most distal site, such as the hand, and move up the arm.
- Larger veins are used for irritating or concentrated medications and solutions.
- The venous access device is removed if the area is red, tender, or edematous.
- Intermittent infusions are used when drugs or fluids need to be administered periodically.
- IV fluids may be used to maintain volume or to correct an existing fluid or electrolyte imbalance.
- In addition to medication, fluids, blood, and blood products are administered IV.

Complications of Peripheral IV Therapy

- Circulatory overload is a potential complication of peripheral intravenous infusions and is noted by jugular vein distention, crackles, and hypertension.
- Signs and symptoms of nerve, tendon, or ligament damage with peripheral IV therapy include extreme pain (similar to electrical shock when the nerve is punctured) and numbness and muscle contraction.
- Intravenous sites are rotated according to policy, usually within 48 to 72 hours.
- Intravenous solutions can hang no more than 24 hours.
- Documentation of intravenous sites is completed each shift.

Extravasation

- Leakage of solution or medication from a vein into the surrounding tissue.
- The result of a needle puncturing the vessel wall or leakage around a venipuncture site and causes local pain and itching, edema, blanching, and decreased skin temperature in the affected extremity.
- Extravasation of a small amount of isotonic fluid or nonirritating drug usually causes only minor discomfort.

- Extravasation of some medications can severely damage tissue and cause necrosis.
- Antidotes may be necessary for many drugs to prevent tissue damage including vasoactive medications and chemotherapy. Check hospital policy for application of heat or cold therapy.

Bolus Intravenous Injection

- Bolus injection allows rapid drug administration and peak blood levels to be reached more quickly.
- An IV bolus may be used for drugs that can't be given IM or a client's ability to absorb intramuscular medication.
- Bolus doses may be injected through an existing intravenous access or through an implanted port.

TOTAL PARENTERAL NUTRITIONAL (TPN) THERAPY

About TPN

- Is a highly concentrated, hypertonic nutrient solution administered by an infusion pump through a large central vein.
- Provides calories, restores nitrogen balance, and replaces essential fluids, vitamins, electrolytes, minerals, and trace elements.
- Clients receiving TPN ideally should gain 1 to 2 pounds (0.5 to 1 kg)/week; weight gain greater than 1 pound (0.5 kg)/day indicates fluid retention.
- Monitor blood urea nitrogen and creatinine levels; increases may indicate excess amino acid intake and renal status.
- Albumin levels may drop initially in a client receiving TPN as hydration is restored.
- Document any adverse reaction or complications including signs of inflammation or infection at the intravenous site, nursing interventions (including infusion rate and the client's response), time and date of administration set changes, specific dietary intake, and any client teaching.
- Refeeding syndrome is a potentially fatal shift in fluids and electrolytes that may occur in malnourished clients and can occur; this includes a rapid drop in potassium, magnesium, and phosphorus levels. TPN is slowed and essential electrolytes are replaced.
- Clients at risk for refeeding syndrome are those who have not had food for 5 days or more.
- A PICC can be used for total parenteral nutrition.

TPN Administration

- Check the TPN label against the practitioner's order.

☐ Assess the solution bag for cloudiness or particulate matter. If found, return the solution to the pharmacy.

☐ Never add medications to TPN solution container. Some medications (such as insulin and famotidine) can be mixed by the pharmacist as ordered by the practitioner.

☐ TPN expires within 24 hours the administration set is attached. Discard remaining fluid in bag.

☐ Use a 1.2-micron filter when administering total parenteral nutrition containing an IV fat emulsion.

☐ Use a 0.2-micron filter when administering a total parenteral nutrition solution that does not contain an IV fat emulsion.

Lipids

☐ Support hormone and prostaglandin synthesis and prevent essential fatty acid deficiency.

☐ Assist in wound healing, red blood cell production, and prostaglandin synthesis.

☐ May be administered piggyback with TPN, given alone or mixed with amino acids and dextrose in one container (total nutrient admixtures), and infused over 24 hours.

☐ Should not be administered to clients who have conditions that disrupt normal fat metabolism, such as pathologic hyperlipidemia or lipid necrosis.

☐ Should be given cautiously to clients with hepatic or pulmonary disease, acute pancreatitis, anemia, or a coagulation disorder and to clients at risk for developing a fat embolism.

Peripheral Parenteral Nutrition (PPN)

☐ Prescribed for clients who have a malfunctioning GI tract and need short-term nutrition lasting less than 2 weeks.

☐ Infused peripherally in various combinations of lipid (fat) emulsions and amino acid-dextrose solutions.

☐ To ensure adequate nutrition, PPN solutions in final concentrations of less than or equal to 10% dextrose and less than or equal to 5% protein should not be administered for longer than 10 days unless they are supplemented with oral or enteral feedings.

TPN Monitoring

☐ Carefully monitor clients receiving TPN to detect early signs of complications such as hyperglycemia, infection, metabolic problems, heart failure, pulmonary edema, or allergic reactions.

☐ Signs and symptoms of electrolyte imbalances caused by TPN include abdominal cramps, lethargy, confusion, malaise, muscle weakness, tetany, convulsions, and cardiac arrhythmias.

☐ Acid-base imbalances can occur as a result of TPN content.

☐ Assess the client receiving total parenteral nutrition for thirst and polyuria, which are indications that the client may have hyperglycemia.

☐ Monitor glucose levels in a client receiving total parenteral nutrition every 6 hours initially and then once a day or according to institution policy.

☐ Monitor protein levels twice a week in a client receiving TPN.

Discontinuing TPN

☐ Weaning the client from TPN usually takes place over 24 to 48 hours, but it can be completed in 4 to 6 hours if the client receives sufficient oral or IV carbohydrates.

☐ When discontinuing, decrease the infusion slowly, depending on current glucose intake; this minimizes the risk of hyperinsulinemia and resulting hypoglycemia.

☐ If the TPN must be discontinued emergently due to nonintact IV bag or the TPN is not delivered as ordered, D10 must be administered until the TPN can be infused.

☐ TPN must be ordered daily based on lab results. This traditionally means the TPN will not be available until afternoon.

ADMINISTRATION OF BLOOD AND BLOOD PRODUCTS

Blood Administration

☐ Institutional policy should be checked: Generally, two licensed professionals need to identify the client and blood products at the bedside before administering a transfusion, to prevent errors and a potentially fatal reaction.

☐ Highly effective leukocyte removal filters are available for use when transfusing blood and packed red blood cells (PRBCs) to postpone sensitization to transfusion therapy.

☐ A Y-type set gives the nurse the option of adding normal saline solution to packed cells—decreasing their viscosity—if the client can tolerate the added fluid volume.

☐ Tubing can be used for two units of blood and then must be discarded.

☐ Prior to administration, the expiration date on the bag is checked, and the bag is assessed for color, clumping, bubbles, and extraneous materials and returned to the blood bank if found.

☐ The name and identification number on the clients name band must match the information in the blood bag label.

☐ In addition to name and client identification, the nurse checks the blood bag identification number, the ABO blood group, and Rh compatibility with a second nurse prior to administration of the blood product.

- □ Blood products should be obtained from the blood bank no more than 30 minutes prior to the start of the transfusion. Blood cannot be stored in the refrigerator on the nursing unit.
- □ A 20-gauge or larger catheter should be used to prevent destruction of cells during infusion.
- □ When infusing multiple units, the filter and tubing should be replaced if more than 1 hour elapses between units.
- □ When administering multiple units of blood under pressure, a warmer is used to prevent hypothermia.

Albumin
- □ Albumin transfusions are used to treat hypoproteinemia, volume loss, and shock due to burns, trauma, surgery, and infection.
- □ Administered with the set supplied by the manufacturer, with the rate and volume dictated by the client's condition and response.
- □ Reactions to albumin infusion (fever, chills, nausea) are rare.
- □ Can be transfused as a volume expander until the laboratory completes crossmatching for a whole blood transfusion.
- □ Infusion is contradicted in severe anemia and is administered cautiously in cardiac and pulmonary disease as heart failure may result from circulatory overload.

Cryoprecipitate
- □ Used to treat bleeding associated with hypofibrinogenemia or dysfibrinogenemia as well as to prevent or treat factor XIII deficiency.
- □ The insoluble portion of plasma recovered from fresh frozen plasma (FFP) containing fibrinogen, factor VIII:c, factor VIII:vwf, factor XIII, and fibronectin.
- □ Cryoprecipitate transfusion is administered with a blood transfusion set.
- □ Normal saline solution can be added to each bag as needed to facilitate transfusion.
- □ Cryoprecipitate must be administered within 6 hours of thawing.
- □ Prior to administration, the nurse assesses labs to confirm a deficiency of one of the specific clotting factors in cryoprecipitate.
- □ Clients with hemophilia A or von Willebrand disease should only be treated with cryoprecipitate when appropriate factor VIII concentrates are not available.

Fresh Frozen Plasma (FFP)
- □ A straight-line IV set is used to administer FFP, and it is administered rapidly.
- □ Is rich in coagulation factors V, VIII, and IX.

☐ Large-volume transfusions of FFP may require correction for hypocalcemia because citric acid in FFP binds calcium.

☐ Transfusions are used to treat coagulation factor deficiencies and thrombotic thrombocytopenic purpura (a rare blood disorder resulting in clotting in small vessels).

Packed Red Blood Cells (PRBCs)

☐ Administration requires a Y-type intravenous solution set and in-line filtration.

☐ PRBCs are used when decreased RBC levels accompany normal blood volume, to avoid possible fluid and circulatory overload.

☐ Washed PRBCs commonly used for clients who were previously sensitized to transfusions, are rinsed with a special solution that removes white blood cells (WBCs) and platelets, thus decreasing the chance of a transfusion reaction.

Platelets

☐ The client may be ordered premedication with antipyretics and antihistamines if they have a history of a platelet transfusion reaction.

☐ Platelet counts are checked on hour after transfusion to determine further therapy.

☐ Transfusion is used to treat bleeding resulting from critically decreased circulating platelet counts or functionally abnormal platelets to prevent bleeding caused by thrombocytopenia.

☐ Platelet transfusion is generally started with a platelet count less than 50,000/μL before surgery or a major invasive procedure.

☐ When administering platelets, a filtered component drip administration set is used to infuse 100 mL over 15 minutes.

White Blood Cells

☐ WBCs are used to treat sepsis unresponsive to antibiotics (especially if the client has positive blood cultures or a persistent fever greater than 101°F [38.3°C]) and granulocytopenia (granulocyte count usually less than 500 mcg/L).

☐ If a transfusion of WBCs causes fever and chills, an antipyretic is administered and the flow rate is slowed.

☐ Prior to infusing WBCs, the container is agitated to mix cells.

☐ One unit daily is administered for 5 days or until the infection resolves.

Whole Blood

☐ Transfusion requires an in-line filter.

☐ Whole blood transfusion replenishes the volume and the oxygen-carrying capacity of the circulatory system by increasing the mass of circulating red blood cells.

- ☐ Each unit of whole blood or PRBC contains enough hemoglobin to raise the hemoglobin level in an average-sized adult 1 g/L, or by 3%.
- ☐ Whole blood is generally only used for hemorrhage.

Immune Globulin

- ☐ Immune globulin is processed human plasma from multiple donors that contains 95% IgG, less than 2.5% IgA, and a fraction of IgM.
- ☐ The administration set supplied by the manufacturer is utilized for infusion after the lyophilized power is reconstituted with 0.9% sodium chloride injection, 5% dextrose, or sterile water.
- ☐ Used to treat primary and secondary immunodeficiencies, Kawasaki syndrome, idiopathic thrombocytopenia purpura, and neurologic disorders such as Guillain-Barré syndrome, dermatomyositis, and myasthenia gravis.
- ☐ Administered at the minimal concentration available and at the slowest practical rate.

ANTIDOTES AND POISONING

- ☐ Activated charcoal is used to treat poisoning or overdose with many orally administered drugs.
- ☐ See Table 5.3 for other common antidotes.

TABLE 5.3	Common Antidotes
Antidote	**Drug/Poison**
Deferoxamine mesylate	■ Adjunctive treatment of acute iron intoxication (will turn the urine rose colored)
Aminocaproic acid	■ Alteplase ■ Anistreplase ■ Streptokinase ■ Urokinase
Amyl nitrite	■ Cyanide poisoning
Atropine sulfate	■ Anticholinesterase toxicity ■ Organophosphate poisoning
Digoxin immune Fab (ovine)	■ Potentially life-threatening digoxin intoxication
Edetate calcium	■ Lead poisoning in clients with blood levels >50 mcg/dL

TABLE 5.3 Common Antidotes (*Continued*)	
Antidote	Drug/Poison
Nalmefene	■ Known or suspected opioid overdose, in adults only ■ Preferred to naltrexone because of its longer half-life, oral bioavailability, and little to no dose-dependent liver toxicity
Pralidoxime chloride	■ Organophosphate poisoning ■ Cholinergic overdose
Protamine sulfate	■ Heparin overdose
Vitamin K	■ Warfarin overdose

CARDIAC MEDICATIONS

Alpha-Blockers

☐ Medications include prazosin and doxazosin.

☐ Alpha-blockers, also called alpha-adrenergic antagonists, treat high blood pressure, benign prostatic hyperplasia, and Raynaud disease.

☐ May cause severe orthostatic hypotension and syncope, especially with the first few doses, an effect commonly called the "first-dose effect."

☐ The most common adverse effects of $alpha_1$ blockade are dizziness, headache, drowsiness, somnolence, and malaise.

☐ May cause reflex tachycardia (due to blood vessel relaxation and hypertension control), palpitations, fluid retention (from excess renin secretion), nasal and ocular congestion, and aggravation of respiratory tract infection.

☐ Teach clients about the hypotensive effects to minimize injury. Take medication at bedtime.

☐ Alpha-adrenergic blockers relax the smooth muscle of the bladder and prostate.

Angiotensin-Converting Enzyme (ACE) Inhibitors

☐ Medication name often ends in -pril.

☐ The most common adverse effects are angioedema of the face and limbs, dry cough, change in taste (dysgeusia), fatigue, headache, hyperkalemia, hypotension, proteinuria, rash, and tachycardia.

☐ ACE inhibitor toxicity may cause severe hypotension. Teach clients about the hypotensive effects to minimize injury.

☐ Should be used cautiously in clients with impaired renal function or serious autoimmune disease and in those taking other drugs known to decrease WBC count or immune response.

- ☐ Administration carries a high risk of fetal morbidity and mortality, particularly in the second and third trimesters.
- ☐ Monitor for dry cough and angioedema. Contraindicated with breast-feeding.
- ☐ Safe use has not been proven with children.
- ☐ Elderly clients may need lower doses due to impaired drug clearance.

Anticoagulant Drugs

- ☐ Warfarin is an oral anticoagulant that prevents vitamin K from synthesizing certain clotting factors.
- ☐ Heparin is a parenteral anticoagulant that interferes with coagulation by readily combining with antithrombin.
- ☐ Target INR for clients on warfarin is 2 to 3.5. Target aPTT for clients on heparin is 45 to 100 seconds.
- ☐ The antidote for heparin is protamine sulfate, and the antidote for coumadin is vitamin K.
- ☐ Warfarin may cause agranulocytosis, alopecia (with long-term use), anorexia, dermatitis, fever, tissue necrosis, or gangrene.
- ☐ Heparin derivatives may cause thrombocytopenia (heparin-induced thrombocytopenia, HIT) and may increase liver enzyme levels.
- ☐ Nonhemorrhagic adverse reactions associated with thrombin inhibitors may include back pain, bradycardia, and hypotension.
- ☐ Teach clients taking warfarin to keep vitamin K intake consistent from day to day to keep PT/INR stable.
- ☐ Assess clients on anticoagulation for bleeding such as nosebleeds, hematuria, GI bleeding, change in level of consciousness, and abdominal pain.
- ☐ Teach clients that NSAIDs and alcohol increase the risk of bleeding.

Antiplatelet Drugs

- ☐ Intravenous antiplatelet drugs abciximab, eptifibatide, and tirofiban antagonize the glycoprotein IIb/glycoprotein IIIa (GPIIb/GPIIIa) receptors located on platelets, which are involved in platelet aggregation.
- ☐ The antiplatelet drug clopidogrel inhibits platelet aggregation by inhibiting the binding of adenosine diphosphate (ADP) to its platelet receptor and the subsequent ADP-mediated activation of the GPIIb/GPIIIa complex.
- ☐ Antiplatelet drugs work for the life of the platelet 7 to 10 days. If bleeding occurs correct with a donor platelet infusion.
- ☐ Teach clients to avoid ginkgo, ginger, and garlic that may increase bleeding time.
- ☐ The antiplatelet drug ticlopidine inhibits the binding of fibrinogen to platelets.

- Aspirin has antiplatelet properties to decrease clot formation.
- Monitor for signs and symptoms of bleeding.
- Discontinue 1 week before elective surgery.

Angiotensin II Receptor Blockers (ARBs)

- Medication names often ends in -sartan.
- Used cautiously in clients with renal impairment and hypovolemia.
- Inhibition of angiotensin II decreases adrenocortical secretion of aldosterone, lowering sodium and extracellular fluid volume.
- ARBs block the vasoconstriction effect of the renin-angiotensin system, decreasing blood pressure.
- Used to treat clients with hypertension, diabetic neuropathy, heart failure, and clients resistant to ACE inhibitors.
- Monitor for hypotension, tachycardia, edema, and hyperkalemia.
- Teach clients about the hypotensive effects to minimize injury.

Antiarrhythmic Drugs

- Antiarrhythmics may produce central nervous system disturbances, such as dizziness or fatigue as well as hypotension.
- Some antiarrhythmics may worsen heart failure.
- Many antiarrhythmic drugs are contraindicated in cardiogenic shock, digoxin toxicity, and second- or third-degree heart block (unless the client has a pacemaker or implantable cardioverter-defibrillator).
- Most antiarrhythmics may cause new or worsened arrhythmias (proarrhythmic effect) and must be used with caution and with continual cardiac monitoring and client evaluation.
- Lidocaine hydrochloride is an antiarrhythmic and a local anesthetic agent. It is commonly used for ventricular dysrhythmias.
- Common adverse effects of lidocaine include dizziness, tinnitus, blurred vision, tremors, numbness and tingling of extremities, excessive perspiration, hypotension, seizures, and finally coma.
- Digoxin is commonly used to slow conduction through the atrioventricular node in treating rapid atrial dysrhythmias such as fibrillation and flutter.
- Atropine is used to decrease vagal tone and increase heart rate in bradycardia and AV block.
- See Table 5.4 for classifications of antiarrhythmic drugs.

Beta-Adrenergic Blockers (BB)

- Medication names often end in -lol.
- Used to treat hypertension and dysrhythmias.

TABLE 5.4	Classification of Antiarrhythmic Drugs
Class	Drugs
Class IA	■ Disopyramide procainamide hydrochloride ■ Quinidine gluconate ■ Quinidine sulfate
Class IB	■ Lidocaine hydrochloride ■ Mexiletine hydrochloride
Class IC	■ Flecainide acetate ■ Propafenone hydrochloride
Class II	■ Beta-blockers (include amiodarone hydrochloride, dofetilide, esmolol hydrochloride, ibutilide fumarate, and sotalol hydrochloride)
Class IV	■ Calcium channel blockers (verapamil hydrochloride)

☐ Suppresses glycogenolysis, limiting the body's ability to correct hypoglycemia and masks signs and symptoms of hypoglycemia.

☐ May cause bradycardia, cough, disturbing dreams, dizziness, dyspnea, fatigue, heart failure, hypotension, lethargy, peripheral edema, and bronchospasm.

☐ Teach clients to how to take their pulse, not to abruptly discontinue this medication, and change position slowly.

☐ Beta-blockers are contraindicated in clients with cardiogenic shock, sinus bradycardia, and heart block greater than first degree.

☐ Recommendations for using BBs during breast-feeding vary by drug.

☐ The client's apical pulse should always be assessed before giving any BB. A heart rate below 55 bpm is cause for further assessment.

☐ Older BBs are nonselective and may block beta 2 receptors in the lungs and cause bronchoconstriction. Use cautiously in clients with asthma and other respiratory diseases.

Calcium Channel Blockers (CCBs)

☐ Medication names may end in -pine except diltiazem and verapamil!

☐ The main physiologic action is to inhibit calcium influx across the slow channels of myocardial and vascular smooth muscle cells, which reduces intracellular calcium levels, which in turn dilates coronary arteries, peripheral arteries, and arterioles and slows cardiac conduction.

☐ Verapamil and diltiazem have the greatest effect on the atrioventricular node, slowing the ventricular rate in atrial fibrillation or flutter and converting supraventricular tachycardia to a normal sinus rhythm.

- ☐ May cause bradycardia, confusion, depression, dizziness, dyspepsia, edema, transient elevations in liver enzyme levels, fatigue, flushing, headache, hypotension, insomnia, nervousness, and rash.
- ☐ The most common adverse reactions to diltiazem are anorexia and nausea.
- ☐ Contraindicated in clients with severe hypotension or heart block greater than first degree (except with functioning pacemaker).
- ☐ Cautiously used in clients with hepatic or renal impairment.
- ☐ Recommendations for breast-feeding vary by drug.
- ☐ Prolonged oral verapamil therapy may cause constipation.
- ☐ Diltiazem reduces the incidence of coronary artery spasm and assists to control Prinzmetal angina.

Dopamine

- ☐ Dopamine, a sympathomimetic drug, is the drug most commonly used to treat cardiogenic shock.
- ☐ Improves myocardial contractility and blood flow through vital organs by increasing perfusion pressure.
- ☐ Is dose dependent, and at lower doses increases renal perfusion so is assessed by urinary output increases and at higher doses is assessed by blood pressure increases.
- ☐ Monitor urine output, ECG monitor, and vital signs.

Cholesterol-Lowering Medications and Antilipemics

- ☐ Antilipemics commonly cause GI upset, including nausea, vomiting, abdominal pain, and increased risk for gallstones.
- ☐ Antilipemics can also interact with anticoagulants causing bleeding.
- ☐ Use of gemfibrozil with lovastatin may cause myopathy.
- ☐ Bile-sequestering drugs (cholestyramine and colesevelam) lower the low-density lipoprotein level by forming insoluble complexes with bile salts, thus triggering cholesterol to leave the bloodstream and other storage areas to make new bile acids.
- ☐ Bile-sequestering drugs are contraindicated in clients with complete biliary obstruction and only used cautiously in clients who have constipation.
- ☐ Fibric acid derivatives (fibrates) are used cautiously in clients with peptic ulcer and contraindicated in clients with primary biliary cirrhosis or significant hepatic or renal dysfunction.
- ☐ Gemfibrozil, a fibrate, reduces cholesterol formation, increases sterol excretion, and decreases lipoprotein and triglyceride synthesis.
- ☐ Fibrates may cause cholelithiasis and have other GI or central nervous system effects.

- ☐ Statins or HMG-CoA reductase inhibitors (atorvastatin, fluvastatin, lovastatin, pravastatin, rosuvastatin, simvastatin) interfere with the activity of enzymes that generate cholesterol in the liver.
- ☐ Statins and cholesterol absorption inhibitors are contraindicated in clients with active liver disease or persistently elevated transaminase levels.
- ☐ Use statins cautiously in clients who consume large amounts of alcohol or in those who have a history of liver or renal disease.
- ☐ Statins may affect liver function or cause rash, pruritus, increased creatinine kinase levels, rhabdomyolysis, and myopathy.
- ☐ Myopathy is a potential side effect. Instruct clients to report muscle aches and pains when taking statins.
- ☐ Ezetimibe, a selective cholesterol absorption inhibitor, inhibits cholesterol absorption by the small intestine, reducing hepatic cholesterol stores and increasing cholesterol clearance from the blood.

Inotropic Agents

- ☐ Positive inotropic agents increase the force of contraction of the heart.
- ☐ Inotropic agents may cause arrhythmias, nausea, vomiting, diarrhea, headache, fever, mental disturbances, visual changes, and chest pain.
- ☐ Teach clients to take their own radial pulse for a full minute.
- ☐ Digoxin is contraindicated in ventricular fibrillation and should be held for a heart rate less than 60 bpm.
- ☐ Digoxin is used cautiously in clients with sinus node disease or atrioventricular block because of the potential to worsen heart block.
- ☐ The therapeutic range for digoxin 0.5 to 2 ng/mL.
- ☐ Hypokalemia can potentiate dig toxicity and cause lethal dysrhythmias.
- ☐ Digoxin is used cautiously in clients with renal insufficiency because of the potential for toxicity.
- ☐ Inamrinone is contraindicated in clients with a sulfite allergy and severe aortic or pulmonic valve disease and acute myocardial infarction.
- ☐ Inamrinone and milrinone may cause thrombocytopenia, hypotension, hypokalemia, and elevated liver enzymes.
- ☐ Dobutamine is used in short-term management of heart failure (intravenously) and increases cardiac output by decreasing peripheral vascular resistance, reducing ventricular filling pressure, and increasing atrioventricular node conduction.

Nitrates

- ☐ Nitrates are commonly administered in PO, IV, sublingual, buccal, translingual, and transdermal routes.

☐ Before giving nitroglycerin, obtain the client's baseline blood pressure and then obtain blood pressures frequently after administration.

☐ Teach client to have a nitro-free period of 10 hours per day to prevent tolerance.

☐ Teach the client to notify the practitioner with severe headache, dizziness, and blurred vision.

☐ If the client's blood pressure has dropped after applying nitroglycerin ointment but is not symptomatic, the client should lie still until the blood pressure returns to normal.

☐ Nitrates may cause flushing, headache, orthostatic hypotension, reflex tachycardia, rash, syncope, and vomiting.

☐ Isosorbide dinitrate can cause hypotension and decreased cerebral perfusion and should not be used in a client who has had a stroke.

☐ Nitrates are contraindicated in clients with severe anemia, cerebral hemorrhage, head trauma, glaucoma, or hyperthyroidism.

☐ Nitrates are contraindicated in clients using phosphodiesterase type 5 inhibitors (sildenafil, tadalafil, vardenafil).

☐ Nitrates are used cautiously in clients with hypotension or recent myocardial infarction.

IMMUNE SYSTEM MEDICATIONS

Highly Active Antiretroviral Therapy (HAART)

☐ Usually consists of two nucleoside analogues and a protease inhibitor.

☐ Antiviral drugs inhibit DNA or RNA replication in the virus, preventing replication and leading to death of the virus.

☐ Nucleoside reverse transcriptase inhibitors suppress human immunodeficiency virus (HIV) replication by inhibiting HIV DNA polymerase.

☐ Protease inhibitors bind to the protease active site and inhibit HIV protease activity.

☐ Zidovudine is an antiviral drug that suppresses the replication of HIV.

☐ Zidovudine helps prevent maternal-fetal transmission of HIV.

☐ Therapeutic effects of HAART include increased CD4 count and T-cell count.

☐ Protease inhibitors can cause soft tissue deformities (such as buffalo hump).

☐ Client assessment when on HAART includes hepatitis panel, liver function tests, and assessment for toxoplasmosis and CMV.

☐ HAART is started with a CD4 count less than 350 cells/mm^3.

- □ HAART is started regardless of CD4 count in pregnant women, hepatitis B infection, and HIV nephropathy.
- □ Client assessment during HAART includes monitoring for (and teaching client to assess for) signs of myelosuppression, opportunistic infections, anorexia, and adverse reactions.
- □ Postexposure prophylaxis (PEP) of HIV infection is designed to prevent transmission to health care workers.
- □ PEP pharmacologic treatment regimen includes two drug therapy over a 4-week period (commonly zidovudine, lamivudine, or emtricitabine).
- □ PEP is recommended with substantial exposure risk within 72 hours of exposure.

RESPIRATORY MEDICATIONS

Short-Acting Bronchodilators
- □ Medications include albuterol, levalbuterol, and terbutaline.
- □ Side effects include hyperglycemia, tachycardia, tremor, angina, and palpitations. Use cautiously in clients with heart disease, diabetes, and glaucoma.
- □ If the client has heart disease, use caution because it can potentiate angina, arrhythmias, or hypertension. If paradoxical bronchospasm occurs, discontinue the drug and call the health care provider.
- □ Common adverse effects include tachycardia, nervousness, tremors, insomnia, irritability, and headache.
- □ If the client is using a bronchodilator and a corticosteroid inhalers, have the client use the bronchodilator first, wait 5 minutes, and then use the corticosteroid. The bronchodilation allows the corticosteroid to enter the respiratory tract (BC—bronchodilate, corticosteroid).

Long-Acting Bronchodilators
- □ Medications include tiotropium, salmeterol, and formoterol.
- □ Should not be used in acute episodes of bronchoconstriction.

Combination Long-Acting Bronchodilator and Steroid Inhalers
- □ Medications include fluticasone/salmeterol and budesonide/formoterol combinations.
- □ Manages inflammation and bronchodilation, and can be used with exercise induced bronchospasm.
- □ Should not be used in acute episodes of bronchoconstriction.
- □ Side effects include tachycardia and palpitations.

Aminophylline

- ☐ Aminophylline dilates the bronchioles by inhibiting cyclic adenosine monophosphate (cAMP) relaxing bronchial smooth muscle.
- ☐ Levels of aminophylline below 10 mcg/mL are considered to be less than therapeutic.
- ☐ Symptoms of aminophylline toxicity, such as nausea, tachycardia, and irritability, can appear when levels exceed 20 mcg/mL.
- ☐ Levels of aminophylline greater than 30 mcg/mL can cause seizures and arrhythmias.
- ☐ Nicotine-containing products increase the hepatic metabolism of the drug requiring higher dosages of aminophylline and theophylline. If the clients stop using nicotine, their dose must be decreased or they are at risk for toxicity.

Antitubercular Drugs

- ☐ Mycobacterial studies and susceptibility tests are performed before starting antitubercular drug therapy.
- ☐ An acid-fast bacilli (AFB) culture and smear is used to diagnose mycobacterium tuberculosis or tubercular bacillus in the sputum.
- ☐ Multiple antitubercular drugs are administered together to prevent the development of resistant strains of bacteria.
- ☐ Assessment of visual function is performed during therapy due to the risk of optic neuritis. Clients should be instructed to report blurred vision and changes in color perception.
- ☐ If clients complain of gastric irritation, administer antitubercular drugs with foods.
- ☐ Teach clients that rifampin turns urine, feces, sputum, tears, and sweat orange. Soft contacts may be permanently discolored.
- ☐ The most common adverse reactions to rifampin include epigastric pain, nausea, vomiting, flatulence, abdominal cramps, anorexia, and diarrhea.
- ☐ Isoniazid may precipitate seizures in clients with a seizure disorder and produce optic or peripheral neuritis, as well as elevated liver enzymes.
- ☐ Ethambutol can cause hepatitis and optic neuritis as well, and the potential is increased with other neurotoxic agents.

NEUROLOGIC MEDICATIONS

Antiseizure Medications, Antiepileptic Drugs (AEDs), or Anticonvulsants

- ☐ Assess clients for seizures during any change or start of medication therapy.

- ☐ Documentation of seizure activity includes onset, timing, characteristics, loss of consciousness, loss of bowel or bladder function, and postictal period.
- ☐ Anticonvulsants include six classes of drugs: hydantoin derivatives, barbiturates, benzodiazepines, succinimides, iminostilbene derivatives (carbamazepine), and carboxylic acid derivatives.
- ☐ Miscellaneous anticonvulsants include magnesium, gabapentin, lamotrigine, pregabalin, and topiramate.
- ☐ Assess for CNS depression and fall safety when giving seizure medications.
- ☐ Carbamazepine may cause bone marrow suppression and fluid retention.
- ☐ Other complications of carbamazepine include reduced oral contraceptive effectiveness and multiple other drug interactions, diplopia, dizziness, ataxia, and rash.
- ☐ Some barbiturates and succinimides limit seizure activity by increasing the threshold for motor cortex stimuli.
- ☐ Selected benzodiazepines and carboxylic acid derivatives may increase inhibition of γ-aminobutyric acid in brain neurons.

Phenytoin

- ☐ Alcohol decreases phenytoin activity, diminishing its effectiveness.
- ☐ Carbamazepine decreases blood levels of phenytoin and hormonal contraceptives.
- ☐ Nutritional supplements and milk interfere with the absorption of phenytoin, decreasing its effectiveness.
- ☐ Intravenous phenytoin is compatible only with saline solutions; dextrose causes an insoluble precipitate to form.
- ☐ Changing phenytoin brands may alter the therapeutic effect.
- ☐ When given through an IV catheter in the hand, phenytoin may cause purple glove syndrome.
- ☐ Abrupt phenytoin withdrawal may trigger status epilepticus; therefore, a client should be warned not to stop taking the drug unless the health care provider instructs them to do so.
- ☐ Rapid intravenous administration of phenytoin can depress the myocardium.
- ☐ Adverse effects of phenytoin include sedation, somnolence, gingival hyperplasia, blood dyscrasia, and toxicity.
- ☐ A phenytoin therapeutic level is 10 to 20 mcg/mL, and a level of greater than 30 mcg/mL indicates toxicity.
- ☐ Symptoms of phenytoin toxicity include confusion and ataxia.

Alzheimer Medications

☐ Alzheimer disease drugs are not recommended for clients with severe hepatic impairment or severe renal impairment (creatinine clearance less than 9 mL/min).

☐ Alzheimer disease drugs are used cautiously with medications that slow heart rate; there is an increased risk for heart block.

☐ Drugs used to treat Alzheimer disease may cause weight loss, diarrhea, anorexia, nausea, vomiting, dizziness, headache, bradyarrhythmias, and hypertension.

☐ Using Alzheimer disease drugs with nonsteroidal anti-inflammatory drugs (NSAIDs) increases gastric acid secretion and increases the risk of gastric bleeding and ulcers.

☐ Alzheimer disease drugs may exaggerate neuromuscular blocking effects of succinylcholine-type neuromuscular blocking agents used during anesthesia.

☐ Cholinesterase inhibitors (donepexil, galantamine, and rivastigmine) slow the breakdown of acetylcholine, and are used to improve cognition and functional autonomy in mild to moderate dementia of the Alzheimer type.

☐ Memantine also delays symptoms by blocking NMDA receptors and reduces brain levels of glutamate.

Antidepressant Medications

☐ Results of antidepressant therapy generally take 4 weeks. Encourage the client to stay on the medications even though results are not immediate.

☐ Many antidepressants can cause GI upset. Clients should be instructed to take with food.

☐ Safety is also a concern with antidepressants. Teach the client to report self-harm impulses, and do not stop abruptly.

☐ Monitor for orthostatic blood pressure changes. Teach client to rise slowly.

☐ Teach clients to report nervousness, insomnia, sexual dysfunction, and worsening depression.

☐ Bupropion should be used cautiously in clients with a history of seizure.

☐ Selective serotonin reuptake inhibitors (SSRIs) can cause insomnia, instruct to take in the morning. Also monitor for hyponatriema and signs of serotonin syndrome.

☐ Tricyclic antidepressants may cause anticholinergic effects. Teach client to increase exercise, fluids, and fiber. Also teach clients to take at night due to daytime drowsiness.

□ Tricyclic antidepressants are used to decrease the frequency of re-enactment of the trauma for the client with posttraumatic stress disorder and clients with memory and sleeping problems.

□ Other antidepressants are contraindicated within 2 weeks of monoamine oxidase inhibitor (MAOI) therapy.

□ Clients taking MAOIs should avoid foods containing tyramine such as cheese, chocolate, and pickled, aged, and smoked meats.

Antiparkinsonian Medications

□ Include synthetic anticholinergics, dopaminergics, and the antiviral amantadine.

□ Anticholinergics (benztropine) may be given alone or with other anti-Parkinson drugs like levodopa/carbidopa. Usually given for tremor.

□ Dopamine agonists (Ropinirole) directly stimulate dopamine receptors in the brain.

□ Dopamine replacement drugs (levodopa/carbidopa) crosses the blood-brain barrier and then is converted to dopamine.

□ Amantadine is an antiviral and antidyskinetic medication. It is thought to increase dopamine release in the substantia nigra and increases muscle control and decreases stiffness.

□ Long-term therapy with levodopa-carbidopa can result in drug tolerance requiring the client to take a "drug holiday."

□ Antiparkinsonian medications side effects include orthostatic hypotension and anticholinergic effects.

□ Teach clients to rise slowly, be aware of decreased mental alertness, and be careful when combining with other CNS depressants like alcohol.

Antipsychotic Drugs

□ Medications include clozapine, risperidone, and amisulpride.

□ Results of psychotropic drug therapy generally take 1 to 3 weeks. Encourage the client to stay on the medications even though results are not immediate.

□ Monitor for side effects including agranulocytosis, tardive dyskinesia, extrapyramidal symptoms, sedation, and constipation.

□ Client will need weekly CBC with absolute neutrophil count (ANC) weekly for the first 6 months.

□ Neuroleptic malignant syndrome is a life-threatening adverse effect characterized by muscle rigidity, confusion, and hyperthermia. Treated with dantrolene.

□ Haloperidol is used for agitation, aggression, hallucinations, thought disturbances, and wandering.

MUSCULOSKELETAL MEDICATIONS

Antirheumatic Drugs
- [ ] The most serious adverse reactions associated with the antirheumatic drugs (such as abatacept and adalimumab) include serious infections and malignancies.
- [ ] Before starting therapy test for tuberculosis infection.
- [ ] Teach client to avoid large crowds and avoid people given live vaccines (MMR, varicella, and rotavirus).
- [ ] Serious adverse reactions to gold therapy include anaphylactic shock, bradycardia, and angioedema.
- [ ] The most common adverse reactions to gold therapy include dermatitis, pruritus, and stomatitis.

Muscle Relaxants
- [ ] Skeletal muscle relaxants (baclofen and cyclobenzaprine) may reduce impulse transmission from the spinal cord to skeletal muscle.
- [ ] Baclofen is used to decrease spasms in a client recovering from a spinal cord injury over other muscle relaxants.
- [ ] Dantrolene acts directly on skeletal muscle to decrease excitation and reduce muscle strength by interfering with intracellular calcium movement.
- [ ] Teach clients to not drink alcohol with muscle relaxants and to be careful with driving or other activities while taking medication.

GASTROINTESTINAL/GENITOURINARY MEDICATIONS

Antacids
- [ ] Many drugs interact and decrease efficacy of medications if taken with or around the same time. Avoid other medications for 2 hours after taking antacids PO.
- [ ] Antacids may decrease digoxin, warfarin, phenytoin, tetracyclines, NSAIDs, and ciprofloxacin absorption.
- [ ] Teach client to chew antacid tablets thoroughly and drink a full glass of water.
- [ ] Monitor for constipation with aluminum and calcium antacids, and diarrhea with magnesium antacids.
- [ ] Teach signs and symptoms of GI bleed and occult bleeding.

Histamine-2 (H$_2$) Receptor Antagonists
- [ ] Medications include famotidine, ranitidine, cimetidine, and nizatidine.

- ☐ Inhibit gastric parietal cells from producing HCl, reducing gastric acid output and concentration, regardless of stimulants, such as histamine, food, insulin, and caffeine, or basal conditions.
- ☐ Teach signs and symptoms of GI bleed and occult bleeding.
- ☐ Though not as severe as other histamine blockers, these may cause CNS depression. Monitor for lethargy, depression, restlessness, and seizure.

Proton Pump Inhibitors (PPIs)

- ☐ Proton pump inhibitors reduce stomach acid production by combining with hydrogen, potassium, and adenosine triphosphate in parietal cells of the stomach to block the last step in gastric acid secretion.
- ☐ Medications include esomeprazole, pantoprazole, and omeprazole.
- ☐ Long-term use of PPIs could lead to bone loss. Teach client to use for a short duration or have regular bone mineral density testing.
- ☐ Take before first meal of the day with plenty of fluids.
- ☐ Teach clients to monitor for signs and symptoms of a GI bleed.

Thiazide Diuretics

- ☐ Medications include hydrochlorothiazide and chlorothiazide. Thiazide-like included in this class are metolazone and chlorthalidone.
- ☐ Thiazide and thiazide-like diuretics interfere with sodium transport across the tubules of the cortical diluting segment in the nephron, thereby increasing renal excretion of sodium, chloride, water, potassium, and calcium.
- ☐ Thiazide diuretics also exert an antihypertensive effect; although the exact mechanism is unknown, direct arteriolar dilation may be partially responsible.
- ☐ Cause excretion of electrolytes, especially potassium. Monitor for potassium loss.
- ☐ Teach the client to eat a diet high in potassium such as citrus fruit, potatoes, and bananas.
- ☐ May increase blood sugar especially in diabetics. Teach client to take blood sugar.
- ☐ Should not be used for clients with hyperparathyroidism because they decrease renal excretion of calcium, thereby raising serum calcium levels even higher.

Potassium-Sparing Diuretic

- ☐ Medications in this class include spironolactone, amiloride, and triamterene.
- ☐ Also used in clients with hyperaldosteronism.

☐ The client taking spironolactone should avoid potassium-rich foods and potassium supplements.

☐ Monitor signs of hyperkalemia including palpitations, nausea, fatigue and muscle weakness.

☐ The diuretics hydrochlorothiazide and spironolactone are often given together because hydrochlorothiazide is potassium depleting and spironolactone is potassium sparing.

Loop Diuretics

☐ Loop diuretics inhibit sodium and chloride reabsorption in the ascending loop of Henle, thus increasing excretion of sodium, chloride, and water.

☐ Medications for this class include furosemide, bumetanide, and torsemide.

☐ Commonly causes metabolic and electrolyte disturbances, particularly potassium depletion.

☐ May cause hyperglycemia, hyperuricemia, hypochloremic alkalosis, and hypomagnesemia.

☐ Rapid parenteral administration of a loop diuretic may cause hearing loss (including deafness) and tinnitus.

☐ High doses of a loop diuretic can produce profound diuresis, leading to hypovolemia and cardiovascular collapse.

☐ Photosensitivity may occur with high doses of a loop diuretic.

☐ Spironolactone is often given with a potassium-depleting diuretic to offset side effects.

☐ Other adverse reactions to loop diuretics include increased blood sugar, increased uric acid levels, ototoxicity, and hypotension.

☐ Encourage a diet high in potassium including salt substitutes which are generally high in potassium.

ENDOCRINE MEDICATIONS

Insulin

☐ Insulin is clear. Adding impurities and making it "cloudy" are ways to delay absorption and prolong action. (See Table 5.5 for the types of insulin.)

☐ Insulin glargine cannot be mixed in the same syringe with other insulins.

☐ Routine blood glucose is tested before the insulin is injected.

☐ Make certain the client's food is available prior to administering rapid-acting insulin.

☐ Clients should eat as the insulin is starting to work (onset of action).

TABLE 5.5	Types of Insulin		
Insulin Type	Onset	Peak	Duration
Rapid-acting insulin (lispro, aspart, glulisine)	15 min	Up to 90 min	3–5 h
Short-acting insulin (Humulin R, Novolin R)	30 min	2–4 h	Up to 8 h
Intermediate-acting insulin (Humulin N)	Up to 2 h	4–12 h	Up to 24 h
Long-acting insulin (glargine, detemir)	1–2 h	Even control of blood sugars	Up to 24 h

☐ The peak of action is the most likely time for a hypoglycemic reaction.

☐ Duration of action tells you when the next dose will be due.

☐ When combining insulins in a syringe, the clear insulin is put into the syringe before the cloudy to avoid contaminating the clear vial of insulin with the cloudy longer-acting insulin.

☐ Insulin is stable at room temperature for up to 18 months but degrades when exposed to heat.

☐ Rotation of injection sites is necessary to prevent lipodystrophy (atrophy and hypertrophy).

☐ Lipodystrophy causes uneven absorption of insulin and fluctuations in blood glucose.

Oral Antidiabetic Agents

☐ Used for type 2 diabetes mellitus.

☐ Normal doses of glyburide normalize the glucose level, but higher doses can produce hypoglycemia.

☐ Meglitinides are nonsulfonylurea antidiabetic agents that stimulate the release of insulin from the pancreas.

☐ Sitagliptin increases insulin release by inhibiting the enzyme dipeptidyl peptidase-4.

☐ Metformin decreases hepatic glucose production, reduces intestinal glucose absorption, and improves insulin sensitivity by increasing peripheral glucose uptake and utilization.

☐ With metformin therapy, insulin secretion remains unchanged, and fasting insulin levels and all-day insulin response may decrease.

☐ The most serious adverse reaction linked to metformin is lactic acidosis; although rare, it's most likely to occur in clients with renal dysfunction.

☐ Other reactions to metformin include dermatitis, GI upset, megaloblastic anemia, rash, and unpleasant or metallic taste.

- Alpha-glucosidase inhibitors, such as acarbose and miglitol, delay digestion of carbohydrates, preventing a spike in glucose levels.
- Pramlintide, a human amylin analogue, slows the rate at which food leaves the stomach, decreasing postprandial increases in glucose level, and reduces appetite.
- Rosiglitazone and pioglitazone are thiazolidinediones, which lower glucose levels by improving insulin sensitivity.
- Thiazolidinediones are potent and highly selective agonists for receptors found in insulin-sensitive tissues, such as adipose tissue, skeletal muscle, and liver.
- Thiazolidinediones may cause fluid retention leading to or exacerbating heart failure.
- Sulfonylureas cause dose-related reactions that usually respond to decreased dosage: anorexia, headache, heartburn, nausea, paresthesia, vomiting, and weakness.
- Alpha-glucosidase inhibitors can cause abdominal pain, diarrhea, and flatulence.

Corticosteroids

- Suppress cell-mediated and humoral immunity.
- Reduce inflammation by preventing hydrolytic enzyme release into the cells, preventing plasma exudation, suppressing polymorphonuclear leukocyte migration, and disrupting other inflammatory processes.
- Steroid use tends to increase blood glucose levels, particularly in clients with diabetes and prediabetes.
- Steroids (like opioids, BB, alcohol, and SSRIs) cause increased waking after sleep onset and can cause mood swings.
- Steroids cause adrenal insufficiency and must be weaned slowly to prevent adrenal crisis.
- Teach clients to take steroids with food to reduce gastric irritation.

ANTIBIOTICS AND ANTIFUNGALS

Overview

- Teach clients to take full prescription even if the client is feeling better.
- Cultures are collected prior to starting antibiotic therapy.
- Empiric therapy: starting antibiotic therapy with a broad-spectrum antibiotic prior to the identification of the organism.
- If a client is colonized, they are not showing systemic signs of infection and antibiotic therapy might not be started.

- ☐ Peak blood levels are usually drawn 30 minutes after administration of the medication.
- ☐ Trough levels are drawn right before the drug is administered.

Aminoglycosides

- ☐ Medications in this class include amikacin, gentamicin, and tobramycin.
- ☐ Ototoxicity (assess for ringing in the ears) and nephrotoxicity (assess BUN and creatinine) are the most serious complications of aminoglycosides.
- ☐ Oral forms of aminoglycosides most commonly cause diarrhea, nausea, and vomiting.
- ☐ Parenteral forms of aminoglycosides may cause vein irritation, phlebitis, and sterile abscess.
- ☐ Aminoglycosides are used cautiously in neuromuscular disorders, renal impairment, pregnancy, breast-feeding, elderly, and infants.
- ☐ Monitor renal function, hearing, appetite, mucus membranes, CBC, and electrolytes.

Cephalosporins

- ☐ First-generation cephalosporins (including cefazolin, cephalexin, and cefadroxil) do not reach therapeutic levels in the central nervous system, but second- and third-generation drugs do.
- ☐ First-generation cephalosporins act against many gram-positive cocci, including penicillinase-producing *Staphylococcus aureus* and *S. epidermidis*, *Streptococcus pneumoniae*, group B streptococci, and group A beta-hemolytic streptococci.
- ☐ Second-generation cephalosporins (including cefotetan, loracarbef, cefprozil, and cefaclor) are effective against all organisms attacked by first-generation drugs and have additional activity against *Moraxella catarrhalis*, *Haemophilus influenzae*, *Enterobacter*, *Citrobacter*, *Providencia*, *Acinetobacter*, *Serratia*, and *Neisseria*.
- ☐ Third-generation cephalosporins (ceftriaxone, cefdinir, cefixime, and cefditoren) are primarily used against gram-negative organisms.
- ☐ Clients who have an allergy to penicillins may have cross sensitivity with cephalosporins due to similar chemical structures.
- ☐ Monitor client for bleeding, colitis, and liver and kidney impairment.
- ☐ Teach clients that cephalosporins can cause birth defects and can cause birth control pills to be less effective.

Metronidazole and Antifungals

- ☐ Metronidazole is given for bacterial and parasitic infections such as amoebas and protozoa.

- When mixed with alcohol, metronidazole causes a disulfiram-like reaction involving nausea, vomiting, and other unpleasant symptoms.
- Teach client to avoid alcohol because antifungal medications may cause hepatotoxicity.
- Many antifungals make the client photosensitive.
- Antifungal side effects such as diarrhea, vomiting, and stomach pain, are rare and usually occur at large doses.

Tetracycline

- Treats various unusual organisms and diarrhea, nausea, and vomiting are common.
- Permanent discoloration of teeth occurs if tetracycline is given during tooth formation in children younger than age 8.
- Teach client to take on an empty stomach and avoid dairy and iron products for 2 hours before and after taking.
- Teach clients that tetracyclines cause photosensitivity.
- Monitor for severe diarrhea and renal and liver impairment.

Chemotherapy

- Often ordered based on body surface area, based on client's height and weight.
- Two RNs must check the medication order for chemotherapy is administered.
- Premedication therapy is used to prevent nausea, vomiting, and allergic reactions.
- Antiemetics may cause fatigue, dizziness, headache, insomnia, and various other side effects.
- Routes oral, intramuscular, intravenous, intra-arterial, intraperitoneal, intrathecal, and implantable devices.
- Continuous chemotherapy infusions must be administered via an infusion pump.
- Vesicant chemotherapy means tissue necrosis can result if the medication extravasates into the tissue.
- If chemotherapy drug extravasates into the tissues, tissue necrosis may result. Antidotes may be necessary for different drugs.
- Assessment for extravasation includes pain or burning, edema, loss of blood return, redness, and decreased intravenous flow.
- Common chemotherapeutic drugs that are vesicants include doxorubicin (Adriamycin, Caelyx-Canada), mechlorethamine (nitrogen mustard), cisplatin, and vincristine.
- Blood return must be checked prior to any administration of intravenous chemotherapy: "No Blood no drug."

☐ Toxic effects of chemotherapy are assessed based on timing: acute (immediately after treatment), chronic (prolonged side effects that may be permanent), and latent (occurs months to years after therapy).

☐ Bone marrow suppression resulting in lowered blood counts is a dose-limiting factor with chemotherapy treatment.

☐ Prior to administration of chemotherapy, hematologic parameters are assessed. Absolute neutrophil count (ANC) should be over 1,000 and platelets higher than 100×10^3, and institutional parameters and protocols need to be followed.

☐ ANC of less than 500 indicates a severe risk of infection in clients receiving chemotherapy.

☐ ANC of 500 to 1,000 is a mild or moderate risk, and ANC greater than 1,000 no risk.

☐ Colony-stimulating factors (filgrastim and erythropoietin) must be stopped 24 hours prior to chemotherapy and given no sooner than 24 hours after chemotherapy.

☐ Filgrastim is a granulocyte colony-stimulating factor and commonly causes bone pain.

☐ Neutropenic precautions in chemotherapy includes private room, no fresh fruit or vegetables, no live plants or flowers, client wears a mask when they leave the room.

☐ The risk of bleeding from thrombocytopenia is substantial under 20,000—clients should be assessed head to toe for bleeding.

☐ Fatigue in chemotherapy is not relieved by sleep, as it is generally caused by anemia.

☐ Nausea and vomiting can be acute (less than 24 hours post chemo), delayed (greater than 24 hours post chemo), and anticipatory (before the administration of chemo).

☐ Not all chemotherapy agents has the same "emetic" potential or potential to cause vomiting. Cisplatin and mechlorethamine have high emetogenic potential.

☐ Clients who have nausea and vomiting are sensitive to smells; cold foods smell less; avoid fatty, greasy, spicy, and sweet foods.

☐ Alopecia is distressing for clients. Reassure them that hair regrowth starts 4 to 6 weeks after therapy.

☐ Clients need to remain well hydrated and urinate frequently to prevent the metabolites of drug therapy to sit in the bladder and cause damage.

☐ Hemorrhagic cystitis commonly occurs with ifosfamide and is treated by administering mesna to protect the bladder.

PHARMACOLOGIC PAIN MANAGEMENT

Overview

- [ ] Adjuvant medications are medications given for pain control that are not technically pain medications or weren't originally developed for pain control.

- [ ] Adjuvant pain medications include anticonvulsants, antidepressants, corticosteroids, muscle relaxants, alpha 2 adrenergic agonists.

- [ ] Breakthrough pain refers to pain that "breaks through" before the next dose of medication is due. It is treated with quick-acting medication.

- [ ] See Table 5.6 for the WHO's 3-step "ladder" of pain treatment.

Opioid Agonists

- [ ] Work by blocking the release of neurotransmitters that are involved in transmitting pain signals to the brain.

- [ ] Medications include codeine, morphine, fentanyl, hydrocodone, and oxycodone.

- [ ] Level of consciousness and vital signs are assessed with all narcotic pain medications.

- [ ] Clients on intravenous pain medications should be kept on bed rest due to safety risks.

TABLE 5.6 WHO's 3-Step Ladder of Pain Treatment	
Pain Level	Treatment
Mild	Aspirin Acetaminophen NSAIDs ■ If indicated add an adjunct such as an anti-depressant or anticonvulsant.
Moderate	Codeine Hydrocodone Oxycodone Tramadol ■ Add or continue adjuncts, if appropriate. Opioids can be combined with a non-opioid like acetaminophen.
Severe	Morphine Hydromorphone Methadone Fentanyl Oxycodone ■ Switch to an opioid that is not combined with acetaminophen. Add or continue adjuncts, if appropriate.

- ☐ Clients receiving epidural analgesia are generally paralyzed below the epidural.
- ☐ PCA means patient-controlled analgesia. Clients need to be taught how to utilize the pump, amount of medication they can receive, and to never turn off the alarm!
- ☐ Codeine may delay gastric emptying and interfere with hepatobiliary imaging studies.
- ☐ Fentanyl is used cautiously in elderly or debilitated clients and in those with head injuries, increased cerebrospinal fluid pressure, respiratory disease, cardiac disease, and hepatic disease.
- ☐ Opioid agonists are used to relieve or decrease pain without causing the client to lose consciousness.
- ☐ Opioid agonists can cause constipation and respiratory depression because of their binding to receptor sites in the peripheral and central nervous system.
- ☐ Opioid agonists are classified as pregnancy category C, and most appear in breast milk; recommend that the client wait 4 to 6 hours after ingesting before breast-feeding.
- ☐ A common adverse reaction to opioid agonists is a decreased rate and depth of respirations that worsens as the dose is increased.
- ☐ Mixed opioid agonist-antagonists are administered to relieve pain while reducing the toxic effects and dependency associated with opioid agonists.
- ☐ Some commonly used mixed opioid agonist-antagonists are butorphanol, nalbuphine, and pentazocine, which do not give euphoric effects as other narcotics.
- ☐ The client with a history of opioid abuse should not receive any mixed opioid agonist-antagonists because they can cause withdrawal symptoms.
- ☐ Barbiturates are general central nervous system depressants and used as sedatives, hypnotics, anesthetics, and antiepileptics.
- ☐ See Table 5.7 for more information on controlled substance schedule.

Opioid Antagonists

- ☐ Opioid antagonists block the effects of opioids and are given for overdose.
- ☐ Common opioid antagonists are naltrexone and naloxone.
- ☐ Naloxone is the drug of choice for managing an opioid overdose by reversing respiratory depression and sedation and helps stabilize the client's vital signs within seconds after administration.
- ☐ Naloxone dosing may need to be repeated as the peak is shorter than most narcotics.

| TABLE 5.7 | Controlled Substance Schedule | |
Schedule	Description	Examples
I	■ High abuse potential ■ No accepted medical use	■ Heroin ■ Marijuana ■ LSD
II	■ High abuse potential ■ Severe dependence liability	■ Opioids ■ Amphetamines ■ Some barbiturates
III	■ Less abuse potential than schedule II drugs ■ Moderate dependence liability	■ Nonbarbiturate sedatives ■ Nonamphetamine stimulants ■ Anabolic steroids ■ Limited amounts of certain opioids
IV	■ Less abuse potential than schedule III drugs ■ Limited dependence liability	■ Some sedatives ■ Anxiolytics ■ Nonopioid analgesics
V	■ Limited abuse potential	■ Mainly small amounts of opioids, such as codeine, used as antitussives or antidiarrheal

☐ The adverse effects of opioid agonists may trigger narcotic withdrawal until med wears off. May also trigger an asthma attack in a susceptible client.

☐ An unconscious client abruptly returned to consciousness after naloxone administration may hyperventilate and experience tremors.

Nonopioid Medications and Nonsteroidal Anti-inflammatory Drugs (NSAIDs)

☐ Nonopioids are the first choice for managing mild pain because they decrease pain by inhibiting inflammation at the injury site.

☐ Examples of nonopioids are acetaminophen, NSAIDs such as ibuprofen, salicylates, cox-2 inhibitors (celecoxib), salicylic acid derivatives (diflunisal), and naproxen.

☐ NSAIDs have an analgesic ceiling or point where increased dose has no more effect.

☐ Common side effects of NSAIDs are gastric irritability and renal insufficiency; clients need to maintain adequate hydration.

☐ Acetaminophen adverse effects include liver toxicity and should not exceed 3 g/day (4 g under supervision).

☐ Hypersensitivity to aspirin is a contraindication for the use of NSAIDs as reactions may occur.

☐ NSAIDs can cause a prolonged bleeding time.

☐ Monitor clients for hepatic and renal problems. Monitor for signs and symptoms of hemorrhage, such as petechiae, bruising, coffee-ground emesis, and black, tarry stools.

☐ Acetylcysteine is used to treat acetaminophen toxicity but should never be given with activated charcoal.

☐ Salicylates are contraindicated in clients with glucose-6-phosphate dehydrogenase deficiency or bleeding disorders, such as hemophilia, von Willebrand disease, or telangiectasia.

☐ Use cautiously in clients with GI lesions and peptic ulcer disease due to increased risk of bleeding.

☐ In a client taking salicylates, periodically monitor the complete blood count, platelet count, prothrombin time, blood urea nitrogen level, serum creatinine level, and the results of liver function studies.

☐ Use acetaminophen cautiously in clients with chronic or heavy alcohol use because hepatotoxicity has occurred.

☐ Teach clients to read labels to avoid the use of multiple acetaminophen-containing drugs.

☐ Monitor the prothrombin time and international normalized ratio values in clients who are receiving oral anticoagulants and long-term acetaminophen therapy.

☐ Aspirin is contraindicated in children or young adults with viral illnesses due to the danger of Reye syndrome.

REVIEW QUESTIONS ▮▮▮▮▮▮▮

1. When infusing total parenteral nutrition (TPN), the nurse should assess the client for which complication?
   1. Essential amino acid deficiency
   2. Essential fatty acid deficiency
   3. Hyperglycemia
   4. Infection

2. Which of the following findings would **most** concern the nurse with a client initially receiving an intravenous infusion of lidocaine hydrochloride?
   1. Palpitations
   2. Tinnitus
   3. Urinary frequency
   4. Lethargy

3. A nurse is teaching a client, newly diagnosed with chronic obstructive pulmonary disease (COPD), about the use of a respiratory inhaler. Which statement demonstrates understanding of the medications?

1. "Prednisone is always used first in an acute exacerbation."
2. "Press the canister down with your finger as you breathe in and then quickly exhale the drug."
3. "Albuterol followed by beclomethasone is the correct administration."
4. "Wait 2 to 3 minutes between puffs if more than one puff has been prescribed."

4. When preparing the teaching plan for a client who is to start clozapine, which of the following is crucial to include?

1. Description of akathisia and drug-induced parkinsonism
2. Measures to relieve episodes of diarrhea
3. The importance of reporting insomnia
4. An emphasis on the need for weekly blood tests

5. The nurse knows which factor **best** indicates that a client is complying with digoxin therapy?

1. Client reports counting the radial pulse for 1 minute before taking.
2. Weight measurement reflects a gain of 2.2 pounds (1 kg) in less than a week.
3. Vital signs reflect an apical heart rate of 101 bpm.
4. Client reports an absence of chest pain during moderate activity.

Chapter References

Acosta, W. A. (2012). *Pharmacology for health professionals* (2nd ed.). Philadelphia, PA: Lippincott Williams & Wilkins.

Golan, D. E., Tashjian, A. H. Jr, Armstrong, E. J., & Armstrong, A. W. (2011). *Principles of pharmacology: The pathophysiologic basis of drug therapy* (3rd ed.). Philadelphia, PA: Lippincott Williams & Wilkins.

Karch, A. (2012). *Focus on pharmacology* (6th ed.). Philadelphia, PA: Lippincott Williams & Wilkins.

Karch, A. (2015). *Lippincott nursing drug guide*. Philadelphia, PA: Wolters Kluwer.

Nursing2016 drug guide (2016) (36th ed.). Philadelphia, PA: Wolters Kluwer.

6

Management of Care

ADVANCE DIRECTIVES

KEY TERMS
- A **living will** is a legal document that authorizes the attending practitioner to withhold or discontinue certain lifesaving procedures under specific circumstances.
- An **advanced directive** is a written directive that allows people to state in advance what their choices for health care would be if certain circumstances should develop.

Living Will
- A legal document that authorizes the attending practitioner to withhold or discontinue certain lifesaving procedures under specific circumstances.
- May also address treatment options, such as enteral feedings, blood transfusion, antibiotic administration, and dialysis.

Durable Power of Attorney
- A durable power of attorney for health care document differs from the usual power of attorney, which requires the client's ongoing consent and deals only with financial issues.
- Most states and provinces have laws authorizing durable power of attorney for the purpose of initiating or terminating life-sustaining medical treatment.

CLIENT ADVOCACY

KEY TERMS
- **Advocacy** is the protection and support of another's rights.

Advocacy
- Advocacy is the protection and support of another's rights.
- Clients with special advocacy needs include those who are uninformed about their rights and opportunities, those with sensory impairment, those who do not speak English well or at all, the very young and the elderly, those who are seriously ill, those who are

mentally or emotionally impaired, those with physical disabilities, and those who lack adequate financial or human resources.

☐ Incorporating services such as an interpreter or social worker in the plan of care (POC) are examples of advocacy.

☐ To be an effective advocate, a nurse must understand the ethical and legal principles of informed consent and that the client's consent isn't valid unless the client understands their condition, the proposed treatment, treatment alternatives, potential risks and benefits, and relative chances of success or failure.

Standards of Care

☐ Standards of care are the basis for providing safe, competent nursing care and set minimum criteria for proficiency on the job, enabling the nurse and others to judge the quality of care provided.

☐ The nurse has a responsibility to assess, monitor, and communicate the status of a client under the nurse's care.

☐ Failure to act as a client advocate has been recognized by the courts when the nurse fails to develop and implement nursing diagnoses and fails to exercise good judgment on the client's behalf.

☐ Failure to communicate with the client refers to not adequately educating the client about care, procedures, or discharge instructions.

☐ Failure to protect from harm occurs when health care providers must protect a client because of the client's vulnerable state and inability to distinguish potentially harmful situations.

☐ Assessment of the client's strengths and weaknesses in coping mechanisms and the presence of support systems is needed to formulate an appropriate POC.

Ethical Decisions

☐ When a client must make an ethical decision, the nurse should help the client resolve the moral dilemma in ways that enhance personal values, priorities, freedom, dignity, and the quality of life.

☐ By listening carefully to the client and asking thoughtful questions, the nurse may be able to help the client and family make ethical decisions with which they are most comfortable. The nurse needs to understand what the practitioner told the client about the situation.

☐ The most difficult ethical decisions in health care involve whether to initiate or withhold life-sustaining treatment for clients who are irreversibly comatose, vegetative, or suffering with end-stage terminal illness.

Life-Sustaining Treatment

☐ The nurse may feel caught in the middle frustrated and demoralized by the demands of caring for an unresponsive client who had expressly wished to withhold life-sustaining treatment.

□ The nurse cannot make the ultimate medical decisions to initiate or limit treatment, but the nurse can help the client express wishes about their health care and guide them in translating these desires into advance directives.

□ The nurse needs to pay attention to the client's questions and misunderstandings and be especially alert for unexpressed fears.

□ Despite the nurse's best efforts to provide objective advice, the client may not be able to reach a decision about initiating or terminating care.

□ The substituted judgment test professes to make the same decision the client would, if the client were capable (the principle of autonomy).

□ The decision may be based on the best interest standard, or deciding what is best for the client, given the client's current circumstances (the principle of beneficence).

□ Effective communication is essential when helping families decide whether to limit or withhold treatment.

□ Create a quiet, private, and unhurried environment and keep all communication to the family simple, factual, and direct.

□ Encourage decision makers in the family to ask questions.

□ Clarify missing or misunderstood information for the client and family.

ASSIGNMENT, DELEGATION, AND SUPERVISION

Nurse-Manager

□ The nurse-manager must assign responsibility, identify the task to be accomplished, explain what outcomes are needed, and determine the time frame for completing the work.

□ The nurse-manager's responsibilities typically include policy and decision making, prodding adequate staffing for safe and effective client care, and evaluating client care.

□ In a crisis situation, the nurse-manager should take command for the benefit of the client.

□ The nurse-manager is responsible for providing client-teaching activities and coordinating nursing services with other client care services.

□ As part of the health care team, the nurse-manager supervises and guides staff members, evaluates staff performance, and participates in staff recruitment and retention.

□ The nurse-manager needs to provide new staff members with an adequate, individualized orientation and also needs to ensure that staff members participate in continuing education.

□ Making sure that staff education is appropriate for each member's assigned responsibilities, planning and implementing budgets are part of the nurse-manager's responsibilities.

- The nurse-manager encourages staff participation in policy and procedure development and quality monitoring.
- Each manager directs staff using a different management style; an effective manager commonly uses more than one style.
- At times, staff should participate in decision making; at other times, staff participation isn't appropriate.
- If a serious problem occurs on the unit, the nurse-manager should be notified as soon as possible.
- If the nurse-manager of a unit isn't on duty when a staff nurse makes a serious medication error, the nursing supervisor on duty will call the nurse-manager at home with details of the problem.
- Scheduling may be safely and appropriately delegated by the nurse-manager to a staff member.
- Termination, disciplinary action, and salary increases shouldn't be delegated to staff that don't have the power and authority to take such actions.
- Planning vacation time and evaluating procedures and client resources require staff input characteristic of a democratic or participative manager.

Delegation

- The state Nursing Practice Act must permit delegation and outline the authorized task(s) to be delegated or authorize the RN to decide delegation.
- The person making the delegation has the appropriate qualifications: appropriate education, skills and experience, as well as current competency.
- The person receiving the delegation must have the appropriate qualifications: appropriate education, training, skills and experience, as well as evidence of current competency.
- Teaching and assessment cannot be delegated by the RN unless to another RN.

Safety

- Being aware of factors that affect delegation, such as developmental level, lifestyle, mobility, sensory perception, knowledge level, communication ability, physical health state, and psychosocial state allows nurses to identify potential hazards and promote wellness.
- Notify your immediate supervisor if you believe an assignment is unsafe.
- Inspect all equipment and machinery regularly, and make sure that subordinates use them competently and safely.

☐ If someone under your supervision isn't familiar with a piece of equipment, teach how to properly operate it before the subordinate uses it for the first time.

☐ Report incompetent health care personnel to superiors through the institutional chain of command.

☐ Don't prescribe or dispense medication without authorization.

Nurse Roles

☐ The primary role of the nurse as caregiver is given shape and substance by the interrelated roles of communicator.

☐ These roles include teacher, counselor, leader, researcher, advocate, and collaborator.

Nursing Care Delivery Systems

☐ Nursing care delivery systems dictate how nursing care is delivered on a nursing unit.

☐ Each delivery system has a unique design that must outline who has the responsibility for making client care decisions, the duration for which client care decisions remain in effect, work distribution among staff, and procedures for communicating client care.

☐ The nurse-manager should understand the individual delivery systems and choose one that's best for the unit or facility; after a delivery system is chosen, the nurse-manager should evaluate the system regularly to make sure the system meets the needs of the clients.

☐ The selection of a nursing care delivery system is critical to the success of a nursing area.

☐ The factor that is essential to the evaluation of a nursing care delivery system is identifying who will be responsible for making client care decisions.

☐ Although dress code, salary, and scheduling planned staff absences are important to any organization, they aren't actually determined by the nursing care delivery system.

The Nursing Process

☐ The nursing process is a continuous, interdependent, systematic organization of cognitive behaviors designed to resolve problems and promote well-being.

☐ The essential steps of the nursing process include assessment, planning, implementation, and evaluation.

☐ Assessment begins with the nurse's initial contact with the client and involves collecting systematic data, identifying the client's needs, and determining the nursing diagnosis.

☐ Implementation involves coordination, performing, or delegating activities specified in the nursing care plan and recording results.

- ☐ Evaluation includes collecting data, measuring outcomes against outcome criteria, and altering the nursing care plan by continuation of the nursing process.
- ☐ Pertinent data are collected using appropriate evidence-based assessment techniques and instruments; analytical models and problem-solving tools are used.
- ☐ RNs are responsible for all phases of the nursing process, including assessing a client's pain and evaluating a client's response to treatment.
- ☐ The RN should assess the client's need for nursing care in all settings in which nursing care is to be provided.
- ☐ The care, treatment, and rehabilitation planning process should ensure that care is appropriate to the client.

CASE MANAGEMENT

Case Management

- ☐ Case management is the process by which a designated health care professional, usually a nurse, manages all health-related matters of a client.
- ☐ The case management model promotes communication, teamwork, and collaboration among caregivers, improves efficiency, and increases better client outcomes by focusing care on mutually developed outcomes.
- ☐ Case managers develop a plan to use health care resources efficiently and achieve the optimum client outcome in the most cost-effective manner.
- ☐ The case manager explores resources available to assist the client in achieving or maintaining a level of independence.
- ☐ The client in the case management system is provided with information on discharge procedures, depending on the location of discharge (home, hospice, or community setting), and plans are made accordingly.
- ☐ The case manager initiates, evaluates, and updates the POC.

Disaster Coordination

- ☐ As the nurse works with the community in the post disaster cycle, a variety of prevention measures may be employed for the community.
- ☐ Primary prevention focuses on keeping the crisis or disaster from happening within the community.
- ☐ The goal of secondary prevention is to reduce the duration and intensity of the disaster or crisis.
- ☐ Tertiary prevention involves reducing the degree and quantity of injury, disability, and damage after a disaster or crisis.

☐ Providing counseling and support for families who have lost their homes is an example of the level of prevention called tertiary prevention.

Health Care Delivery Systems

☐ Health care delivery systems provide payment for health care.

☐ There are three basic types of health care systems: health maintenance organization (HMO), preferred provider organization (PPO), and managed care organizations.

☐ HMOs provide comprehensive health services for a designated payment; fixed payment is given to the health care provider periodically to cover the costs of health care for each individual enrolled in the HMO.

☐ PPOs negotiate special, reduced rates to attract insurance plan beneficiaries; members' care is paid for if they use a health care provider who's under contract to the PPO.

☐ In Canada Health Act, the federal government ensures that the provinces and territories meet certain requirements, such as free and universal access to publicly insured health care.

Clinical Pathways

☐ Clinical pathways provide sequences of multidisciplinary interventions that incorporate teaching, consultation, discharge planning, medications, nutrition, diagnostic testing, activities, treatments, and therapeutic modalities.

☐ The goal of a clinical pathway is to achieve realistic expected outcomes for the client and family members.

☐ Clinical pathways promote a professional and collaborative goal for care and practice and assure continuity of care.

☐ Clinical pathways should also guarantee appropriate use of resources, which reduces costs and hospital lengths of stay while also providing the framework for quality management.

☐ Clinical pathways are clinical tool used by case managers to achieve better quality and cost outcomes by outlining and sequencing the usual and desired care for particular groups of clients.

☐ Clinical pathways incorporate care requirements from preadmission through postdischarge.

Nursing Management

☐ In nursing, management involves coordinating staff to accomplish the facility's objectives in the most efficient, most cost-effective manner.

☐ The nurse-manager is responsible for the effectiveness of discharge planning and client teaching.

☐ The nurse-manager must collaborate with all members of the interdisciplinary health care team so that all clients attain their maximum state of wellness.

Plan of Care

- ☐ The POC can be affected by the specific client diagnosis, prescribed treatments, and self-care ability of the client.

- ☐ Care maps may be used in planning for the client, or other plans of care such as a clinical pathway, to guide and evaluate client care.

- ☐ Evidence-based practice (EBP) and research are utilized when the case manager is providing care.

- ☐ Data collection is systematic and ongoing, involving the client, partners, and health care providers when appropriate.

- ☐ Nursing diagnoses are derived from the assessment data; diagnoses are validated with the client, partners, and health care providers when possible.

- ☐ Diagnoses are documented in a manner that facilitates the determination of expected outcomes and POC.

Client Outcomes

- ☐ Outcomes are culturally appropriate and are derived from the nursing diagnoses when formulating a care plan.

- ☐ Outcomes for the client are formulated taking into account any associated risks, benefits, costs, current scientific evidence, and clinical expertise.

- ☐ Outcomes include a time estimate for attainment.

- ☐ Outcomes provide direction for continuity of care and are modified based on the client's status.

- ☐ Outcomes are documented as measurable goals.

CLIENT RIGHTS

Right to Die

- ☐ The right to die involves whether to initiate or withhold life-sustaining treatment for a client who is irreversibly comatose, vegetative, or suffering with end-stage terminal illness.

Organ and Tissue Donation

- ☐ The federal Omnibus Reconciliation Act of 1986 mandates that all hospitals establish written protocols for the identification of potential organ and tissue donors.

- ☐ An organ procurement coordinator is knowledgeable about the organ donation process and should have exceptional interpersonal skills for dealing with grieving family members.

Right to Refuse Treatment

- ☐ A psychiatric inpatient usually receives a copy of the bill of rights for psychiatric clients, which includes the right to refuse treatment, the right to a written treatment plan, the right to confidentiality, and the right to personal mail.

☐ Any mentally competent adult may legally refuse treatment if the client is fully informed about their medical condition and about the likely consequences of refusal.

☐ Some clients may refuse treatment on the grounds of freedom of religion or cultural beliefs.

☐ The client's right to refuse treatment may be challenged if compelling reasons exist to overrule the client's wishes, such as when the refusal endangers the life of another, when a parent's decision to withhold treatment threatens a child's life, when a client makes statements indicating that the client wants to live, and when public interest outweighs the client's right.

☐ If the client is a critically ill minor, the court may deny the parents' request to refuse treatment.

☐ The courts also recognize several compelling circumstances that justify overruling a client's refusal of treatment. These include when refusal endangers the life of another, when a parent's decision to withhold treatment threatens a child's life, when despite refusing treatment the client makes statements indicating that the client wants to live, and when the public interest outweighs the client's right.

☐ If the client is going to refuse treatment or the client simply refuses to give consent, you should stop preparations for treatment at once, notify the practitioner immediately, and report your client's decision to your supervisor promptly.

Religious Freedom

☐ Jehovah's Witnesses oppose blood transfusions based on their interpretation of a biblical passage that forbids "drinking" blood.

☐ Some Jehovah's Witnesses believe that even a lifesaving transfusion given against their will deprives them of everlasting life.

☐ Most religious freedom court cases involve Christian Scientists, who oppose many medical interventions, including medicines.

☐ The right-to-die laws recognize the client's right to choose death by refusing extraordinary treatment when the client has no hope of recovery.

Refusing Pain Medication

☐ The most appropriate action when the client refuses injections for pain is to call the practitioner to request an oral pain medication; by doing so, the nurse is adhering to the client's wishes.

☐ Administering an injection without client consent is considered battery and may lead to a lawsuit.

☐ When the client refuses injections for pain, withholding the medication without providing an alternative would violate the standards of care.

☐ Any attempt to manipulate the client into taking the medication also would violate the standards of care.

Teenage Client

☐ A teenage client should be kept informed about medical decisions, but until the teen is an adult or emancipated, a parent must give consent for the child's care.

☐ A pregnant teen is medically emancipated.

Client Right to View the Chart

☐ The client has a legal right to see their chart. The nurse should first ask the client if he or she has any questions about their care and try to clear up any confusion.

☐ The nurse should check the facility's policy to see whether the chart must be read in the nurse's presence when the client wishes to view it.

☐ The nurse should inform the practitioner and nurse-manager of the client's request to see the chart.

Discharge Against Medical Advice

☐ If a client requests a discharge against medical advice, the nurse should notify the practitioner immediately.

☐ If the practitioner can't convince the client to stay, the practitioner will ask the client to sign an against medical advice form, which releases the facility from legal responsibility for any medical problems the client may experience after discharge.

☐ If the practitioner isn't available, the nurse should discuss signing against medical advice form with the client and obtain the client's signature.

☐ A client who refuses to sign against medical advice form shouldn't be detained because this would violate the client's rights.

☐ After the client leaves, the nurse should document the incident thoroughly and notify the practitioner that the client has left.

Means of Medical Treatment

☐ Ordinary means of medical treatment are medications, procedures, and surgeries that offer the client some hope of benefit without incurring excessive pain or expense.

☐ Extraordinary means, sometimes called heroic measures, merely maintain or prolong a client's life, usually at great expense and suffering for the client and family.

☐ Because of continuing advances in medicine and technology, the distinction between ordinary and extraordinary treatments is becoming less defined.

Terminating Life-Sustaining Treatment
- ☐ When deciding whether to terminate life-sustaining treatment, health care providers face incredible emotional pressure; a client can't be brought back after treatment stops.
- ☐ Because the nursing profession is oriented to saving and prolonging lives, the nurse may find it difficult to go along with a client's decision to withhold life-sustaining treatment.
- ☐ A client who has chosen to forgo life-sustaining treatment still has the right to receive care that preserves comfort, hygiene, and dignity; in particular, the client has the right to adequate pain control.

Autonomy
- ☐ The right to refuse treatment is based on the ethical principle of respect for the autonomy of the individual.
- ☐ The principle of autonomy has led to the concept of informed consent—the obligation of health care providers to inform the client of the risks and benefits of a procedure and to obtain permission before the procedure is carried out.
- ☐ If the nurse believes that the client's decision will violate the nurse's own values by implementing a certain treatment, the nurse has an obligation to arrange for the transfer of the client's care to another provider.

Conscience Clause
- ☐ The conscience clause, or conscientious objection, applies to the nurse who does not wish to assist in abortions as well as to the nurse who does not wish to cooperate in noninitiation or withdrawal of life-sustaining treatment or euthanasia.

Client Rights
- ☐ The client has the right to refuse treatment to the extent permitted by law and to be informed of the medical consequences of the action.
- ☐ The client has the right to considerate and respectful care, as well as the right to obtain from the practitioner complete current information about their diagnosis, treatment, and prognosis in terms he can reasonably understand.
- ☐ The client has the right to know, by name, the practitioner responsible for coordinating care.
- ☐ The client has the right to every consideration of privacy concerning their own medical care program.
- ☐ Case discussion, consultation, examination, and treatment are confidential and should be conducted discreetly; those not directly involved in the case must have permission of the client to be present.
- ☐ The client has the right to expect that all communications and records pertaining to their care should be treated as confidential.

- [ ] The client has the right to expect that within its capacity, a hospital will make reasonable response to the client's request for services.
- [ ] The client has the right to obtain information about the existence of any professional relationships among individuals, by names, who are treating the client.
- [ ] The client has the right to be advised if the hospital proposes to engage in or perform human experimentation affecting care or treatment; the client has the right to refuse to participate in such research projects.

Client Bill of Rights

- [ ] The Client's Bill of Rights is also known as the Patient Care Partnership and includes the client's rights and responsibilities.
- [ ] Many hospitals in the United States have used the American Hospital Association's Client Bill of Rights as a model for formulating their own bills of rights.
- [ ] Canadian hospitals use the Patient's Bill of Rights, and these rights are enforced through federal-provincial agreements.

COLLABORATION WITH INTERDISCIPLINARY TEAM

Staff Nurse

- [ ] A staff nurse on a busy unit can act as an excellent role model for the unit and hospital staff.
- [ ] The staff nurse can encourage colleagues to participate in the unit's decision-making process and help them improve their clinical skills.
- [ ] The nurse can function effectively in the role as leader.
- [ ] A leader doesn't always have formal power and authority but influences the success of a unit by being an excellent role model and by guiding, encouraging, and facilitating professional growth and development.

Nurse-Manager

- [ ] A manager has formal power and authority from the status within the organization, and such power and authority are detailed in the manager's job description.
- [ ] Authority, a characteristic of a managerial position, is given by virtue of position within an organization.
- [ ] In participative management, the staff is encouraged to share their ideas, but the manager retains the authority to make final decisions.
- [ ] Resentment and frustration can come from the fact that the actual decision made by the manager may not include input from the staff.
- [ ] A nurse-manager assumes 24-hour accountability for the nursing care delivered in a specific nursing area.

Plan of Care (POC)

- ☐ Should be individualized to the client's condition or needs.
- ☐ Is developed with the client, partners in care, and health care providers.
- ☐ Includes strategies that address each of the nursing diagnoses.
- ☐ Should provide for continuity of care and should also include a pathway or timeline.
- ☐ Provides directions to other health care providers.
- ☐ Reflects current statutes, rules and regulations, and standards, as well as current trends and research.
- ☐ The economic impact of the POC needs to be considered.
- ☐ Should be documented using standardized language and terminology.
- ☐ The nurse coordinates implementation of the POC, and coordination of care should be documented.
- ☐ Evaluation of the POC is systematic, ongoing, and criteria based.
- ☐ The client, partners, and providers are involved in the evaluation process of the POC.
- ☐ Results of the evaluation of care should be disseminated to the client and other health care providers involved with the client's care in accordance with all laws and regulations.

Nurses Role

- ☐ Nurses interact with and contribute to the professional development of peers and colleagues.
- ☐ Nurses and other health care professionals frequently confer in groups to plan and coordinate client care.
- ☐ Nurses share knowledge and skills with colleagues and others through such activities as client care conferences and presentations.
- ☐ Nurses provide peers with constructive feedback regarding their practice.
- ☐ Nurses interact with colleagues to enhance the nurse's own professional practice.
- ☐ Nurses maintain compassionate and caring relationships with peers and colleagues.
- ☐ Nurses contribute to an environment that is conducive to education of health care professionals.
- ☐ Nurses contribute to a supportive and healthy work environment.

CONCEPTS OF MANAGEMENT

Nurse-Manager

- ☐ Must assign responsibility, identify the task to be accomplished, explain what outcomes are needed, and determine the time frame for completing the work.

☐ Responsibilities typically include policy and decision making, providing adequate staffing for safe and effective client care, and evaluating client care.

☐ In a crisis situation, the nurse-manager should take command for the benefit of the client.

☐ Responsible for providing client-teaching activities and coordinating nursing services with other client care services.

☐ As part of the health care team, the nurse-manager supervises and guides staff members, evaluates staff performance, and participates in staff recruitment and retention.

☐ Needs to provide new staff members with an adequate, individualized orientation and also needs to ensure that staff members participate in continuing education.

☐ Making sure that staff education is appropriate for each member's assigned responsibilities and planning and implementing budgets are part of the nurse-manager's responsibilities.

☐ Encourages staff participation in policy and procedure development and quality monitoring.

☐ Each manager directs staff using a different management style; an effective manager commonly uses more than one style.

☐ At times, staff should participate in decision making; at other times, staff participation is not appropriate.

☐ If a serious problem occurs on the unit, the nurse-manager should be notified as soon as possible.

☐ If the nurse-manager of a unit is not on duty when a staff nurse makes a serious medication error, the nursing supervisor on duty will call the nurse-manager at home and apprise the manager of the problem.

☐ Scheduling may be safely and appropriately delegated by the nurse-manager to a staff member.

☐ Termination, disciplinary action, and salary increases shouldn't be delegated to staff that do not have the power and authority to take such actions.

☐ Planning vacation time and evaluating procedures and client resources require staff input characteristic of a democratic or participative manager.

☐ If a nurse-manager has received complaints from discharged clients about inadequate instructions for performing home care, knowing the importance of good, timely client education, the nurse-manager should work with the staff to evaluate current client education practices and revise as needed.

Management

☐ An effective nurse-manager knows that to evaluate risk management findings accurately, the manager must look at the entire process and circumstances surrounding each incident.

☐ There are many management styles including autocratic, laissez-faire, democratic, transactional, quantum, transformational, and participative. (See Table 6.1 for characteristics of each management style.)

TABLE 6.1 **Types of Management Styles**	
Management Style	**Characteristics**
Autocratic	■ Decisions are made with little or no staff input. ■ Manager doesn't delegate responsibility and staff dependence is fostered. ■ High staff turnover and burnout are more common with this style of leadership.
Laissez-faire	■ Manager provides little direction, structure, or support. ■ Manager abdicates responsibility and decision making whenever possible and staff development isn't facilitated. ■ Most effective when all staff are clinical experts with a deep understanding of both clinical and administrative processes.
Democratic	■ Staff members are encouraged to participate in the decision-making process whenever possible. ■ Most decisions are made by the group, not the manager. ■ Group satisfaction and motivation are excellent benefits of this style.
Transactional	■ Style is based on a task-and-reward orientation. ■ Team members agree to a satisfactory salary and working conditions in exchange for commitment and compliance to their leader.
Quantum	■ Views an organization and its members as interconnected and collaborative ■ A helpful approach when unpredictable events and changing environments present themselves.

(Continued)

TABLE 6.1 Types of Management Styles (*Continued*)	
Management Style	Characteristics
Transformational	■ Can create revolutionary change ■ Often described as charismatic, these leaders are unique in their ability to inspire and motivate others. ■ They create intellectually stimulating practice environments and challenge themselves and others to grow personally and professionally and to learn.
Participative	■ Problems are identified by the manager and presented to the staff with several solutions. ■ Staff members are encouraged to provide input. ■ Manager makes the final decision.

CONFIDENTIALITY/INFORMATION SECURITY

Confidentiality

☐ All members of the health care team are responsible for keeping the client's health care records private, including facilities, nursing homes, pharmacies, and clinics; practitioners and dentists; laboratories and radiology centers; insurance companies, HMOs, and most employer group health plans; and certain government programs that pay for health care, such as Medicare and Medicaid.

☐ The nurse may lawfully disclose confidential information about a client when the welfare of a person is at stake.

☐ All types of health information are considered confidential, including the client's chart or medical record, conversations about a client's care or treatment, information in the facility's computer system, and billing information.

☐ Breeches in confidentiality are subject to fines. Specific protected health information that falls under the privacy rule includes individually identifiable information (such as the client's name, date of birth, and Social Security number); past, present, and future health information; demographic information (address, phone number, fax number, or e-mail address); billing and payment information; and information about the client's relatives, household members, and employers.

Health Insurance Portability and Accountability Act (HIPAA)

☐ The HIPAA protects the privacy and security of medical information.

- ☐ Under the HIPAA, only those who have a "need to know" are authorized to access client information.
- ☐ Personal Health Information Protection Act (PHIPA) is an example of a provincial health information privacy law established in Ontario, Canada.

Privacy Rule
- ☐ The privacy rule, which is part of the HIPAA, consists of national standards that protect all oral, written, and electronic (computer and fax) health information.
- ☐ The privacy rule allows health care providers to share any information they need to give high-quality health care at the same time that it protects the public by granting client's rights over their health information.

Photographing
- ☐ Photographs of clients are considered protected health information, so the same protections that apply to written information apply to photos.
- ☐ Permission is needed when the client's name, face, or a unique feature (such as a tattoo) are shown.
- ☐ However, permission isn't required when pictures are taken as part of the client's medical record or when the photo doesn't show enough information to identify the client.

Deidentified Health Information
- ☐ Any health or health care information that doesn't reveal a client's commonly identifiable information (including information that could identify the client through relatives, household members, and employers) is considered deidentified health information.
- ☐ One example of deidentified health information is a case study presented at a conference that uses a fictitious name in place of the client's real name.
- ☐ There are no limits on the use of deidentified health information; it isn't protected by the privacy rule.

Safeguards
- ☐ To ensure that privacy standards are maintained, health care providers must implement specific strategies to protect their clients' medical information.
- ☐ Strategies to protect clients' medical information include such safeguards as not posting lists of clients' names where the public can see them, not allowing staff to discuss client information in public areas where others can overhear, and disposing of protected health information in a proper and confidential manner, usually by shredding it.

Electronic Information

☐ Electronic information requires special safeguards to ensure that it's protected, such as assigning computer passwords that allow each employee access only to information necessary to do the employee's job, forbidding employees from sharing or posting passwords, and instructing them to log out of the computer immediately after each use.

Written Permission

☐ Prior written permission is required when a provider must give information to a client's employer such as in a drug test for employment.

Protected Health Information

☐ Protected health information can be shared without the client's written permission during the course of treatment to coordinate care with other health care providers and services, in the case of a medical emergency, or to aid in accurate diagnosis and treatment.

☐ Protected health information can be shared without the client's written permission for payment (to bill and collect payment for treatment and services provided) and for health care operations—for quality assessment and improvement, legal issues, auditing, training, and evaluating the performance of health care providers.

☐ The facility may also decide to release information to the client's relatives or significant others if the client can't agree to release information because of illness or injury.

Minors

☐ Minors have the right to privacy, but in most situations, a parent or legal guardian is authorized to receive and release the minor's protected health information.

☐ In some circumstances, the parent isn't considered the minor's personal representative and therefore doesn't control the minor's protected health information.

☐ Parents cannot control the minor's public health information when there's a reasonable suspicion of parental abuse, neglect, or endangerment; when state (or other applicable) law stipulates that the minor doesn't require the consent of a parent or other person before the minor can obtain a particular health care service; when a court determines someone other than the parent must make treatment decisions for the minor; and when a parent agrees to a confidential relationship between the minor and the practitioner.

☐ The Center for Adolescent Health and the Law has stated that it's appropriate for a minor to exercise privacy rights under HIPAA.

☐ It isn't appropriate for the nurse (or the practitioner) to discuss the client's information with the client's caregiver without the client's permission.

☐ The Family Educational Rights and Privacy Act (FERPA) protects the confidentiality of minors by defining the term "education records" to include all material containing information related directly to a student and by giving the parents' permission to have some control over disclosure of this information; it doesn't apply to health care situations.

☐ The neonate's safety and protection is the first priority when the nurse observes an abusive action by the caregiver.

CONTINUITY OF CARE

Types of Nursing
☐ Nursing can be performed as team nursing, modular nursing, primary nursing, total client care nursing, and functional nursing. (See Table 6.2 for characteristics of each type of nursing.)

Case Management
☐ Case management is a form of primary nursing that involves an RN who manages the care of an assigned group of clients; this nurse coordinates care with the entire health care team.

☐ The case management nurse helps develop protocols, policies, and procedures and develops a plan to achieve client outcomes.

Client Teaching
☐ If the client is admitted to the hospital as an emergency, client teaching should begin as soon as the client's condition stabilizes.

☐ RNs teach clients, and licensed practical nurses (LPNs) and aides can reinforce teaching.

Discharge Planning
☐ Discharges and admissions are completed by the RN.

☐ Discharge planning should begin before hospitalization for clients with planned admissions. For example, a client planning to undergo a nonemergency surgical procedure should be taught about the procedure and postoperative care in the practitioner's office before admission to the hospital.

☐ Discharge planning should begin as soon as the client is admitted.

☐ Beginning the planning for discharge as soon as possible gives the staff time to allocate necessary resources the client will require at discharge.

☐ Waiting until the client stabilizes, the day before discharge, or after the order is written doesn't allow adequate time for planning for the client's discharge.

☐ Many clients are discharged from acute care settings so quickly that they don't receive complete instructions.

TABLE 6.2 Types of Nursing	
Type	Characteristics
Team nursing	■ An RN leads nursing staff who work together to provide care for a specific number of clients. ■ The team typically consists of RNs, LPNs, and client care attendants. ■ The team leader assesses client needs, plans client care, and revises the care plan based on changes in the client's condition for continuity of client care. ■ The team leader assigns tasks to team members as needed.
Modular nursing	■ The modular nursing system is similar to team nursing, but the team is typically smaller, and an RN is assigned to a group of clients in a specific geographic location. ■ Typically, in modular nursing, an RN is paired with an LPN to provide continuity of care for a small group of clients.
Primary nursing	■ An RN plans and organizes care for a group of clients and cares for this group during their entire hospitalization. ■ The RN assumes 24-hour accountability for the group of clients in the nurse's care and delegates care in the nurse's absence to other staff members. ■ The RN who cares for the clients in the absence of the primary nurse is called an associate nurse; the associate nurse follows the care plan developed by the primary nurse.
Total client care nursing	■ An RN plans, organizes, and delivers client care for a specific group of clients. ■ If an LPN is caring for a group of clients, an RN assesses the clients and plans the care delivered by the LPN.
Functional nursing	■ Each caregiver on a specific nursing unit is given specific tasks that fall into their scope of practice. For example, an RN may administer medications to the entire unit while an LPN performs treatments and the client care attendants provide physical care.

Documentation

- ☐ Complete, accurate, and timely documentation is crucial to the continuity of each client's care.

- ☐ A well-documented record allows interdisciplinary exchange of information about the client and reflects professional and ethical conduct and responsibility.

- ☐ A well-documented record provides evidence of the nurse's legal responsibilities toward the client and also demonstrates standards, rules, regulations, and laws of nursing practice.

- ☐ A well-documented record supplies information for analysis of cost-to-benefit reduction analysis.

- ☐ A well-documented record furnishes information for continuing education, risk management, diagnosis-related group assignment and reimbursement, continuous quality improvement (QI), case management monitoring, and research.

Documentation Errors

- ☐ Common documentation errors include omissions, personal opinions, vague entries, late entries, improper corrections, unauthorized entries, erroneous or vague abbreviations, illegibility, and lack of clarity.

- ☐ If the medication administration record doesn't provide space to document the drug omission, the nurse should document the reason in the progress notes.

- ☐ Any time a drug is omitted, the reason for withholding the medication must be documented.

Evidence-Based Practice

- ☐ EBP in nursing is a problem-solving approach to making clinical decisions, using the best evidence available.

- ☐ EBP blends both the science and the art of nursing so that the best client outcomes are achieved.

- ☐ Guidelines written by a panel of experts that combine information from multiple studies and recommend best practices to treat clients with a disease, a symptom, or a disability are called EBP guidelines.

ETHICAL PRACTICE

Ethical Conflicts

- ☐ At times, the nurse may not know what the right or ethical course of action should be.

- ☐ There are no automatic guidelines for solving all ethical conflicts.

- ☐ In the assessment process, the nurse gathers facts, perceptions, and opinions about the ethical problem and talks with the client and family, other health care providers, and anyone who may be familiar with the client's values.

☐ Identify the people involved in any problem, and assess their roles, responsibilities, authority, and decision-making abilities.

☐ When making an ethical decision, identify available resources; these may include the ethics committee, chaplain, nurse ethicist, counselors, and facilitators; resources may also include institution policies, as well as literature on similar cases.

☐ Help decision makers participate in values clarification.

☐ Investigate the nature of the conflict by examining the rights, duties, and values that are in dispute; identify possible courses of action, along with their probable and possible risks and benefits.

Nurse Practice Act

☐ The nurse practice act is a series of statutes, enacted by each state legislature, that outline the legal scope of nursing practice within a particular state.

☐ The nurse practice act sets educational requirements for the nurse, distinguishes between nursing practice and medical practice, and defines the scope of nursing practice.

☐ Facility policies and procedures govern the practice in that particular facility.

☐ Standards of care, which are criteria that serve as a basis for comparison when evaluating the quality of nursing practice, are established by federal, accreditation, state, and professional organizations.

☐ Each state has a nurse practice act designed to protect both the nurse and the public by defining the legal scope of nursing practice and excluding untrained or unlicensed people from practicing nursing.

☐ Your state's nurse practice act is the most important law affecting your nursing practice.

☐ You're expected to care for clients within defined practice limits; if you give care beyond those limits, you become vulnerable to charges of violating your state's nurse practice act.

☐ Make sure that you're familiar with the legally permissible scope of your nursing practice as defined in your state's nurse practice act and that you never exceed its limits; otherwise, you're inviting legal problems.

Rules of Conduct

☐ Legally, nurses are responsible for using their knowledge and skills to protect the comfort and safety of their clients.

☐ Laws are binding rules of conduct enforced by authority.

☐ In many situations, laws and ethics overlap; when they diverge, you have to identify and examine the fine lines that separate them.

□ When a law is challenged as unjust or unfair, the challenge usually reflects some underlying ethical principle.

□ When clients believe they haven't been treated with respect and dignity or that their needs and rights have been ignored or violated, they're more likely to initiate legal action.

Dilemmas

□ A nurse who must decide whether to follow a practitioner's prescription to administer an unusually high dose of an opioid faces a moral dilemma—an ethical problem caused by a conflict of rights, responsibilities, and values.

□ An ethical dilemma carries with it a great deal of stress.

□ Moral dilemmas call for ethical choices in the face of profound uncertainty.

□ A moral dilemma may be further complicated by psychological pressures and personal emotions, especially when a choice is a forced one at best and, in many cases, results in an uncomfortable compromise.

□ Many moral dilemmas in nursing involve choices about justice or fairness, when scant resources (such as bed space or limited staffing) must be divided among clients with equal needs.

□ Dilemmas of beneficence are those that involve deciding what is good as opposed to what is harmful; they often occur when health care providers, clients, or family members disagree about what course of action is in the client's best interest.

□ Dilemmas of nonmaleficence are those that involve the avoidance of harm; these issues often involve a nurse's responsibility to "blow the whistle" if the nurse sees others compromising the client's safety.

□ Dilemmas of autonomy are those that involve deciding what course of action maximizes the client's right of self-determination.

□ Autonomy issues are often closely related to beneficence issues, especially when individuals other than the client must determine (or attempt to determine) what is best for the client.

□ Dilemmas of justice are ethical issues of fairness and equality, such as dilemmas that involve dividing limited health care resources fairly.

□ Dilemmas of fidelity are those that involve honoring promises; these include the extent and limits of a nurse's role and duties to a client that might conflict with other duties, such as the nurse's duties to the practitioner.

Fidelity

□ Fidelity involves confidentiality, respecting privileged information; a client's right to privacy must be balanced against society's right to be informed of potential threats to public health.

□ Fidelity involves a commitment to veracity: telling the truth and fully informing a client of their medical condition.

Decisions

□ Active decisions by the nurse are ethical decisions that lead directly to actions and bring about change.

□ Passive decisions are ethical decisions that deny, delay, or avoid action and maintain the status quo by denying or shifting responsibility to avoid change.

□ Programmed decisions are those decisions that use precedents, established guidelines, procedures, and rules to resolve anticipated, routine, and expected types of moral dilemmas.

□ Nonprogrammed decisions are those that require a unique response to complex and unexpected moral dilemmas.

□ Most commonly, a nurse's programmed decisions are also active ones.

Values

□ The nurse is likely to encounter many conflicting sets of values in the course of her professional career. The nurse must choose among competing values to establish her own ethical beliefs.

□ The nurse needs to incorporate chosen values into everyday thoughts and actions, to be better prepared to act on chosen values when confronted with difficult ethical choices.

INFORMED CONSENT

Informed Consent Background

□ Informed consent involves providing the client (or someone acting on their behalf) with enough information to know what the client is getting into if the client decides to undergo the treatment or procedure, as well as the anticipated consequences if consent is refused or withdrawn.

□ Responsibility for obtaining informed consent rests with the person who will perform the treatment or procedure (usually the practitioner).

□ The client must be fully informed regarding treatment, tests, surgery, and the risks and benefits prior to giving informed consent.

□ The client should be told that he has a right to refuse the treatment or procedure without having other care or support withdrawn and that he can withdraw consent after giving it.

□ Carrying out a procedure without informed consent can be grounds for charges of assault and battery.

Elements of Informed Consent
☐ A description of the treatment or procedure
☐ A description of inherent risks and benefits that occur with frequency or regularity (or specific consequences significant to the given client or designated decision maker)
☐ Explanation of the potential for death or serious harm (such as brain damage, stroke, paralysis, or disfiguring scars) or for discomforting adverse effects during or after the treatment or procedure
☐ Explanation and description of alternative treatments or procedures
☐ Name and qualifications of the person who is to perform the treatment or procedure
☐ Discussion of the possible effects of not undergoing the treatment or procedure
☐ An explanation of alternative treatments or procedures

Who Can Sign
☐ The client's next of kin can only sign the consent form if the client is deemed incompetent.
☐ In medical malpractice cases that involve consent issues, expert testimony is usually required to establish whether or not the information given to the client was reasonable, understandable, presented at a time when the client was functionally able to process the information (as opposed to being sedated or medicated), and complete enough to allow the client to knowledgeably agree to proceed.
☐ If the health care practitioner knows that specific consequences are particularly significant to the client, those must be discussed before true informed consent may be obtained.

Nurse's Responsibility
☐ Nurses may provide clients and their families with information that's within a nurse's scope of practice and knowledge base.
☐ A nurse can't substitute their knowledge for the practitioner's input.
☐ The professional nurse only witnesses the informed consent process and doesn't actually obtain the consent.
☐ If you witness a client's signature on a consent form, you attest to three things: The client voluntarily consented, the client's signature is authentic, and the client appears to be competent to give consent.
☐ Except in emergencies, information for informed consent should include but is not necessarily limited to the specific procedure or treatment, the medically significant risks involved, and the probable duration of incapacitation.

Incapacitated/Incompetence

□ If the nurse believes a client is incapacitated (incompetent) to participate in giving consent because of medication or sedation, or the nurse can learn that the practitioner has discussed consent issues with the client when the client was heavily sedated or medicated, you have an obligation to bring it to the practitioner's attention immediately.

□ Legally, the client must be mentally capacitated (competent) to give consent for procedures.

Emancipated Minor

□ Every state allows an emancipated minor to consent to their own medical care and treatment.

□ Most states allow teenagers to consent to treatment, even though they aren't emancipated, in cases involving pregnancy or sexually transmitted infection.

□ Only a minor who is married or emancipated can give informed consent.

INFORMATION TECHNOLOGY

Computerized Record System

□ As with the manual record system, the computerized medical record provides a detailed account of the client's clinical status, diagnostic tests, treatments, and medical history.

□ Unlike the manual system, the computerized record stores all of the client's medical data in a single, easily accessible source.

□ A hospital's computer system typically consists of a large, centralized computer to store information, linked to smaller video display terminals in each work area.

□ The computer recognizes by the signature code that the nurse has authorized access to the information stored in its memory.

□ The nurse can order a printed copy of the client's record.

□ A universal medical record follows a client throughout their life.

□ Some systems provide the nurse with a selection of words and phrases from which she can quickly create a complete narrative note.

Advantages of a Computerized Record System

□ By improving legibility, computers reduce the risk of misinterpretation.

□ A written record of each person who entered and viewed the medical record.

□ Computers reduce misinterpretation by offering standardized, structured input formats and mandatory charting fields for assessment reports, flow charts, and care plans.

Disadvantages of a Computerized Record System

☐ Use of an incorrect descriptive prompt or phrase can give a misleading assessment.

☐ If the prompts aren't exactly descriptive, it's important to type or write out the assessment.

☐ The need for backup records in case computers break down and make information unavailable.

☐ Ensuring completeness and continuity in charting requires a backup system.

☐ The key to avoiding computer problems is for all members of the health care team to know how to use the system.

Verification

☐ Verification is one way of reducing errors in the computerized record.

☐ Verification serves the same purpose as signing off on the manual record of a practitioner.

☐ To use verification, the unit secretary enters the practitioner's order into the computer; the order is held in a "suspense file" until the nurse reviews the entry, verifies the order, and adds it to the active record file.

☐ Many facilities use computerized order entry, which eliminates the verification process.

Liability

☐ Your liability when working with computer documentation is exactly the same as when working with a manual system.

☐ You may be liable for any client injuries associated with charting errors.

☐ To minimize legal risks, always double-check all client information.

☐ Don't divulge signature codes.

☐ Inform your supervisor if you suspect that someone is using your signature code.

State Rules and Regulations

☐ Know your state's rules and regulations and your facility's policies and procedures regarding privileged data, confidentiality, and disclosure.

☐ To learn about state rules and regulations, consult your facility's policy and procedure manual, check with your facility's attorney, or consult your state board of nursing or the state statutory and administrative codes.

Safeguards

☐ The primary safeguard, the signature code, limits access to the records; for example, a nurse's code would call up a client's entire record, but a technician's code would produce only part of the record.

☐ Care must be taken to safeguard client information sent by fax machine.

☐ Policies and procedures should be established to prevent confidential client information, such as a positive result on an HIV test, from being transmitted by fax machine, especially one that's centrally located and easily seen by staff members or the general public.

☐ Hospitals must show that their computer systems are trustworthy enough to be used in court.

☐ The hospital should use software that automatically records the date and time of each entry and each correction, as well as the name of the author or anyone who modifies a record.

LEGAL RIGHTS AND RESPONSIBILITIES

KEY TERMS

☐ **Breach of duty** means that the nurse provided care that didn't meet the accepted standard.

☐ **Negligence** is failure to exercise the degree of care that a person of ordinary prudence would exercise under the same circumstances.

☐ **Malpractice** is a specific type of negligence. It is a violation of professional duty or a failure to meet a standard of care, or failure to use the skills and knowledge of other professionals in similar circumstances.

Nurse's Scope of Practice

☐ A nurse may not knowingly administer or perform tasks that will harm a client.

☐ It's within a nurse's scope of practice to refuse to carry out orders that would harm a client.

☐ Administering medications and initiating IV therapy aren't within the scope of practice for nursing assistants.

☐ A staff nurse is not licensed to fill prescriptions.

☐ The nurse-manager is legally responsible for actions that fall within the scope of practice of the staff members who perform them.

☐ The scope of nursing practice within the facility may be narrower than the scope described in your nurse practice act, but it shouldn't be broader.

☐ Nurses have a legal obligation to practice within your nurse practice act's limits.

☐ Nurses should protect themselves by knowing their facility's policies and the nurse practice act.

☐ Conflicts of duty can arise if the state's nurse practice act disagrees with a facility's policies.

Abuse

☐ A detailed description of physical findings of abuse in the medical record is essential if legal action is pursued.

☐ Assault occurs when a person puts another person in fear of harmful or threatening contact.

☐ Battery is the actual contact with one's body.

☐ The nurse should not report suspicion of abuse when the client is a capacitated (competent) adult who has the right to self-determination; nurses do, however, have a duty to report cases of actual or suspected abuse in children and elderly clients.

☐ Discovery rule is the actual term for the client's discovery of the injury.

☐ Alternative dispute resolution refers to any means of settling disputes outside the courtroom setting.

☐ Indications of elder abuse are often dismissed as normal signs of aging.

☐ Elder abuse can be in the form of emotional, financial, sexual, and physical abuse.

☐ The responsibility of a nurse in a domestic abuse situation is to document the situation and provide support for the victim.

☐ In a case of suspected abuse, the nurse's responsibility is to document the client's statement and complete a body map indicating size, color, shape, location, and type of injuries.

☐ Many facilities have a policy, procedure, or protocol to help nurses and other health care providers make observations that aid the identification of possible abuse victims.

☐ It is the nurse's responsibility to document findings objectively without emotion.

Negligence

☐ Negligence is failure to exercise the degree of care that a person of ordinary prudence would exercise under the same circumstances.

☐ Any professional negligent action must meet four demands—commonly known as the four Ds—to be considered negligence and result in legal action: a duty for the health care professional to provide care to the person making the claim, a dereliction (breach) of that duty, a breach of duty that resulted in damages, and evidence that the damages were a direct result of the negligence (causation).

☐ Malpractice is a specific type of negligence; it is a violation of professional duty or a failure to meet a standard of care or failure to use the skills and knowledge of other professionals in similar circumstances.

Becoming an RN

☐ To become licensed as an RN, you must meet certain qualifications, such as passing the NCLEX.

☐ All states and provinces require completion of a basic professional nursing education program.

☐ Your state or province may have additional requirements to become licensed as an RN, including being of good moral character, in good physical and mental health, free from criminal conviction, fluent in English, and free from drug or alcohol addiction.

Protecting Yourself

☐ It is your responsibility to ask the practitioner if you're confused about an order.

☐ If the practitioner fails to correct the error or answer your questions, inform your immediate supervisor or nurse-manager of your doubts.

☐ Follow the chain of command established in your facility.

☐ Incident reports are internal to the facility and are used to evaluate care, determine potential risks, or examine system problems that could have contributed to the error.

Policies and Procedures

☐ The nursing service department in each facility develops detailed policies and procedures for staff nurses.

☐ Policies and procedures usually specify the allowable scope of nursing practice within the facility.

☐ To align nurse practice acts with current nursing practice, professional nursing organizations and state boards of nursing generally propose revisions to regulations.

☐ Nurse practice acts are statutory laws subject to the inevitably slow legislative process, so the law sometimes has trouble keeping pace with medicine.

Drug Administration Safety

☐ Administering drugs to clients continues to be one of the most important and, legally, one of the riskiest tasks a nurse performs.

☐ When administering drugs, one easy way to guard against malpractice liability is to remember the long-standing "five rights": the right drug to the right client at the right time in the right dosage by the right route.

☐ The law expects nurses to know a drug's safe dosage limits, toxicity, potential adverse effects, and indications and contraindications for use.

☐ The law expects nurses to refuse to accept an illegible, confusing, or otherwise unclear drug prescription and also to seek clarification of a confusing order from the practitioner rather than trying to interpret it.

☐ It is a nurse's responsibility to follow the facility's policies if you question a drug prescription.

☐ If unsure about a medication, the nurse can ask the prescribing practitioner. If the question is not satisfied, the nurse should then talk to their supervisor or get in touch with the facility administration.

☐ The nurse documents that the drug was not given and records the reason for omission in the progress notes.

Right-of-Conscience Laws

☐ Some US states and Canadian provinces have enacted right-of-conscience laws that excuse medical personnel from the requirement to participate in any abortion or sterilization procedure.

☐ Under right-of-conscience laws, the nurse may refuse to give any drug believed it is intended to induce abortion.

Breach of Duty

☐ Breach of duty means that the nurse provided care that didn't meet the accepted standard.

☐ When investigating breach of duty, the court asks: How would a reasonable, prudent nurse with comparable training and experience have acted in comparable circumstances?

Malpractice Trials

☐ During a malpractice trial, the court will measure the defendant nurse's action against the answer it obtains to the following question: What would a reasonable prudent nurse, with like training and experience, do under these circumstances?

☐ The plaintiff client and attorney have the burden to prove that certain standards of care exist and that the defendant nurse failed to meet treatment standards, as well as having to prove the appropriateness of those standards, how the nurse failed to meet them, and how that failure caused the client injury.

☐ When the standard of care is at issue, the plaintiff client must present expert witness testimony to support the claims.

☐ The defendant nurse and attorney need to produce expert witness testimony to support the claim that the nurse's actions didn't fall below accepted standards of care and that the nurse acted in a reasonable and prudent manner.

☐ The court seeks information about all the national and state standards applicable to the defendant nurse's actions.

☐ The court may seek applicable information about the policies of the defendant nurse's employer.

☐ Nurses who perform the same medical services are subject to the same standard of care and liability as practitioner.

☐ During a malpractice trial, nonnursing professionals who are trained and educated in medicine are familiar with standards of nursing care, and delegate nursing orders may provide expert witness testimony with regard to standards of nursing care.

Disciplinary Action

☐ The state board of nursing can take disciplinary action against a nurse for any violation of the state's nurse practice act.

☐ In all states and in Canadian jurisdictions, a nurse faces discipline if she endangers a client's health, safety, or welfare.

☐ Depending on the severity of the violation, a state board may formally reprimand the nurse, place the nurse on probation, suspend or refuse to renew the nurse's license, or even revoke their license.

☐ Other types of disciplinary action include imposing a probationary period, imposing a fine, and restricting the nurse's scope of practice.

☐ The list of punishable violations varies from state to state.

☐ The nurse can be convicted of a crime involving moral turpitude if the offense bears directly on whether the person is fit to be licensed.

☐ The nurse can be punished for habitual use of or addiction to drugs or alcohol.

Unprofessional Conduct

☐ Can include but is not limited to:

   ○ Falsifying, inaccurately recording, or improperly altering client records

   ○ Negligently administering medications or treatments

   ○ Performing tasks beyond the limits of the state's nurse practice act

   ○ Failing to take appropriate action to safeguard the client from incompetent health care and violating the client's confidentiality

   ○ Taking on nursing duties that require skills and education beyond one's competence

   ○ Violating the client's dignity and human rights by basing nursing care on prejudice

   ○ Abandoning a client

   ○ Abusing a client verbally or physically

PERFORMANCE AND QUALITY IMPROVEMENT

Overview

☐ If a nurse-manager has received complaints from discharged clients about inadequate instructions for performing home care, knowing the importance of good, timely client education, the nurse-manager should work with the staff to evaluate current client education practices and revise as needed.

Client Education

☐ Client education is the responsibility of all nurses providing care to the client, and the nurses must work together to establish the best methods.

☐ When providing client education is a concern for discharged clients, the nurse-manager at the facility should be contacted to pursue the concern, not the nursing staff.

☐ Evaluating client education in only one setting doesn't consider the entire process and the staff providing it. No complaint should be ignored.

☐ Client education is an important nursing responsibility.

Budgeting

☐ The nurse-manager provides a unit budget for the next quarter.

☐ In the development of a budget by a nurse-manager, a variance is projected based on personnel costs; to minimize this variance, the nurse-manager is advised to reduce the use of outside agency personnel.

☐ Reducing the use of outside agency personnel is the most appropriate way to minimize costs because there is often an overhead cost of 60% or more for outside agency staff.

☐ It is generally less expensive and in the interest of client safety to rearrange staffing patterns for the usual staff to provide coverage, rather than reducing the client census or increasing the client-to-nurse ratio.

☐ Revenue over expenses in a nonprofit organization is tax-exempt and is usually reinvested in the organization and used to improve services.

Types of Budgets

☐ Nurse-managers must develop three types of budgets: capital, operating, and personnel budgets. (See Table 6.3 for characteristics for each type of budget.)

☐ The nurse-manager compiles the budgets using historical data, client population, staffing needs, equipment needs, and accrediting agency requirements.

Performance Evaluation

☐ Professional growth of staff requires a self-reflective approach, as well as evaluation and goal setting.

TABLE 6.3	Types of Budgets
Budget	**Characteristics**
Capital budget	■ Reviewed annually ■ Outlines a plan for providing equipment needed for the unit that costs more than $500 ■ Nurse-manager determines what large, fixed assets or pieces of equipment that depreciate are needed within a specified budgetary period (usually 3–5 years).
Operating budget	■ Deals with the day-to-day operating expenses of a specified nursing area excluding personnel costs ■ Expenses include medical and nonmedical supplies, certain utilities, small equipment, and funding for the continuing education and professional development of staff.
Personnel budget	■ Identifies the cost for staffing the nursing care unit ■ Based on the number of personnel or full-time equivalents (FTEs) needed to adequately staff the unit; one FTE is equal to one person working 8 hours per day, 5 days per week, for 52 weeks per year. ■ Nurse-manager must include salaries, potential raises, benefits, and anticipated overtime.

□ Performance evaluation is a primary managerial function for nurse-managers.

□ A performance evaluation need not be agreed to in full by staff.

□ An effective performance evaluation provides recognition of strengths, identifies areas for improvement, and clarifies performance expectations.

□ Performance evaluations should be done in private, not in front of others.

□ All components of a performance evaluation should be documented in writing.

□ Although input from staff members can be useful in preparing performance evaluations, delegating all responsibility to others is inappropriate.

□ Peer evaluation is used in some settings but is done in a systematic way with clear criteria rather than informal "vouching."

Staff Development

□ Staff development is usually the responsibility of the employing institution.

Benchmarking

- [ ] Benchmarking is the process of comparing the delivery of client care practices in one organization to those in the best health care organizations.
- [ ] If the nurse-manager has contacts at the best facilities, she's the most appropriate person to obtain the necessary information from those institutions.
- [ ] The nurse-manager should evaluate the policies to determine which ones might be implemented at the facility and then make recommendations for change in conjunction with the staff.
- [ ] Asking the staff to form a task force is a good idea, but benchmarking is a practice that saves time and effort and allows information to be obtained from excellent resources.

Performance Improvement

- [ ] Support should be provided for the graduate nurse with the opportunity to improve performance.
- [ ] Performance improvement is an important component of continuous quality improvement (QI).
- [ ] Providing feedback on strengths as well as areas for improvement and clarifying what the staff member is expected to accomplish before the next performance evaluation are actions an effective nurse-manager takes when conducting performance evaluations.

Quality Management

- [ ] In quality management, there is continuous QI; it is used to continually assess and evaluate the effectiveness of client care.
- [ ] One of the concepts in quality management is benchmarking, whereby the nurse-manager compares best practices from top hospitals with the nurse-manager's unit and adapts the unit's practices as needed.
- [ ] Quality management also involves performance improvement, which establishes a system of formal evaluation of job performance and recommends ways to improve performance and promote professional growth.

Quality Improvement

- [ ] Continuous QI, based on principles from the business world, is a system used to continually assess and evaluate the effectiveness of client care.
- [ ] The nurse-manager uses reports from risk management to assess and evaluate care.

☐ Areas that need improvement can be identified by reviewing such incidents as medication errors, client fall reports, treatment errors, and treatment omissions.

☐ Incidents are investigated and a plan is devised to minimize or eliminate the risk of recurrence.

Managing Resources

☐ The approach to managing resources depends on whether the facility is nonprofit or for-profit.

☐ Traditionally, health care facilities were nonprofit organizations, making them tax-exempt, and excess revenue was recorded as a positive fund balance, or net worth; this revenue was reinvested in the organization and used to expand or improve services.

☐ Many facilities today are for-profit organizations where the excess revenue generated is divided as a dividend among stockholders or reinvested in the organization.

Committees

☐ The performance improvement committee identifies problems that don't meet an established standard and then recommends changes in the facility's policies, procedures, or documentation forms in an effort to improve client care.

☐ The Joint Commission is a private agency that establishes guidelines for the operation of hospitals and other health care facilities.

☐ Unit council is a group of individuals who represent the nursing unit and voice concerns of other staff members.

Roles of the Nurse-Manager

☐ Should meet with the staff nurse to discuss the nurse's performance and ways the nurse can improve.

☐ Shouldn't ignore a nurse's actions that deviate from the accepted policy.

☐ Shouldn't correct the nurse in front of peers because this would embarrass the nurse and isn't professional behavior.

☐ Is responsible for the performance of the staff.

☐ Job description defines the manager's authority over a specified group of employees and describes the job responsibilities.

☐ Must continuously search for methods to improve the quality of client care.

☐ Must think strategically and plan for changes before they arise because change is constant in health care.

Roles of the Nurse

☐ Systematically enhances the quality and effectiveness of nursing practice

- [ ] Demonstrates quality by documenting the application of nursing process in a responsible, accountable, and ethical manner
- [ ] Uses the results of quality-of-care activities to initiate changes in nursing practice and throughout the health care delivery system
- [ ] Uses creativity and innovation to improve care delivery
- [ ] Participates in QI activities
- [ ] Helps identify aspects of care important for quality monitoring
- [ ] Collects data to monitor quality and effectiveness of nursing care and analyzes quality data to identify opportunities for improving care
- [ ] Assists in developing policies, procedures, and practice guidelines to improve quality of care
- [ ] Participates on interdisciplinary teams that evaluate clinical practice or health services
- [ ] Analyzes factors related to safety, satisfaction, effectiveness, and cost/benefit options
- [ ] Analyzes organizational barriers
- [ ] Can help in implementing processes to remove or decrease organizational barriers
- [ ] Incorporates new knowledge to initiate change in nursing practice if outcomes aren't achieved
- [ ] Maintains professional records that evidence competency and lifelong learning
- [ ] Should provide culturally, ethnically sensitive and age-appropriate care
- [ ] Engages in self-evaluation of practice on a regular basis, identifying areas of strength as well as areas where professional development would be beneficial
- [ ] Participates in systematic peer review as appropriate
- [ ] Takes action to achieve goals identified during the evaluation process
- [ ] Provides rationales for practice, beliefs, decisions, and actions as part of the evaluation process
- [ ] Evaluates factors related to safety, effectiveness, availability, cost and benefits, efficiencies, and impact when choosing practice options that would result in the same expected client outcome

REFERRALS

Abuse
- [ ] Many support services have become available for both abusers and their victims.

- ☐ If a female victim of abuse is afraid to return to the scene of her abuse, she may find temporary housing in a women's shelter.
- ☐ The victim may be able to stay with a friend or family member or a shelter if available.
- ☐ Social workers or community liaison workers may also be able to offer the abuse victim suggestions for shelter.
- ☐ The police department should be called to collect evidence if the client wants to press charges against the abuser.
- ☐ If the client is a child, the law requires filing a report with a government family-service agency.
- ☐ The nurse needs to evaluate the abuser's ability to handle stress.
- ☐ In some cases of abuse, the nurse may be able to refer the abuser to an appropriate local or state agency that can offer help.
- ☐ In most cases, an abuser poses a continued threat to others and needs help to understand their behavior and how to change it.

Parents Anonymous
- ☐ For abusive child caregivers, a local chapter of Parents Anonymous may be helpful.
- ☐ Parents Anonymous, a self-help group made up of former abusers, attempts to help abusing parents by teaching them how to deal with their anger.

Self-Help Groups
- ☐ Besides helping short-circuit abusive behavior, a self-help group takes abusing parents out of their isolation and introduces them to individuals who can understand their feelings.
- ☐ A self-help group provides help in a crisis, when members may be able to prevent an abusive incident.

Telephone Hot Lines
- ☐ Telephone hot lines to crisis intervention services give abusers someone to talk with in times of stress and crisis and may help prevent abuse.
- ☐ Commonly staffed by volunteers, telephone hot lines provide a link between those who seek help and trained counselors.
- ☐ By becoming familiar with national and local resources, the nurse will be able to respond quickly and authoritatively when an abuser or victim needs your help.

REVIEW QUESTIONS ||||||||||||

1. A nurse and newly hired nursing assistant are caring for a group of clients. The nurse is administering medications and needs to know the fingerstick glucose results before administering a medication. The nursing assistant has not been validated on obtaining fingerstick glucose readings but states "I've seen it done many times and I know I can do it." What should the nurse do?

   1. Give the nursing assistant the glucose meter, and allow the nursing assistant to perform the fingerstick.
   2. Provide the nursing assistant with an article on the procedure.
   3. Go with the nursing assistant into the client's room, and validate the nursing assistant's ability to perform the procedure.
   4. The nurse should perform the fingerstick glucose testing.

2. An RN and an unlicensed assistive personnel (UAP) are caring for four clients together on the telemetry unit. Which nursing action can safely be delegated to the UAP?

   1. Applying electrodes in the correct position for ECG monitoring
   2. Teaching a client about an echocardiogram
   3. Assessing peripheral pulses on a client status post a coronary angiogram
   4. Monitoring blood pressures on a client who is receiving titrated dopamine

3. The nurse-manager of a home health facility includes which item in the capital budget?

   1. Salaries and benefits for her staff
   2. A $1,200 computer upgrade
   3. Office supplies
   4. Client education materials costing $300

4. A team leader chooses to apply the participative leadership style in managing the team of nurses. What value does this reflect?

   1. Freedom
   2. Justice
   3. Altruism
   4. Equality

5. A home care nurse visits a client with muscular dystrophy. Which comment by the client indicates that he needs more information about an advance directive?

   1. "I'm going to the doctor to get a new brace next week."
   2. "I've got a sore on my heel where my wheelchair rubs."
   3. "My dog is my best friend. I really don't have anyone who can make decisions for me when I no longer can."
   4. "I love apple pie. I don't ever want a feeding tube when the time comes that I can't eat."

Chapter References

American Hospital Association. (n.d.). The patient Care partnership. [Online]. Accessed September 2015 via the web at http://www.aha.org/advocacy-issues/communicatingpts/pt-care-partnership.shtml

Ellis, J. R., & Hartley, C. L. (2012). *Nursing in today's world* (10th ed.). Philadelphia, PA: Lippincott Williams & Wilkins.

Huston, C. (2014). *Professional issues in nursing: Challenges and opportunities.* Philadelphia, PA: Lippincott Williams & Wilkins.

Marquis, B., & Houston, C. (2015). *Leadership roles and management functions in nursing: theory and application.* Philadelphia, PA: Wolters Kluwer.

Mazurek Melnyk, B., & Fineout-Overholt, E. (2015). *Evidence based practice in nursing & health care: A guide to best practice* (3rd ed.). Philadelphia, PA: Wolters Kluwer.

Taylor, C., et al. (2014). *Fundamentals of nursing: The art and science of patient-centered care* (8th ed.). Philadelphia, PA: Wolters Kluwer.

7

Client Safety

ACCIDENT AND INJURY PREVENTION AND HOME SAFETY

Proper Body Mechanics

☐ Poor body mechanics, improper lifting or transfer technique, and workplace injuries can lead to musculoskeletal disorders.

☐ A low center of gravity helps you keep your balance and distributes your weight evenly between the upper and lower parts of your body when lifting objects.

☐ Try to keep your work (such as the client you will transfer or the object you will lift) close to your body, which aligns your back properly and lets your leg muscles—the body's strongest muscle group—do most of the work to avoid undue strain on your back.

☐ A wide base of support lowers your center of gravity and provides lateral (side-to-side) stability.

☐ To widen your base of support, stand with your feet spread about 8 to 12 inches (20.3 to 30.5 cm) apart, or roughly the width of your shoulders.

☐ Proper body alignment helps prevent muscle fatigue and overstretched ligaments; keep your head above your shoulders so your ears line up vertically with the top of your shoulders, and keep the top of your shoulders over your hips.

☐ Clients and their caretakers should also be taught proper body mechanics and encouraged to use special adaptive equipment to minimize bending, twisting, and long reaches.

☐ Maintaining a neutral posture while operating a computer is important, regardless if sitting or standing.

Preventing Back Injuries

☐ Repositioning or physically moving clients are major sources of back injury.

☐ Eliminate or reduce manual lifting and moving of clients whenever possible by using assist device equipment when available that are appropriate for the activity.

- Examples of assist device equipment include transfer boards, drawsheets, roller boards, transfer slings, lifts, lift chairs, lift cushions, push-up bars, trapeze bars, and pivot discs.

- Use a full-sling mechanical lift device for lifting a dependent client from the floor and a full-sling or stand-assist lift when the client can assist.

- When moving a client, engage the clients to help as much as possible by giving them clear simple instructions with adequate time for response.

- Obtain adequate help and utilize the lift team if available within your facility. The primary focus of a lift team is the movement of clients requiring maximum assistance for mobility, including bed repositioning, and transfers to chair, commode, bed, or gurney.

- Use (or modify) chairs, beds, or other surfaces to keep work tasks, equipment, and supplies close and at the correct height (i.e., between the waist and shoulders).

- Make sure brakes hold properly and apply them firmly on beds, gurneys, and wheelchairs.

Moving Large Objects

- Pulling is *not* the preferred method to move large or heavy objects.

- If you must pull a large object, stand close to it; tighten your leg, stomach, and buttock muscles; and keep a low center of gravity over a stable base.

- Never lift more than you're able to; seek help from coworkers, or use appropriate assistive or mechanical devices.

- Always bend at the knees and hips—never at the waist.

- Use your leg muscles, not back muscles, to lift.

- When lifting and carrying a heavy object, keep it close to your body.

- Move heavy objects in one smooth, continuous motion.

- Avoid awkward postures, especially when lifting.

- Avoid repetitive motions. If you can't avoid them, take frequent rests.

Belts

- Back belts may cause problems by giving workers a false sense of security or making the workers think they can lift heavier loads.

- Back belts should not be relied on as personal protective equipment (PPE) and should not be recommended for use in the workplace.

- Gait belts (also called transfer belts) are used to assist a client with walking; they have handles at the waist that the health care worker can grasp to support and stabilize the client.

☐ Gait belts are used for partially dependent clients who can bear weight and need minimal assistance; they should never be used to help lift a client.

Musculoskeletal Disorders

☐ Musculoskeletal disorders are conditions that involve the nerves, tendons, muscles, and supporting structures (such as the disks in the spine).

☐ The nurse can help avoid musculoskeletal disorders by maintaining good posture, practicing good body mechanics, using appropriate assistive and mechanical devices, asking for help from coworkers, exercising regularly, and wearing supportive footwear.

☐ Clients should avoid postures that can lead to injury, which include swayback (exaggerated inward curve of the lower back), slouching, holding the head too high, looking down too much, carrying a heavy object on one side of the body, and cradling a phone between the neck and shoulder.

Using a Walker

☐ If the client uses a walker, make sure that the client moves it about 6 to 8 inches (15 to 20 cm) at a time and then steps forward on to the weaker leg while using arms for support.

☐ Encourage the client to take steps of equal length with each leg.

☐ Instruct the client that to sit down, place the stronger leg against the chair and the weaker leg right in front; then the client can lower into the chair using the stronger leg and the opposite arm.

☐ Instruct the client using a walker to get up from a chair by putting the walker in front of the chair and using both hands on the arms of the chair to push himself up; once standing, the client can support the body with the stronger leg and opposite arm and grasp onto the walker.

Preventing Falls

☐ Many factors contribute to the high incidence of falls in older adults, including changes related to aging such as the spine tends to flex forward, causing a shift in balance and an increased risk for falls.

☐ Other factors include risks from mobility aids, adverse effects from medications, environmental hazards, unsafe caregiving, clothing that trips the client, and the effects of disease.

☐ Medications, particularly those that can cause dizziness, vertigo, drowsiness, orthostatic hypotension, and incontinence (such as antihypertensives, antipsychotics, sedatives, and hypnotics) can increase the risk for falls.

- ☐ A fall risk assessment should be performed on all clients at the time of admission to an acute care facility and then periodically therefore after using a standardized fall assessment scale.

- ☐ Given that about half of all falls happen at home, clients and their caretakers should be encouraged to complete a home safety check to help identify potential fall hazards that need to be removed or changed.

- ☐ Universal fall precautions apply to all clients regardless of fall risk and include items such as orienting the client to the hospital environment and call light system, maintaining the call light and client's personal possessions within their safe reach, keeping floor surfaces clean and dry, maintaining an uncluttered environment, and following safe client handling practices.

- ☐ Encourage the use of handrails, nonslip and well-fitting footwear, and lights.

- ☐ Bed positioning to prevent falls includes keeping the bed in the low position when a client is resting in bed and raising it to a comfortable height when the client is transferring out of bed keeping the bed or wheelchair brakes locked.

- ⊙ ☐ Scripted hourly rounding by hospital staff addressing issues such as pain, toileting, personal needs, positioning, and availability of the call light can decrease the risk of a hospital fall.

Bariatric Care

- ☐ Special equipment may be needed to safely care for bariatric clients.

- ☐ The client's weight, weight distribution, size, and physical needs must be taken into consideration when choosing the right equipment type, such as the correct type of bed.

- ☐ Using equipment that is not built for the task at hand can increase the risk of injury for both the client and health care provider.

- ☐ Make sure you know the capacity or expanded capacity of any equipment, including toilets.

The National Highway Traffic Safety Administration Recommendations for Car Safety

- ☐ Infants should be kept in the back seat, in rear-facing child safety seats, as long as possible up to the height or weight limit of the particular seat; at a minimum, keep infants rear-facing until a at least age 1 and at least 20 pounds (9 kg).

- ☐ When children outgrow their rear-facing seats, they should ride in forward-facing child safety seats, in the back seat, until they reach the upper weight or height limit of the particular seat (usually around age 4 and 40 pounds [18 kg]).

- ☐ Once children outgrow their forward-facing seats, they should ride in booster seats, in the back seat, until the vehicle seat belts fit properly.

- [ ] For a child age 8 or 4 feet 9 inches (145 cm) tall, seat belts fit properly when the lap belt lays across the upper thighs and the shoulder belt fits across the chest.

- [ ] When children outgrow their booster seats, they can use the adult seat belt in the back seat, if it fits properly (lap belt lays across the upper thighs and the shoulder belt fits across the chest).

- [ ] Car safety requires all children aged 12 and under to be buckled in the back seat of the car using the appropriate sized device to reduce injury from an accident and to prevent secondary injury from front seat airbags.

- [ ] Health care providers are often in a position to address the leading cases of preventable injuries due to motor vehicle collisions, such as nonuse or misuse of seat belts, distracted driving, speeding or aggressive driving, and alcohol consumption prior to driving.

- [ ] Many states have mandatory Department of Motor Vehicle reporting by health care providers for disorders or conditions that might interfere with the alertness, strength, physical coordination, agility, judgment, attention, knowledge, or skill necessary to safely operate a motor vehicle, such as dementia or uncontrolled seizure disorder.

- [ ] Clients should be cautioned not to drive when taking medications that cause sleepiness, blurred vision, dizziness, slowed movement, fainting, or the inability to focus or pay attention.

- [ ] Clients undergoing conscious sedation type procedures should not be allowed to drive for remainder of the day, regardless of how they feel.

Using a Cane

- [ ] A person holding a cane should have a 15-degree bend in their elbow.
- [ ] If the client needs a cane to walk, make sure the client holds it close to the body, about 4 inches (10 cm) to the side of the stronger foot.
- [ ] Help the client keep a slow and even pace when walking with a cane.
- [ ] When sitting while using a cane, make sure the client does not lean on the cane for support but stands with the backs of the legs against the chair, holds the arm rests with both hands, and lowers into the seat.

Assisting Clients

- [ ] When transferring a client from the bed to a wheelchair, bring the wheelchair as close to the bed as possible and make sure the wheelchair lock wheels before the client transfers.
- [ ] When assisting a client who is walking, walk beside the client with one arm around their waist for support in the event the client starts to fall.

☐ If a client begins to fall as you are walking beside the client, try to break the client's fall with your body and guide the client to the floor as gently as possible while supporting the upper body and head as best you can.

Preventing Falls in the Home

☐ In the client's home environment, instruct the client to remove clutter from hallways and stairs, secure electrical cords, remove throw rugs, replace burnt-out light bulbs, remove loose stair treads, and trim frayed carpet.

☐ In the client's home bathroom, instruct the client to make sure they use a bath stool or shower chair with nonskid feet, a raised toilet seat, and grab wall bars.

☐ Warn the client against climbing on a chair or an unsteady stool to reach high cabinets; instead use an extended reach tool or grips.

Preventing Fires

☐ Instruct the client to install smoke and carbon dioxide alarms on each level of the home.

☐ Instruct the client to check the alarms once a month and to change the batteries every 6 months whether they work are working.

☐ Electrical safety is an important aspect of preventing fires, especially in the presence of oxygen.

☐ Smoking is prohibited in the presence of oxygen.

☐ Caution clients taking sedatives or hypnotics to be careful with lit cigarettes.

EMERGENCY RESPONSE PLAN

KEY TERMS

☐ **Emergency** is a natural or man-made event that impacts your hospital's ability to provide care, treatment, and services and causes a sudden, major increase in the number of people who need the hospital's services.

☐ **Vertical evacuation** staff, clients, and visitors are moved to a different floor in the facility.

☐ **External evacuation** staff, clients, and visitors are moved to another hospital or site.

☐ **Industrial chemical spill** is an example of an accidental chemical emergency.

☐ **Toxic chemical release** such as by terrorists is an example of a planned chemical emergency.

Emergencies

☐ During an emergency, your hospital must maintain the safety of clients, staff, and visitors, and each worker must respond quickly and efficiently.

☐ If an emergency occurs, listen for the announcement of the disaster code, stay calm, avoid tying up lines of communication, and provide clients, families, and visitors with emotional support.

☐ Steps to an emergency response include preparation, protection, decontamination, treatment, and recovery.

☐ During an emergency, maintain client confidentiality.

☐ Always follow your hospital's emergency operation plan and the instructions of your emergency coordinator.

☐ Instructions to follow during an emergency will originate from the incident commander, located in the command center, who will spread information using the chain of command.

Nurse's Role in Emergencies

☐ The nurse must be able to assess for possible hazards in the work area.

☐ Each health care worker should understand and carry out their role in an emergency.

☐ Health care workers should know how to obtain and use equipment required for their emergency response role.

☐ Health care workers should be able to show correct use of emergency communication equipment, such as emergency phones, fax machines, and radios.

☐ Health care workers should communicate well with other employees, clients, families, and the public in an emergency.

☐ Health care workers should know how to seek help through the chain of command in an emergency.

Hospital's Role in an Emergency

☐ The hospital develops an emergency operation plan that is put into effect by hospital administrators and identifies leadership's role and the chain of command during an emergency.

☐ The hospital develops procedures for establishing a command center, where the incident commander will lead the emergency operation.

☐ The hospital develops procedures for responding to and recovering from the emergency, including the type of evacuation and exit route and ways to notify external authorities of emergencies.

☐ The hospital develops ways to identify and assign staff to cover all vital duties, including accounting for all employees after evacuation.

Emergency Operation Plan

☐ An emergency operation plan identifies procedures for evacuating the entire hospital and ways to establish an alternative care site.

☐ An emergency operation plan identifies roles and responsibilities of staff during emergencies and ways to recognize care providers and other staff during emergencies.

☐ An emergency operation plan identifies plans for combining efforts with other local health care facilities and backup communication systems in case primary communication fails.

☐ An emergency operation plan identifies an alternative plan for meeting utility needs and ways to isolate and decontaminate those exposed to biologic, chemical, and radioactive agents.

☐ Make sure you're familiar with your hospital's emergency operation plan, and be prepared to participate in regular drills.

Personal Protective Equipment (PPE)

☐ PPE helps protect the nurse from illness or injury caused by contact with hazardous materials.

☐ PPE, depending on the situation, may include a face shield, goggles or safety glasses, safety shoes or boots, splash apron or coveralls, hood, gloves, respirator or breathing apparatus, nonencapsulating or fully encapsulating suit, and a radiation-protective suit.

☐ The level of protective PPE for chemical, biologic, radiologic, or HAZMAT-type emergencies is divided into four categories, A, B, C, and D, based on the level of protection afforded (Table 7.1).

☐ All "first responders" and emergency personnel for hazardous materials incidents must meet OSHA requirements for both staff training and response to hazardous materials.

External Emergencies

☐ External emergencies include biologic incidents, chemical incidents, radiation incidents, gas leaks, explosions, power or water outages, water main breaks, and airplane, train, or motor vehicle crashes.

☐ External emergencies include natural disasters and severe weather (for instance, earthquakes, hurricanes, tornadoes, floods, snowstorms, tsunamis, and severe heat or cold) or other mass casualty incidents (including domestic war).

☐ Responses to this type of emergency may require the hospital to defend and or shelter in place.

Internal Emergencies

☐ Internal emergencies include fires, power or water outages, gas leaks, explosions, flooding, internal telephone or communication systems failure, airplane or motor vehicle crashes into the hospital, workplace violence, bomb threats, and hostage situations.

TABLE 7.1	Levels of PPE
Level	**Recommendations**
Level A	■ Provides the greatest level of skin, respiratory, and eye protection ■ Comprised of a totally encapsulated chemical and vapor-protective suit (TECPS) with integrated gloves, visor, and boots and self-contained breathing apparatus (SCBA) with full-face piece
Level B	■ For response to an unknown hazard ■ Includes a positive-pressure self-contained breathing apparatus and splash-protective chemical-resistant clothing.
Level C	■ For hospital-based first receivers, in personnel performing initial triage and decontamination at the hospital ■ Components include full-face mask with sealed visor, air-purifying respirator, hooded chemical-resistant clothing, under-suit clothing (disposable coveralls or surgical scrubs, to prevent wetting), and internal and external gloves
Level D	■ Contamination only. PPE is used for most radiation and biologic incidents. ■ Includes the usual work uniform, with surgical gown and over boots, gloves, safety glasses, splash goggles or face shield, and surgical cap ■ This affords minimal protection and is used for "nuisance."

☐ If an internal emergency occurs, the nurse should remove people from immediate danger, call the appropriate number according to hospital policy, and contact the nursing supervisor.

☐ Follow the hospital internal emergency response plan according to the type of internal emergency.

Evacuation

☐ During some emergencies, staff, clients, and visitors may need to evacuate.

☐ Evacuation may be horizontal, vertical, or external.

☐ In horizontal evacuation, staff, clients, and visitors are moved to a different area on the same floor.

☐ In vertical evacuation, staff, clients, and visitors are moved to a different floor in the facility.

☐ In external evacuation, staff, clients, and visitors are moved to another hospital or site.

Biologic Emergencies

☐ Biologic emergencies are life-threatening diseases or outbreaks resulting from contact with dangerous biologic agents.

☐ Biologic emergencies may be accidental (natural) or planned.

☐ An example of a biologic emergency is the severe acute respiratory syndrome (SARS) outbreak reported in China in 2002.

☐ Bioterrorism is a planned biologic emergency caused by terrorists.

☐ Bioterrorism is also called germ warfare or biologic warfare.

☐ Biologic agents used by bioterrorists include the germs that cause anthrax, botulism, plague, smallpox, tularemia, Ebola virus disease (EVD), Marburg virus infection, and brucellosis.

☐ Biologic emergency victims (and, possibly, caregivers and other persons in close contact with victims) may require immediate decontamination (such as removing the person's clothing and showering with soap and water), isolation precautions, immunization, and treatment that cures the disease or eases symptoms.

Chemical Emergencies

☐ An industrial chemical spill is an example of an accidental chemical emergency.

☐ Toxic chemical release by terrorists is an example of a planned chemical emergency.

☐ Agents that may be involved in chemical emergencies include cyanide, sulfur mustard, ricin, sarin, organophosphates (such as certain insecticides), and other toxins.

☐ In a chemical emergency, exposure occurs when a person breathes air, drinks water, eats food, or touches soil that contains a hazardous agent.

☐ Most deaths from chemical incidents result from inhalation (breathing in the chemical).

☐ Health care workers who care for clients who have been exposed to toxic chemical liquids are at risk when the chemical evaporates if they don't wear the proper PPE.

☐ Depending on their injuries, victims of a chemical emergency may require immediate decontamination before entering the emergency department to remove the hazardous chemical agent, preventing it from being further absorbed into the victim's body and from spreading to other people and surfaces.

☐ Victims of a chemical emergency may require measures to keep their airway open and maintain breathing and circulation, as well as medications to reverse the effects of chemical agents.

☐ Never induce vomiting if the victim ingested a toxic chemical.

☐ If the victim of a chemical emergency enters the hospital before decontamination takes place, be sure to cover the victim with a blanket or sheet right away to keep others and the area from becoming exposed; then take the victim to the decontamination area.

Chemical Decontamination

☐ Chemical decontamination involves three steps: removing clothing, washing the victim, and disposing of clothing and belongings.

☐ In a chemical decontamination, quickly remove any clothing with the toxic chemical on it and cut away clothing that would have to be pulled overhead.

☐ In a chemical decontamination, if solid material remains on the skin, brush or wipe it off (some materials react with water) and then quickly wash the area with running water for at least 15 minutes.

☐ In a chemical decontamination, if the eyes are burning or vision is blurred, rinse the eyes with water or an approved eyewash solution for 15 minutes and wash the victim's eyeglasses or remove contact lenses, as applicable, but don't put contacts back in the eyes.

☐ In a chemical decontamination, place the victim's clothing and belongings in a plastic bag, being careful not to touch any contaminated areas as you do this; then seal the bag, place it inside another bag, and (if appropriate) dispose of it according to your hospital's policy.

☐ In a chemical decontamination, you must maintain the chain of custody for all clothing and valuables, keeping in mind that these articles may be evidence if the contamination was crime related.

Radiation Emergencies

☐ Radiation emergencies can result from release of or exposure to radioactive material, as in explosion of a nuclear device, nuclear weapons testing, or nuclear power plant accidents.

☐ Radiation emergencies can result from radioactive material in the food or water supply, accidental release of radioactive material from a medical or industrial device, or accidental overexposure to a client undergoing radiation therapy.

☐ Radiation emergencies can result from accidents involving the transport of radioactive materials or terrorist acts, such as blowing up a truck carrying radioactive material, bombing a nuclear facility, or blowing up a "dirty" bomb.

☐ Radiation emergencies may contaminate or expose hundreds of people to radioactive material.

☐ If the radiation emergency involves an explosion, thermal burns and blast injuries also may occur.

□ If a radiation victim is admitted to your hospital, a radiologic emergency response team or radiation officer should manage the response.

□ The radiation victim should be checked using a radiation meter to determine if the client is contaminated.

External Radioactive Contamination

□ External radioactive contamination occurs when a radioactive material lands on a person's hair, skin, or clothing.

□ People with external radioactive contamination may contaminate other people or surfaces they physically contact, caregivers who touch or move the client, equipment used to assess and treat the client, and the surrounding area.

□ People with external radioactive contamination may also contaminate the air itself (although rare), if they are covered with dust or powder that contains radioactive particles.

Internal Radioactive Contamination

□ Internal radioactive contamination occurs when a person breathes in or swallows radioactive material, or absorbs such material through the skin or an open wound.

□ People with internal radioactive contamination may expose others to radiation; if their body fluids (such as blood, sweat, and urine) contain radioactive materials, anyone who comes in contact with these fluids may be exposed to or contaminated with radiation.

Radiation Decontamination

□ A person contaminated with radioactive material must be decontaminated to prevent or reduce internal contamination, to reduce the radiation dose from the contaminated site, and to prevent radioactive material from spreading to other people.

□ Before radioactive decontamination, the victim's clothing and belongings are removed and double bagged.

□ The bags containing the radioactive decontaminated victim's clothing are sealed, a radioactive material label is placed on the outside bag, and the bag is then placed in a designated storage area until it can be properly discarded.

□ To decontaminate a person with radioactive contamination, clean wounds and body openings first, followed by intact skin areas; then wash each area gently under a stream of warm tap water while scrubbing gently with a surgical sponge or soft brush.

□ If plain water washing is ineffective when decontaminating a person with radioactive contamination, use a mild soap or surgical scrub soap.

Natural Disasters

- ☐ To help keep the facility functioning during an emergency, you must know your responsibilities for reporting to work during a natural disaster.
- ☐ To help keep your facility functioning during an emergency, you must plan other ways to get to work and be prepared to report to another area in the facility, depending on where your skills are needed most.
- ☐ Know which types of natural disasters are most likely to strike your area.

Emergency Preparedness

- ☐ Participate in emergency preparedness drills to gain knowledge and experience.
- ☐ Learn how to use emergency communication equipment in case land and cell phone lines are overloaded during the disaster.
- ☐ During high-wind weather, such as a tornado or hurricane, keep all exterior doors and windows closed, unplug unnecessary equipment, keep people and vital equipment away from doors and windows, and be prepared to move clients to hallways or the basement, if ordered.
- ☐ Make sure key equipment is connected to an emergency (red) power outlet at all times.
- ☐ Know where to locate and how to use an alternative communication method, such as a two-way radio or an emergency phone system.
- ☐ Although most health care facilities have backup generators, these generators may not meet all energy needs (such as air conditioning).

Hospital Fire

- ☐ If a fire occurs in your hospital, you must act quickly. Use the memory aid RACE to help you remember what to do (Table 7.2).
- ☐ Be sure to close all fire and smoke barriers to buy precious time.
- ☐ During a fire remember to use the stairs—not the elevator.
- ☐ If not in immediate danger, do not remove clients from oxygen.

Bomb Report

- ☐ If a telephone caller reports a bomb in your hospital, stay calm and try to have someone else notify security while you stay on the line with the caller.
- ☐ In the event of a bomb threat, prepare to evacuate—usually a distance of at least 300 to 400 feet (92 to 122 m) from the bomb's location.
- ☐ In the event of a bomb threat, don't touch or move any suspicious packages or objects you encounter while evacuating. Instead, notify authorities of the location.

TABLE 7.2	R.A.C.E. for Fire
R = *Rescue*	■ Rescue anyone in danger, and move clients to a safe area.
A = *Alarm*	■ Activate the fire alarm system, and call the phone number chosen by your hospital to report the fire.
C = *Contain*	■ Contain the smoke and fire by closing all doors and windows in both client and nonclient areas.
E = *Extinguish* or *Evacuate*	■ Extinguish the fire, if possible. ■ Evacuate clients (if you can't extinguish the fire) starting with those nearest the fire.

☐ In the event of a bomb threat, don't reenter the hospital until you get permission from law enforcement personnel.

Hostage Situation

☐ If someone has been taken hostage in the nurse's workplace, the nurse should notify security personnel immediately (if this hasn't been done already) and try to stay calm and reassure others.

☐ Expect the hospital to be either evacuated or "locked down" (meaning no one can enter or leave).

☐ If there is an active shooter in the workplace area, the nurse should implement the phrase RUN, HIDE, FIGHT. The nurse should call the emergency number when it is safe to do so. If the nurse cannot speak, they should dial the number and set the phone down. If the nurse is not in immediate danger, provide the following information: location, number of shooters, physical description, number and type of weapons, and number of victims and hostages, if applicable.

☐ Most facilities have special procedures or an infant or child abduction as well other types of abductions (such as dependent adults). It is important that staff execute protocols quickly.

ERROR PREVENTION

Allergy Prevention

☐ Always ask the client about allergy to any medications, plants, or herbal supplements, even if the client is in distress.

☐ A client who has a peanut allergy could have an anaphylactic reaction to ipratropium given by a metered-dose inhaler because it contains soy lecithin.

□ Special precautions may be needed for clients with latex allergy and tropical fruits.

Client Teaching

□ Client teaching is a crucial aspect of the client's responsibility in minimizing medication errors and their consequences.

□ Teach the client about the diagnosis and the purpose of the drug therapy and provide this information in writing.

Drug-Related Problems

□ Always ask clients if they take over-the-counter medications, herbal remedies, or nutritional supplements in addition to the client's prescribed drugs.

□ Instruct the client what types of drug-related problems warrant notifying their health care practitioner.

□ Encourage the client to report anything about their drug therapy that is of a concern or worry.

Client Identification

□ Always check the client's identification using two client identifiers according to facility policy every time a medication is given or procedure is performed on a client.

□ In addition to the traditional "five rights" of medication administration, best practice researchers have added three additional "rights": the right reason, the right response, and the right documentation to help prevent medication errors.

Preventing Medication Errors

□ Always verify that the drug prescribed is appropriate to treat the client's condition.

□ Monitor the client's response to the drug administered.

□ Completely and accurately document in the client's medical record the drug administered; the monitoring of the client, including the client's response; and any other nursing interventions.

□ Safety procedures used with high-alert medications include double-checking with another licensed health care professional when preparing, administering, or handing off a high-alert medication and medication-specific competency checks.

□ The Joint Commission (TJC) has a list of problem-prone abbreviations that should be avoided when prescribing medications.

□ Technology and automation to help prevent medication errors include point-of-care bedside medication charting systems and bar coding; computer physician order entry (CPOE) systems that are integrated with pharmacy, laboratory, and nursing documentation systems; and decentralized automated dispensing systems.

Medication Error

□ The National Coordinating Council for Medication Error Reporting and Prevention defines a medication error as "any preventable event that may cause or lead to inappropriate medication use or client harm while the medication is in the control of the health care professional, client, or consumer."

□ Medication errors can occur from process problems within any one stage or within multiple stages of drug administration.

□ Medication errors that occur as part of ordering or prescribing can include incomplete or illegibly written orders by the prescriber; prescription of contraindicated drugs (such as drugs to which the client is allergic); prescription of the wrong drug, dose, route, or frequency; or using inappropriate or inadequate verbal orders to prescribe drugs.

□ Medication errors that occur as part of transcribing and verifying include transcribing the incorrect drug, dose, route, time, or frequency into the medication administration record (MAR) by the pharmacist or nurse or inadequate drug verification and documentation in the MAR by the pharmacist or nurse.

□ Medication errors that occur as part of dispensing include incorrect filling of the prescribed drug and failure to deliver the right drug to the right place for the right client.

□ Medication errors that occur as part of administering include giving the wrong drug to the wrong client by the nurse or other licensed professional; the nurse or other licensed professional calculating and giving or infusing the wrong dose, or preparing the right drug incorrectly (such as crushing a drug that shouldn't be crushed).

□ Medication errors that occur as part of administering can also include the nurse or other licensed professional administering the correct drug by the wrong route (such as an oral drug that is injected intravenously) and the nurse or other licensed professional giving the correct drug at the wrong time or frequency.

□ Medication errors that occur as part of monitoring and reporting include inadequate monitoring of the client by the nurse before and after medication administration and inadequate documentation and reporting of the client's condition by the nurse before and after medication administration.

□ Medication errors that occur as part of monitoring and reporting can also include inadequate handoff communication between licensed professionals and inadequate reporting of medication errors.

☐ Medications that have a heightened potential for causing client harms when misused are broadly defined as high-alert medications.

☐ Verbal orders are to be used infrequently and limited to those situations in which it is impossible or impractical for the ordering health care provider to enter the order in the client's records.

☐ Medication errors are more detrimental in children. Many medications must be adjusted based on weight or body surface area. For many clinical purposes, BSA is a better indicator of metabolic mass than body weight because it is less affected by abnormal adipose mass.

HANDLING HAZARDOUS MATERIALS

KEY TERMS

☐ **Carcinogens** are substances that can cause cancer.

☐ **Combustibles** are substances that burn, but don't easily catch on fire.

☐ **Corrosives** are substances that cause damage and burns when they contact the skin or eyes.

☐ **Explosives** are substances that can cause a sudden release of pressure and heat that's harmful.

☐ **Flammables** are substances that easily catch on fire.

☐ **Hazardous materials** are only dangerous when they come in contact with and enter the body.

☐ **Infectious wastes** place you at risk for getting an infection.

☐ **Irritants** are substances that cause redness or swelling of the skin or eyes on contact.

☐ **Organic peroxides** are substances that contain oxygen, which may cause other substances to burn.

☐ **Oxidizers** are substances that cause other substances to change and burn.

☐ **Physical hazards** threaten a person's safety; the most common types of physical hazards include materials that are likely to burn, explode, or react with water.

☐ **Pyrophoric substances** can spontaneously burst into flames.

☐ **Sensitizers** are substances that cause allergic reaction after repeat contact.

☐ **Teratogens** are substances that may cause birth defects.

☐ **Toxic** or **highly toxic agents** are substances that cause health problems with even the smallest exposure.

☐ **Unstable reactives** are substances that may react with pressure, moisture, a container, or temperature changes.

☐ **Water reactives** are substances that may explode or release a gas that easily burns when in contact with water.

Hazard Communication Standard

☐ OSHA created the Hazard Communication Standard, which protects workers who use or come in contact with hazardous materials in their workplace.

☐ The Hazard Communication Standard states that workers must be taught about hazardous materials and their proper use.

☐ The Hazard Communication Standard states that workers have the "right to know" about the possible risks to their health and safety and the right to tell their physician this information.

☐ The manufacturer who makes the hazardous materials must label the material with the product name, a warning, and the manufacturer's name and address.

☐ The manufacturer who makes the hazardous materials must provide information about how to safely use the product.

Hazard Material Coding System

☐ Hospitals often purchase hazardous materials in large volumes and then transfer them to smaller containers. All secondary containers must be adequately labeled.

☐ New labeling requirements require product identifier information, signal words (a single word used to indicate the relative level of severity of the hazard), a pictogram, hazard statement regarding the nature of the hazard, a precautionary statement describing the recommended measures to be taken or minimized to prevent an adverse effect resulting from exposure, and contact information of the manufacturer or distributor.

Safety Data Sheet (SDS)

☐ SDS is an updated format of the Material Safety Data Sheet (MSDS).

☐ The SDS has 16 sections in strict ordering that contains the name of the substance, the physical and health hazards associated with the substance, and ways in which the substance can enter the body.

☐ Hazardous materials are any substances or chemicals that pose a physical or health hazard and include hazardous chemicals (including some drugs), infectious wastes, and radioactive materials, all of which can be found in your workplace.

Hazards

☐ OSHA's Hazard Communication Standard classifies hazards into two major categories: health hazards and physical hazards.

☐ Hazardous materials can get into your body if you breathe them in, if you eat or drink them, or if your skin absorbs them.

☐ Your hospital's respiratory protection program helps to protect you from hazards that can be breathed in, such as vapors, gases, fumes, dusts, and infections (such as tuberculosis).

☐ OSHA requires that respirators be "fit-tested" every year.

☐ To protect yourself from contact with hazardous materials, clean work surfaces before and after working with hazardous materials, wash your hands before eating, don't eat or drink near hazardous materials, and dispose of all sharp instruments immediately.

☐ Treat batteries as hazardous waste, and do not dispose of them into normal trash, red bags, or sharps containers.

☐ As part of national efforts to decrease medical waste, most hospitals eliminated mercury thermometers and blood pressure cuffs.

Health Hazards

☐ Health hazards may cause serious health problems.

☐ Health hazards include carcinogens, teratogens, toxic or highly toxic agents, irritants, corrosives, and sensitizers.

☐ Carcinogens are substances that can cause cancer.

☐ Teratogens are substances that may cause birth defects.

☐ Toxic or highly toxic agents are substances that cause health problems with even the smallest exposure.

☐ Irritants are substances that cause redness or swelling of the skin or eyes on contact.

☐ Corrosives are substances that cause damage and burns when they contact the skin or eyes.

☐ Sensitizers are substances that cause allergic reaction after repeat contact.

Physical Hazards

☐ Physical hazards threaten a person's safety; the most common types of physical hazards include materials that are likely to burn, explode, or react with water.

☐ Physical hazards include flammables, combustibles, pyrophoric, explosives, water reactives, unstable reactives, oxidizers, and organic peroxides.

Radioactive Materials

☐ Radioactive materials may be present in health care workplace.

☐ Nurses may be exposed to radioactive materials through contact with X-ray machines and other testing equipment, through contact with clients who need radioactive materials for testing or treatment (also known as *brachytherapy*), and through radioactive materials that have spilled.

☐ When working with radioactive materials, observe the principles of time (limiting the amount of time exposed to the material), distance (keeping distance between you and the radioactive material), and shielding (using a lead barrier between the nurse and the radioactive material whenever possible).

☐ When working with radioactive materials, wear a personal radiation dosimeter, such as a film badge, to monitor exposure to radiation and wear lead protection whenever handling radioactive wastes.

☐ Place all radioactive waste in a special radiation container with a radiation label; immediately notify the appropriate person in your hospital to help clean up a radiation spill or other accident with radioactivity.

☐ Clients and visitors must also be protected from overexposure to radioactive materials.

Magnetic Resonance Imaging (MRI)

☐ MRI uses magnetic fields and radio frequencies instead of radiation to produce medical images.

☐ MRI poses specific safety hazard in that any magnetic object within the high magnetic field of the magnet can be pulled into the scanner itself, which could cause severe injuries to or even death of a client or staff member as well as considerable damage to MRI equipment.

☐ All medical personnel working in MRI environment must prevent metal objects (such as gurneys, oxygen tanks, infusion pumps, tools, and other client-use items containing metal [jewelry, hairpins, glasses, hearing aids, nonpermanent dentures, etc.]) from entering the MRI environment.

☐ A handheld magnet scanner can help detect metal objects such as noncompatible pacemakers and defibrillators, prosthesis, pumps, surgical clips, or metal fragments that cannot be imaged.

Compressed Gas Cylinders

☐ Transport gas cylinders larger than lecture bottle size with a hand truck or cylinder cart. Never roll or "walk" a cylinder.

☐ If not in use, never transport a cylinder with a regulator attached. Always protect the valve during transport by replacing the valve cover.

☐ Always store cylinders in an appropriate stand, a cart, or a cylinder storage rack in a well-ventilated area aware from ignition sources.

Eyewash Stations

☐ Eyewash stations should be located in hospital areas where there is a risk of eye contamination, such as the laboratory and emergency department.

☐ If the eye comes in contact with a hazardous material, go immediately to the nearest eyewash station and flush the eye with clear water or an approved eyewash solution for 15 minutes while holding the eyelid open and moving the eyes so the water or solution flows onto the entire surface of the affected eye and into the surrounding folds.

INFECTION CONTROL

Hospital-Acquired Infection (HAI)

☐ An infection acquired during treatment at a hospital or medical facility, also known as a nosocomial infection.

☐ Associated with increased morbidity, mortality, and cost; making them a major concern for both health care providers and clients.

☐ Health care workers play an important role in stopping the spread of infection.

☐ Universal steps to reduce the risk of a HAI include handwashing for the proper length of time and frequency, cleaning and sterilization of the client's environment, proper staff attire, and reduction in invasive procedures and operations.

☐ Follow standard precautions at all times with all clients and especially whenever you might come in contact with blood, body fluids, broken skin, or mucous membranes.

☐ Contact the infection control or employee health department for treatment options if you are exposed to an infectious agent.

Infection

☐ One of the most important things that nurses must do as a health care worker is to keep infection from spreading.

☐ Infections can increase the amount of time that clients spend in the hospital, increase health care costs, and cause workers to miss time at work.

☐ An infection occurs when an organism enters the body and the body's immune system is unable to fight it off, causing illness.

☐ Infections can be caused by different types of organisms, including bacteria, viruses, fungi, protozoa, and parasites as well as prions.

☐ Health care providers should receive vaccinations toward preventable diseases at high risk for nosocomial transmission and should avoid work when sick.

☐ Pathogens with high transmission potential from health care providers to clients include norovirus, respiratory infections, measles, and influenza.

Chain of Infection

☐ For an infection to occur, a six-part chain, known as the chain of infection, must be present (Table 7.3).

TABLE 7.3	Chain of Infection
Infectious agent	The organism responsible for the infection
Reservoir	The place where the infectious agent lives and grows, such as food, water, soil, an animal, an insect, or a human
Exit route	The way in which the infectious agent leaves the living being, such as through secretions, excretions, skin, or droplets
Mode of transmission	The way in which the infectious agent spreads to another location, such as by direct contact, through droplets in the air, by eating or drinking contaminated food or water, or through insect or animal bites
Portal of entry	Where the infectious agent finds its way onto or into another person, such as through an opening in the skin or through the airway or eyes
Susceptible host	A person who is at risk for getting the infection

☐ Two major types of infection control procedures can help you break the chain of infection: standard and expanded (formally transmission-based) precautions.

Controlling the Chain of Infection

☐ The best way to control the spread of infection is to break the weakest link in the chain of infection, which is usually the mode of transmission, or the way in which the infectious agent spreads.

☐ You can break the weakest link by performing good hand hygiene; using barriers, such as PPE; and following isolation precautions.

☐ Performing hand hygiene is one of the most important things you can do to prevent the spread of infection.

Performing Hand Hygiene

☐ Wash your hands with soap and water whenever they are visibly soiled, before eating, and after using the restroom.

☐ Before and after direct client contact.

☐ Before putting on sterile gloves to perform any procedure.

☐ After removing gloves.

☐ If moving from one body site to another during client care.

☐ After contact with any object that is near a client, including when entering and leaving the client's room.

Using an Alcohol-Based Hand Rub

☐ When using an alcohol-based hand rub, first apply the product to the palm of your hand and rub your hands together, covering all surfaces, until they're completely dry.

☐ Be sure to get the alcohol-based hand rub under your fingernails.

☐ Alcohol-base hand rubs do not kill all microorganisms such a *Clostridium difficile*, which are protect by a spore coating.

Washing Your Hands with Soap and Tepid Water

☐ When washing your hands with soap and tepid water, first wet your hands with water and then apply soap to your hands; rub your hands together briskly for at least 15 seconds, covering all surfaces of the hands and fingers; and then rinse your hands with water while pointing them downward.

☐ After washing your hands with soap and water, dry them with a paper towel and use another paper towel to turn off the faucet.

☐ Handwashing cannot be substituted if the hands are visibly soiled or the nurse has come in contact with a spore-protected microorganism.

☐ The WHO describes the five moments of hand hygiene to include before touching a client, before clean/aseptic procedures, after body fluid exposure/risk, after touching a client, and after touching client surroundings.

Preventing Infection

☐ Nurses should not wear artificial nails if they have direct contact with client equipment or clients who are at risk for infection, or if they prepare food.

☐ Keep natural nail tips less than ¼ inches (6 mm) long.

☐ Nail polish is discouraged and should be removed if chipped.

☐ Avoid using hot water when washing your hands; repeated use of hot water may increase your risk of developing skin problems.

☐ Use hospital-supplied hand lotions and creams to prevent your skin from drying and cracking.

Personal Protective Equipment (PPE)

☐ PPE can help prevent the spread of infection by acting as a barrier against the infectious agent.

☐ PPE includes gloves, gowns, eye and face shields, surgical mask, a particulate respirator such as the N95 respirator, hoods, caps, and shoe covers.

☐ Particulate respirator must be fit tested initially and then annually.

Gloves

☐ Choose the right size and type of gloves (gloves that contain powdered latex can cause allergic reactions in clients or staff with latex allergies).

☐ Check to see that there are no holes or tears in the gloves when first putting them on.

☐ Change gloves whenever moving from one body site to another.

☐ If gloves become torn, remove them, perform hand hygiene, and put on a new pair.

☐ Avoid touching your face and adjusting other PPE.

☐ Wash your hands (if visibly soiled) or use an alcohol-based hand rub (if not visibly soiled) right after discarding gloves.

Gown

☐ When wearing a gown, make sure the gown covers your torso, fits well when it's tied in the back at the waist and neck, and the sleeves fit snugly at the wrist.

☐ Remove the gown right before leaving the client's room by untying the waist strings first, then the neck strings, and then allowing the gown to fall forward (down toward your wrists), turning it inside out as it falls.

☐ When removing a gown, make sure the soiled portion of the gown doesn't touch your clothing.

☐ Place a used gown in a laundry bag or discard a disposable gown in an appropriate container inside the client's room.

☐ Wash your hands or use an alcohol-based hand rub right after removing a gown.

Goggles

☐ Goggles protect your eyes and the areas just above, below, and next to them.

☐ Goggles should fit snugly over and around your eyes (or eyeglasses).

Eyewear

☐ A face shield protects your skin as well as your eyes, nose, and mouth; the shield should cover your forehead, extend below your chin, and wrap around the side of your face.

☐ When removing eyewear, make sure you don't touch the outer surface; if eyewear is reusable, clean it after use according to your hospital's policy.

☐ Wash your hands or use an alcohol-based hand rub right after removing the eyewear.

N95 Respirator

☐ Always wear an N95 respirator to protect yourself against airborne diseases, and make sure it fits properly before each use.

☐ Avoid touching the N95 respirator once it's in place and change it when it becomes damaged.

- ☐ Remove the N95 respirator outside the client's room when the door is closed, touching only the straps of the N95 respirator during removal.
- ☐ Wash your hands or use an alcohol-based hand rub right after removing the N95 respirator.

Surgical Mask
- ☐ When wearing a regular surgical mask to protect against diseases that require droplet precautions, always make sure the mask fits properly before use.
- ☐ When wearing a surgical mask, avoid touching the face mask once it's in place and change it when it becomes damp.
- ☐ Touch only the straps or strings of the mask during removal; remove the face mask when you exit the client's room and discard it in the appropriate waste container.
- ☐ Wash your hands or use an alcohol-based hand rub right after removing a face mask.

When to Wear PPE
- ☐ During mouth-to-mouth resuscitation, use a mouthpiece or a pocket mask.
- ☐ When there's a risk that blood or body fluids could be splashed or sprayed, you may need to use a hood, surgical cap, shoe covers, face mask, or eye shield in addition to a gown and gloves.
- ☐ If you're wearing several types of PPE at once, always remove gloves first because they're the most contaminated items.

Removing PPE
- ☐ First remove gloves.
- ☐ Second, remove face shield or goggles.
- ☐ Third, remove the gown by peeling away from neck and shoulders and turning inside out as you disrobe.
- ☐ Fourth, remove the mask.
- ☐ Fifth, perform hand hygiene.
- ☐ When removing PPE, remove the face mask or N95 respirator last, making sure to remove the N95 respirator when you are outside of the client's room. If only gloves are worn, you can safely remove and discard them in the client's room.
- ☐ A gown can be safely removed inside the client's doorway just before exiting the room or removed in the anteroom (for contact and droplet isolation precautions only).
- ☐ Masks used for droplet precautions can be removed when you exit the client's room.

Standard Precautions

☐ Standard precautions are based on the idea that the blood and body fluids of any client may carry infection.

☐ Health care workers must follow standard precautions whenever they may come in contact with blood, body fluids (breast milk, feces, fluid from the lungs, saliva, semen, urine, vaginal secretions, wound drainage, and other fluids, such as excretions and secretions except sweat), broken skin, and mucous membranes.

"Always" in Performing Standard Precautions

☐ Always perform hand hygiene.

☐ Always wear gloves when touching blood, body fluids, broken skin, or soiled items.

☐ Always change gloves between clients.

☐ Always wear a mask and eye protection or a face shield to protect the eyes, nose, and mouth when splashing is likely.

☐ Always wear a gown to protect skin and prevent soiling of clothing when splashing or spraying is likely.

☐ Always use hospital safety sharps and dispose them in a puncture-resistant sharps container.

☐ Always use mouthpieces or resuscitator bags when cardiopulmonary resuscitation is needed.

☐ Always clean and disinfect equipment and surfaces.

☐ Always handle soiled linen away from your body.

Expanded Precautions

☐ Formerly called transmission-based precautions are used in addition to standard precautions for clients with certain types of infections.

☐ These include airborne infection isolation precautions, droplet precautions, and contact precautions.

Airborne Infection Isolation Precautions

☐ Used for clients with known or suspected diseases that spread through the airborne route.

☐ An airborne isolation room is a special isolation room with negative pressure.

☐ Diseases that spread through the airborne route: tuberculosis, varicella (chickenpox), measles (rubeola), and SARS.

☐ Diseases that spread through the airborne route are spread through small droplet nuclei that float in the air or attach to dust; the droplet nuclei exit the body when an infected person coughs, sneezes, or speaks.

During Airborne Infection Isolation Precautions

☐ The client must be placed in an airborne isolation room.

☐ The door of the room must be kept closed except when entering or exiting the room.

☐ Everyone who enters the room must wear an N95 respirator that has been properly fit tested.

☐ The N95 respirator should be removed outside of the client's room when the door to the isolation room is closed.

☐ Procedures and treatments should be done in the client's room, if possible.

☐ If the client needs to go to another area, the client should wear a surgical mask; if the client can't wear a mask, the client should be taught to cover their mouth with a tissue with coughing or sneezing.

☐ Teach client to perform frequent hand hygiene.

Droplet Precautions

☐ Droplet precautions are used to prevent the spread of infections through droplets.

☐ The client should be placed in a private room; if one isn't available, he or she can be placed in a room with another client who has the same infection.

☐ The door to the client's room may be open or closed.

☐ Everyone who enters the client's room must wear a regular surgical mask and other PPE according to hospital policy.

☐ The client must stay in the room except when special testing or a procedure is needed; then the client should wear a surgical mask, if able.

☐ If the client can't wear a mask, the client should be taught to cover their mouth with a tissue with coughing or sneezing.

☐ Teach client to perform frequent hand hygiene.

Contact Precautions

☐ Contact precautions reduce the spread of infectious agents through direct (skin-to-skin) or indirect contact (by touching surfaces or client care items that contain the germ).

☐ Make sure the client is placed in a private room; if one isn't available, the client can be placed in a room with someone who has the same infection.

☐ Put on gloves and a gown before entering the client's room.

☐ Make sure gloves cover the cuffs of the gown; none of your hand, wrist, or arm should be exposed.

☐ Change gloves after contact with germ-containing material.

☐ Remove gloves before leaving the client's room.

☐ Remove your gown just before leaving the client's room or in the anteroom, making sure your clothing doesn't touch anything that may contain germs after the gown is removed.

Protecting Yourself

☐ You must wash your hands or use an alcohol-based hand rub after removing PPE.

☐ Always wear gloves when handling used client items because many different client items, including towels, bed linens, and used dressings, tubing, or equipment, could contain infectious agents.

Sharps

☐ A sharp is anything that could cut or puncture someone who handles it, such as a needle, scalpel, scissors, or broken glass.

☐ Never bend, break, or shear a contaminated sharp.

☐ Never place a sharps container in a biohazard plastic bag for disposal.

☐ Never reach into a sharps container.

☐ Always use tongs to pick up a contaminated sharp.

☐ Change out sharps containers when they are three-quarters full.

☐ Discard contaminated sharps as soon as possible in a rigid, puncture-resistant container. These containers must be marked with a biohazard symbol and clearly labeled as a sharps container.

☐ If you experience a needlestick injury or a cut from a sharp, flood the needlestick or cut with water, and clean the wound with soap and water.

Immunization

☐ The CDC recommends that all health care workers get immunized against influenza, hepatitis B (only if at risk for blood or body fluid exposure), and varicella (chickenpox).

☐ A varicella vaccine is necessary with a negative immune titer result even if a person had a previous varicella (chickenpox) infection.

Exposure to Blood or Body Fluid

☐ If you become exposed to blood or body fluid splashes to the nose, mouth, or skin, flush with water and then wash your skin with soap and water.

☐ If your eyes become exposed to blood or body fluid, flush them with clean water or another approved eyewash fluid using the nearest eyewash station.

☐ If you become exposed to blood or body fluids, seek medical care as soon as possible after you have cleaned the exposed site.

☐ Report any exposure to blood or body fluids right away to the appropriate supervisor and to your employee health coordinator, risk management coordinator, or both.

☐ If you become exposed to blood or body fluids, complete the proper forms according to your hospital's policy and follow your hospital's policy concerning treatment options.

Exposure to Tuberculosis (TB)

☐ If you think you've been exposed to TB in the workplace, notify the appropriate supervisor and the infection control or employee health department right away, and fill out reports according to your hospital's policy.

☐ If you think you've been exposed to TB in the workplace, notify the employee health department in your hospital to schedule a TB skin test right away; they will notify the local or state health department as required by law.

☐ If the TB skin test taken after exposure to TB is negative, you'll need to schedule repeat testing and symptom screening in 8 to 10 weeks after exposure.

☐ If the TB skin test is positive or you have symptoms, you'll need to have a chest X-ray; make sure you report any symptoms right away.

☐ If you don't know that you've been exposed and the employee health department is informed that a client you had contact with was diagnosed with TB, your hospital must notify you right away to schedule testing.

SPECIFIC HOSPITAL-ACQUIRED INFECTION (HAI)

☐ In addition to the standard and expanded precautions, there are several bundle strategies that target specific HAIs of importance.

☐ Bundles are series of interventions that when implemented *together* achieve significantly better outcomes than when implemented individually.

Ventilator-Associated Pneumonia (VAP)

☐ The best way to prevent VAP is to prevent intubation and reintubation whenever possible.

☐ Noninvasive ventilation should be considered whenever possible.

☐ If intubation is necessary, oral intubation is preferred to nasal intubation unless otherwise contraindicated.

☐ Once the client is intubated, the VAP prevention bundle consists of the following:

○ Elevation of the head of bed at 30 to 45 degrees in the semirecumbent body position

- ○ Daily oral care with chlorhexidine solution of strength 0.12%
- ○ Daily sedation vacation if feasible and assessment of readiness to extubate
- ○ Peptic ulcer disease prophylaxis
- ○ Deep vein thrombosis (DVT) prophylaxis

- ☐ Other good ventilator care management requires health care providers to monitor endotracheal tube cuff pressure (keep it greater than 20 cm H_2O) to avoid air leaks around the cuff, which can allow entry of bacterial pathogens into the lower respiratory tract and to periodically drain and discard the condensate that collects in the ventilator tubing.

- ☐ Endotracheal tubes with a subglottic suction port to prevent pooling of secretions around the cuff leading to micro-aspiration and closed suctions systems should be used when available.

Central Line–Associated Bloodstream Infection (CLABSI)

- ☐ CLABSI prevention bundles are divided into those taken during insertion and those taken after insertion.

- ☐ During insertion, the subclavian vein is preferred (avoid the femoral vein whenever possible due to lower flora concentrations); use maximal sterile barrier precautions (cap, mask, sterile gown, and sterile gloves) and a sterile full-body drape, cleanse the insertion site with appropriate solution (such as a chlorhexidine preparation with alcohol), and apply a sterile gauze or sterile, transparent, semipermeable dressing to cover the catheter site.

- ☐ A chlorhexidine/silver sulfadiazine or a minocycline/rifampin-impregnated catheter should be considered when the catheter is expected to remain in place for more than 5 days and if the bloodstream infection rates are high in the unit despite successful implementation of measures to reduce CLABSI.

- ☐ After insertion and with every catheter use, wear gloves and clean the catheter opening with an antiseptic solution.

- ☐ The need for the catheter should be assessed daily; remove the catheter when not required.

- ☐ As with all intravenous systems, use of closed catheter and needleless systems should be used. Stopcocks should be avoided.

Catheter-Associated Urinary Tract Infection (CAUTI)

- ☐ CAUTI can be avoided by using urinary catheter only for appropriate indications; following aseptic insertion of the catheter; maintaining a closed drainage system; maintaining unobstructed urine flow and keeping the urinary drainage bag below the level of the bladder and of the floor; changing the system if compromised; and removing the catheter when it is no longer needed.

Surgical Site Infection (SSI)

☐ The SSI prevention "bundle" applies to all surgical procedures. It includes initiating antibiotics immediately prior to surgery and stopping antibiotics within 24 hours after the surgery, limited or minimal hair removal at the surgical site using clippers and avoidance of razors, antimicrobial washes by clients the night before and the morning of surgery in order to reduce bacteria on the client's skin, and use of antiseptic scrub in the operating room, immediately prior to surgery.

☐ Additional bundle measures include maintenance of tight glucose control for all clients undergoing cardiac surgery procedures and maintenance of normal temperature postoperatively for all clients immediately following certain types of gastrointestinal procedures.

RESTRAINT USE

KEY TERMS

☐ **Restraint** is defined as the direct use of force against a person's body; the force may be applied by the use of hands, mechanical devices, seclusion, or a combination of each.

☐ **Restraint** in the health care setting is commonly defined as use of any single or combined force that limits a client's freedom of movement, access to the client's own body, or access to the environment.

☐ **Clinical restraints** can be further classified as treatment restraints and behavioral restraints.

☐ **Treatment restraint** is the use of soft restraints, waist belts, bed enclosures, and other forms of restraints to protect a client who is confused, disoriented, unable to call for assistance, or unable to follow personal safety instructions or from dislodging a medical device; or from interfering with the integrity of a dressing or wound.

☐ **Behavioral restraint** is the use of a physical or mechanical device to involuntarily restrain the movement of all or a portion of a client's body as a means of controlling violent or assaultive behavior with the intent to prevent client from harming self or others.

☐ **Seclusion** is described as involuntary confinement of a person to a room or a specific area from which he is told not to leave or is physically prevented from exiting.

☐ **Chemical restraint** can include drugs that are used to restrict or manage a client's behavior or restrict freedom of movement.

Seclusion

☐ Seclusion is used to provide a safe, desensitized environment to support the client's efforts to regain control over unacceptable behavior.

☐ Seclusion eliminates stimulation when less restrictive approaches have failed and imminent danger to the client or staff is likely.

☐ According to Centers for Medicare & Medicaid Services (CMS) standards, seclusion may only be used for the management of violent or self-destructive behavior that jeopardizes the immediate physical safety of the client, staff members, or others.

Restraint Use

☐ Restraint can happen with or without the client's permission.

☐ Less restrictive measures should be attempted before resorting to the use of restraint.

☐ The goal is to use restraints only when absolutely necessary.

☐ Restraint use has many associated risks for the client, including death, neurovascular injury, fractures, psychological harm, bruising, skin breakdown, loss of dignity, and violation of the client's rights.

☐ Restraints can be used in acute medical-surgical care for the nonviolent, non–self-destructive client during treatment of certain conditions, such as acute brain injury.

☐ Restraints can be used in acute medical-surgical care for the nonviolent, non–self-destructive client during certain clinical procedures, such as endotracheal intubation.

☐ Restraints can be used in acute medical-surgical care for the nonviolent, non–self-destructive client to prevent client injury (e.g., to prevent the client from discontinuing treatment or dislodging medical equipment that is necessary for client care).

☐ Restraints and seclusion can be used for behavioral health purposes for the violent or self-destructive client to protect the client from injuring himself or to prevent the client from injuring others.

☐ When restraint is the only alternative, maintain the client's safety, protect the client's rights, preserve the client's dignity, and preserve the client's physical and psychological well-being.

☐ Using a restraint solely to keep a client in bed or to keep the client from falling is not an acceptable use.

☐ Always document what the client is doing and why the behavior presents a safety risk to the client and requires the use of restraint or seclusion.

Initiation of Restraint

☐ When restraints are initiated, the registered nurse caring for the client must immediately notify the physician or licensed independent practitioner (LIP), who will evaluate the situation and who must see the client face to face within 24 hours.

☐ When the initiation of restraints is warranted because of a significant change in the client's condition, the registered nurse caring for the client must immediately notify the physician or LIP, who will then evaluate the client.

Restraint Order

☐ If the physician or advanced practitioner is unavailable to give an order, the registered nurse can initiate restraints based on her assessment of the client; the physician or LIP must be notified of the restraint use immediately, and a written or telephone order must be obtained.

☐ If a telephone order is obtained for restraint use, the order must be signed within 24 hours of the initiation of restraint.

☐ The order for restraint use cannot be written as a standing order or on an as-needed basis (PRN).

☐ If medical-surgical restraint is necessary beyond the 24 hours authorized by the original order, the physician or LIP must provide a new order.

☐ Renewal of the restraint order must occur each calendar day that the restraint is needed after the client is examined by the physician or advanced practitioner.

☐ When behavioral restraint or seclusion is necessary, an order must be obtained from the physician or LIP responsible for the client's care as soon as possible, but no longer than 1 hour after the initiation of restraint use.

Face-to-Face Assessment

☐ The physician or LIP must perform a face-to-face assessment of the client placed in behavioral restraints or seclusion within 4 hours of initiation of restraint use or seclusion for clients age 18 and older and within 2 hours of initiation of restraint for children and adolescents age 17 and younger.

☐ The physician or LIP must perform a face-to-face assessment of the client placed in behavioral restraints or seclusion within 1 hour if the hospital is required to follow guidelines established by the CMS.

☐ At the time of the face-to-face assessment, the physician or LIP must collaborate with the client and staff to identify measures to help the client gain control of the client's behavior.

☐ At the time of the face-to-face assessment, the physician or LIP must collaborate with the client and staff to revise the client's plan of care and provide a new written order, if indicated.

Limitations of Orders

☐ According to TJC and CMS standards, verbal and written orders for restraint and seclusion are limited to 4 hours for adults age 18 and older, but these time limits may vary by state.

- ☐ According to TJC and CMS standards, verbal and written orders for restraint and seclusion are limited to 2 hours for children and adolescents ages 9 to 17, but these time limits may vary by state.

- ☐ According to TJC and CMS standards, verbal and written orders for restraint and seclusion are limited to 1 hour for children under age 9, but these time limits may vary by state.

- ☐ If the client's condition changes, the restraint can be discontinued before the order expires.

Mechanical Extremity Restraints

- ☐ Mechanical extremity restraints may be applied to the wrists and ankles.

- ☐ Commonly used mechanical extremity restraints include soft restraints and leather restraints.

Soft Restraints

- ☐ Soft restraints are commonly made of foam or lamb's wool and are applied over padded bony prominences.

- ☐ When applying soft or leather restraints, make sure that two fingers can be inserted between the wrist or ankle and the restraint.

Leather Restraints

- ☐ Leather restraints are padded devices that lock in place with a key.

- ☐ Leather restraints are used only when soft restraints aren't sufficient and sedation is dangerous or ineffective.

Upper Extremity Restraints

- ☐ Upper extremity restraints include elbow restraints and hand mitts.

Elbow Restraints

- ☐ Elbow restraints are commercially made devices that keep the elbow immobilized.

- ☐ Elbow restraints are especially helpful in protecting the surgical incision in small children after cleft lip or palate repair.

Hand Mitts

- ☐ Hand mitts are netted devices that may be tied down and are used to restrain the client's hands.

- ☐ Hand mitts prevent the client from scratching or removing invasive equipment or dressings and also prevent combative clients from hurting themselves or others.

- ☐ Hand mitts are considered restraints regardless of whether they are tied down because they prevent the client from having normal access to the body.

Other Types of Restraints

☐ A roll belt restraint may be used to prevent falls from a bed or chair while permitting movement of the arms and legs; they allow the client to turn freely in bed.

☐ Belt restraints are used to prevent falls from a chair and can also be used as a seatbelt for the client who is out of bed in a wheelchair.

Bed Side Rails

☐ Bed side rails can be considered another form of restraint.

☐ Maintaining all of the client's bed side rails in the "up" position limits the client's movement within the environment, making the side rails a form of restraint.

☐ Keeping one side rail in the "down" position allows the client access to the environment; in this situation, the side rails are no longer considered a form of restraint.

Mummy Restraint

☐ Mummy restraints are commonly used for infants and small children; they help maintain an infant or a small child in a fixed position during examinations or procedures.

☐ When using a mummy restraint on a child or infant, always make sure that the infant's or child's arms are kept in proper alignment with the body.

Client Monitoring

☐ All restraints used for nonviolent, non–self-destructive medical-surgical purposes must be removed at least every 2 hours, or as indicated by your hospital's policy.

☐ A client who is being restrained for medical-surgical purposes must be monitored and assessed at least every 2 hours.

☐ Client monitoring during restraint use is important because it maintains the client's physical and emotional well-being and protects the client's rights, dignity, and safety.

☐ Client monitoring during restraint use allows for periodic inspection of devices to ensure that restraints are secure and properly applied, released, and reapplied as necessary.

☐ Client monitoring during restraint use enables frequent reassessment and opportunities to use less restrictive alternatives whenever possible.

☐ Client monitoring during restraint use allows staff-client interaction and opportunities to assist the client to change behavior so that restraints can be removed.

☐ Clients being restrained for violent or self-destructive behavioral reasons require direct observation by an assigned staff member.

☐ Monitor the restrained client's vital signs and recognize the psychophysiologic effects that restraint or seclusion might have on them.

☐ Monitor the restrained client's nutritional and hydration needs, and ensure that these needs are met.

☐ Check the restrained client's circulation, and perform range-of-motion exercises with each extremity.

☐ Make sure that the restrained client's hygiene and toileting needs are met.

☐ Assess the restrained client's skin for any sign of restraint-related injury, such as bruising or skin breakdown.

☐ The client who is being restrained should be assessed more frequently if policy dictates or the client's condition warrants more frequent assessment; become familiar with your hospital's policy on this issue.

☐ Restraint ties must be secured to the movable portion of the bed frame, not the side rails.

☐ Always use a quick-release knot when tying any type of restraint.

Discontinuing Restraint

☐ Restraints must be discontinued at the earliest possible time, according to the CMS.

☐ According to TJC standards, restraints used for medical-surgical purposes can be discontinued when the client's condition improves and no longer poses a threat to the client's own medical healing, when the client's condition improves and less restrictive measures prove effective, or when the client's medical condition deteriorates and restraints are no longer necessary.

☐ Restraints used for behavioral purposes can be discontinued when the client is able to develop a safety plan, when the client is reoriented to place and time, or when the client is no longer making threats.

☐ After discontinuing restraints or seclusion, a debriefing should occur that should involve the staff, the client, and (if appropriate) the client's family to reduce the risk of recurrent restraint or seclusion use.

Things Not Considered Restraint

☐ Limitation of mobility or temporary immobilization for medical, dental, diagnostic, or surgical procedures, including postprocedure care.

☐ Adaptive support is used in response to a client's assessed need such as braces.

☐ Protective equipment, such as helmets.

☐ Age or developmentally appropriate protective safety interventions (such as stroller safety belts, swing safety belts, high chair lap belts, raised crib rails, and crib covers) that a safety-conscious child care provider outside a health care setting would utilize to protect an infant, toddler, or preschool-age child.

SAFE EQUIPMENT USE

Electrical Shock

☐ Insulated cords and other coverings prevent the electricity inside electrical equipment from touching you; if there's a problem with any of these parts, you might not be able to see it from the outside as the electrical problem may remain hidden until it becomes very dangerous.

☐ Electricity can cause serious or deadly injuries, including electrocution, electrical shock, burns, falls, and blast injuries.

☐ If you find a person who is suffering an electrical shock, don't touch the victim, or you could get shocked, too; unplug the appliance or turn off the power at the control panel.

☐ If you find a person who is suffering an electrical shock and you can't reach the wall outlet to unplug the appliance, use a dry object that isn't made of metal, such as a dry piece of wood, to move the appliance away from the victim; don't pull the appliance away with your hands or kick it away with your shoe because you could get shocked.

Electrical Hazard Areas

☐ Some client care areas pose a high risk for electrical hazards; these include operating rooms, intensive care units, emergency departments, procedure units, and postanesthesia care units.

☐ The operating room is a very high-risk area because electricity travels the path of least resistance, and an open surgical wound would be a path of least resistance.

Using Electrical Equipment

☐ Before using any electrical equipment, read the manufacturer's directions.

☐ Look at electrical equipment before use to see if you notice any problems.

☐ Don't use electrical equipment that isn't grounded.

☐ Keep in mind that even high-quality electrical equipment isn't always hazard-free.

☐ Remove unsafe equipment from use right away, and report it to the engineering department.

☐ If a hazard alarm sounds, unplug the equipment right away and remove it from use; tag it with the date, time, and reason that you are removing it from use and tell the engineering department.

☐ Keep floors and other surfaces dry.

Client Personal Equipment

☐ Don't allow clients to use electrical equipment from home.

☐ If a client's personal equipment is brought to the hospital, it must be checked by the engineering department.

Electrical Outlets

☐ In the hospital, ivory outlets are for general equipment use.

☐ In the hospital, red emergency outlets are for equipment that needs nonstop power.

☐ Only lifesaving equipment (such as ventilators and life safety equipment) should be plugged into red outlets; these outlets connect to generators that operate when the hospital's main electricity system fails.

☐ Electrical equipment used in the hospital should be polarized and grounded.

☐ Outlets, plugs, and power cords used in the hospital should be of heavy-duty, hospital-grade quality.

Electrical Plugs

☐ Hospital-grade plugs are marked with a green dot and are made to hold up under a lot of wear and tear.

☐ Use only polarized plugs.

☐ Never try to force a polarized plug into an outlet the wrong way.

☐ Never try to remove the third prong of a three-prong plug.

☐ Don't use a "cheater" adapter plug because it can overheat or overload a circuit.

☐ Don't use a plug with a bent or broken prong.

☐ Always insert the plug all the way so that no part of a prong is exposed.

☐ Make sure the plug fits into the socket and doesn't become loose or fall out.

Power Cords

☐ A damaged or worn power cord can cause electrocution or shock.

☐ Always check the cord before use, and don't use it if it's cut, frayed, or broken.

☐ Don't roll equipment or furniture over the cord.

☐ Keep the cord out of the path of foot traffic.

☐ Don't attach the cord to a wall, baseboard, or other surface using staples or other fasteners.

- ☐ Keep the cord away from door and window edges, which may cause kinking.
- ☐ Keep some slack in the cord to reduce tension.
- ☐ Clients should be taught proper electrical safety for home use, especially when using equipment usually found in a hospital, such as intravenous pumps or nebulizers.
- ☐ Don't pull on the cord to disconnect a device from an electrical outlet; always grip the plug and then pull it out.
- ☐ Keep cords away from heat sources, moisture, and metal pipes.
- ☐ After use, don't wrap an electrical cord around the equipment until the equipment has cooled.

Extension Cords
- ☐ Avoid using extension cords whenever possible.
- ☐ Extension cords are dangerous because they retain heat when covered, which can lead to fire; are likely to become looped, kinked, or otherwise mangled, causing the wires inside the cord to touch and spark a fire; and often become overloaded, which can overload the circuit.
- ☐ Restrict use to hospital-grade devices.

Water and Electricity
- ☐ Water conducts electricity, making water and electricity a deadly mix.
- ☐ Never use wet electrical equipment or ungrounded equipment near water.
- ☐ Never touch anything electrical if your hands are wet—even if the electrical device is turned off.

Electrical Devices
- ☐ Never use electrical devices or touch switches, wires, or metal when any part of your body is touching water.
- ☐ Don't use electrical equipment, cords, or wall outlets in wet weather or a damp environment.
- ☐ If you can't avoid working in a damp environment, make sure all the equipment is properly grounded.
- ☐ If liquid spills onto an electrical device, unplug the device immediately—if this can be done safely.
- ☐ If an electrical device drops into water, don't touch it until you've unplugged it; after it's unplugged, remove the device from use and notify the engineering department.
- ☐ Stay alert for the warning signs of electrical hazard, which can include flickering lights, warm light switches or wall outlets, loose electrical connections, equipment that "trips" a circuit breaker or blows a fuse, equipment that causes a shock or even a slight tingle, and equipment that smokes, sparks, or emits a burning odor.

Medical Devices

☐ The Food and Drug Administration (FDA) states that a medical device is an item used to help diagnose, treat, cure, or prevent disease.

☐ Examples of medical devices include man-made heart valves, ventilators, X-ray machines, defibrillators, bandages, IV pumps, and hospital beds.

☐ The Safe Medical Devices Act of 1990 requires hospitals to assess the client right away to find the cause of a serious injury or death and report any death or serious injury that may have been caused by a medical device to the FDA and the company that made the device within 10 work days. In addition, the Act requires hospitals to send a yearly review to the FDA about all medical device reports submitted during the previous year.

Client Entrapment

☐ Client entrapment in a bed is rare, but when it occurs, it can be fatal; it involves clients being caught, trapped, entangled, or strangled in hospital beds.

☐ The head, neck, and chest as key body parts at risk for entrapment.

☐ Areas around the head and foot board, between the rails, and between the rails and the mattress are all potential risks for client entrapment in a hospital bed.

Electrical Device Problem

☐ If you find a problem with an electrical device in your hospital, don't use the device, don't let anyone else use the device, and don't try to fix the problem yourself.

☐ Remove the equipment from service, and tag it with the date, time, and reason it is being removed from service; keep the settings the same on the piece of equipment; or if you can't, then write down the original settings; and report the problem to the engineering department right away.

Lockout or Tagout

☐ A lockout or tagout is a system that's used to lock or tag equipment so that it can't cause injury by starting up or releasing energy by mistake.

☐ With a lockout system, a lock is placed on the device to keep it in a safe or "off" position; in a tagout system, a tag is placed on the device warning workers not to use it.

☐ An I.V. pump that doesn't work properly would be "tagged out," but a computed tomography scanner that doesn't work properly would be "locked out."

☐ The OSHA requires putting a lock or tag on any equipment that needs service or repair to help protect workers from injury.

☐ Make sure you know your hospital's policy about using locks or tags and who is allowed to place and remove them.

SECURITY

Workplace Violence
☐ Among hospital settings, the highest rates of workplace violence occur in drug and alcohol rehabilitation units, geriatric units, emergency departments, and mental health departments and in admitting or triage areas.

☐ Types of workplace violence include threats (which may be verbal, written, or expressed through body language); verbal abuse or harassment; sexual harassment; stalking; mugging; hostage taking; physical assaults, such as punching, hitting, biting, pushing, and kicking; rape; homicide; and terrorist attacks.

Hospital Violence
☐ Violence in a hospital may be committed by a client, a worker, a visitor or other stranger, or a worker's relative or friend (when domestic violence spills over into the workplace).

☐ The most common type of violence in health care facilities is client-on-worker violence.

☐ The hospital uses codes to announce emergency security situations. The operator typically announces these codes over the hospital intercom system.

☐ Make sure you know what number to call to report each type of emergency, what each code means, and how to respond to each code.

Hospital Security Measures
☐ If your hospital has other security devices, such as panic buttons or other security alarms, make sure you know where they are located and how to use them.

☐ Security measures include special identification badges for restricted access areas, such as maternity or pediatric units.

☐ Make sure you know your hospital's policies on restricted access areas.

Ensure Your Safety
☐ Allow clients to express their anger verbally as long as their anger is not out of control.

☐ Express empathy for their feelings and situation.

☐ Allow the client to calm down in a "time-out" period if their anger is escalating or they cannot speak rationally.

☐ Never allow yourself to be in a closed space with an angry client; have your back to the exit.

☐ Ask for a security escort when transporting an agitated or hostile client; ask the security officer to stay with you until the client is under control.

☐ Within the hospital and on its grounds, use special care in dimly lit or isolated, out-of-the-way areas, such as stairwells, hallways, elevators, restrooms, and parking lots or garages; avoid being alone in these areas.

☐ Discourage coworkers, clients, and visitors from being alone in dimly lit or isolated, out-of-the-way areas, such as stairwells, hallways, elevators, restrooms, and parking lots or garages.

☐ Don't get into an elevator with someone who behaves in an odd or threatening way or who looks out of place; call security.

☐ If someone on an elevator makes you nervous, get off as soon as possible and call security.

☐ When leaving work, ask a coworker or security officer to escort you to your car if you're working late hours.

☐ If you are working late hours, have your cell phone within easy reach and consider programming security's number for quick access.

Client or Family Member Violence

☐ Stay alert for possible violence in anyone who shows or claims to have a weapon, makes a threat, verbally expresses anger or frustration, looks angry or defiant, paces back and forth, speaks in a loud voice, has clenched fists, has shifting eyes, states that people are out to get him, or shows signs of drug or alcohol use.

☐ In the hospital, some situations can trigger violence in people who might not otherwise become violent.

☐ Clients or family members may turn violent when they are frustrated with treatment delays, don't know the cause of a health problem, don't know if their loved one will recover, or are worried about the cost of treatment.

☐ Certain behaviors may signal whether a person may become violent, including holding grudges, reacting defensively to criticism, becoming easily frustrated or angered, and abusing drugs or alcohol.

NEVER EVENTS

Overview

☐ The CMS recently stopped reimbursing health care facilities for the added cost of treating "never events."

☐ Never events are "reasonably preventable" hospital-acquired conditions such as surgery on the wrong body part, mismatched blood transfusions, certain infections, and stage III and stage IV pressure ulcers.

Surgical Errors
- ☐ To address the problem of surgical site errors, TJC developed the "Universal Protocol for Preventing Wrong Site, Wrong Procedure, and Wrong Person Surgery."
- ☐ This protocol requires preprocedure verification, marking the procedure site clearly, and taking a time-out before the surgery to conduct a final check.

Pressure Ulcer
- ☐ The pressure ulcer bundles starts with a thorough head-to-toe skin assessment on admission and then at least every shift for all clients.
- ☐ This is followed by daily risk assessment. Use of a risk assessment tool, such as the Braden Scale, allows the client's risk to be quantified.
- ☐ Other bundle elements include frequent turning and repositioning, nutritional assessment, minimizing head of bed elevation to less than 30 degrees, incontinence care, and pressure relief.

Work Hours
- ☐ Sleep deprivation and long work hours can result in decreased performance, greater number of medical errors, and increased risk of occupational injury, thus increasing the potential of harm to both clients and health care providers.
- ☐ In efforts to decrease medical errors and occupational injury to health care workers, many states now limit the length of work hours or require prescribed time off between shifts, and several states have mandatory nurse-to-client ratios.

Communication
- ☐ Good communication is required every time information is exchanged, such as client-centered rounds, read-back, and face-to-face conversations.
- ☐ The process of communication when transitioning responsibility for care of a client is known as a handover or handoff.
- ☐ A standard policy for handoffs should be followed that allows for specific client needs.
- ☐ Many organizations have incorporated situational briefing techniques such as situation, background, assessment, and recommendations (SBAR) as a standardized framework for communicating critical information.

REVIEW QUESTIONS ||||||||||

1. A nurse is planning care for a group of clients who have issues with mobility. The nurse wants to ensure that best practices are incorporated in the plan. Which source should the nurse access in order to institute safe quality care?
   1. Evidence-based research
   2. Designated outcome criteria
   3. Approved clinical guidelines
   4. Pertinent assessment data

2. A public health nurse is teaching a community seniors group about the risk of falls. Which aging characteristic increases the risk of falls in elderly individuals?
   1. Forward-flexed posture
   2. Decreased ability to adapt quickly if balance is lost
   3. Inability to take responsibility for care of their daily cleaning
   4. Increased reaction time

3. A nurse is calculating the most accurate dosage of a medication for a child. What parameter should influence this calculation?
   1. Age
   2. Body weight
   3. Developmental stage in relation to age
   4. Body surface area in relation to weight

4. Nurses have instituted a falls prevention program. Which strategy will have the highest likelihood of preventing falls?
   1. Putting a falls risk sign on the clients' doors
   2. Having the client wear a color-coded armband
   3. Making rounds of the unit and clients' rooms
   4. Keeping all beds in low position

5. Which action is **most** appropriate when dealing with a client who is expressing anger verbally, is pacing, and is irritable?
   1. Conveying empathy and encouraging ventilation of feelings
   2. Using calm, firm directions to get the client to a quiet room
   3. Putting the client in restraints
   4. Discussing alternative strategies for when the client is angry in the future

Chapter References

Centers for Disease Control and Prevention (CDC). (2015). Healthcare-associated infections: Preventing HAIs. Retrieved from: http://www.cdc.gov/HAI/prevent/prevention.html

CDC Healthcare Infection Control Practices Advisory Committee. (2009). Precautions to prevent transmission of infection. [Online]. Accessed September 2015 via the web at http://www.cdc.gov/hicpac/2007IP/2007ip_part3.html

Food and Drug Administration and Hospital Bed Safety Workgroup. (2006). Hospital bed system dimensional and assessment guidance to reduce entrapment. [Online]. Accessed September 2015 via the web at http://www.fda.gov/RegulatoryInformation/Guidances/ucm072662.htm

Joint Commission on Accreditation Health. (2012). *2012 Hospital Accreditation Standards*. Terrance, IL: Joint Commission Resources Inc.

Taylor, C., Lillis, C., & Lynn, P. (2014). *Fundamentals of nursing: The art and science of person-centered nursing care* (8th ed.). Philadelphia, PA: Wolters Kluwer.

United States Department of Labor, Occupational Safety & Health Administration. (n.d.). Emergency response program to hazardous substance releases, 1910.120(q). [Online]. Accessed September 2015 via the web at https://www.osha.gov/pls/oshaweb/owadisp.show_document?p_table=STANDARDS&p_id=9765

World Health Organization. (n.d.). Healthcare associated infections: FACT SHEET. [Online]. Accessed September 2015 via the web at http://www.who.int/gpsc/country_work/gpsc_ccisc_fact_sheet_en.pdf

CORRECT ANSWERS AND RATIONALES

CHAPTER 1

1. **2.** Fine crackles are caused by fluid in the alveoli and commonly occur in clients with heart failure. Tracheal breath sounds are auscultated over the trachea. Coarse crackles are typically caused by secretion accumulation in the airways. Friction rubs occur with pleural inflammation.

2. **3.** Suctioning the respiratory tract for prolonged periods depletes the client's oxygen supply and causes hypoxia. It is recommended that each suctioning period not exceed 15 seconds.

3. **3.** The nurse must always palpate for a thrill and auscultate for a bruit in the arm with the fistula and promptly report the absence of either thrill or bruit to the health care provider, because these findings indicate an occlusion. No procedures such as IV access, blood pressure measurements restricting wraps, or blood draws are done on an arm with a fistula because doing so could damage the fistula. The fistula does not need to be kept at hear level.

4. **4.** Hyperkalemia, a life-threatening complication of acute kidney injury, is characterized by tall-peaked T waves on electrocardiogram. Elevated BUN is expected. The other findings are normal.

5. **3.** Risk factors for the development of pressure ulcers include poor nutrition, indicated by a decreased serum albumin level. Other risk factors include immobility, incontinence, and decreased sensation. A client who does not ambulate often can be repositioned frequently to prevent pressure ulcers. Having an indwelling urinary catheter does not normally increase the risk of developing a pressure ulcer unless pressure from the tubing impinges on urethral or other tissue. An elevated white blood cell count does not place a client at risk for pressure ulcers.

CHAPTER 2

1. **2.** At 4 hours postpartum, the fundus should be midline and at the level of the umbilicus. Whenever the placenta is manually removed after birth, there is a possibility that the entire placenta has not been removed. Sometimes small pieces of the placenta are retained, a common cause of late postpartum hemorrhage. The client is exhibiting signs and symptoms associated with retained ̄̄̄̄̄̄̄ments. The client will continue to bleed until the fragn̄ and cervical lacerations are characterized firmly contracted fundus at the level th̄ is characterized by a full bladder, whic̄ fullness just above the symphysis pub̄ be deviated to one side and boggy t̄

2. **3.** After spontaneous rupture of th̄ may carry the umbilical cord out of t̄ of the fetal heart rate comm̄ and/or prolapse of the cord, wh̄ This client is particularly at risk ̄ fetal head may not be engageḡ

is not a priority action. However, changing the client's position would be appropriate if variable decelerations are present. The nurse should assess the color, amount, and odor of the fluid, but this can be done once the fetal heart rate is assessed and no problems are detected. Cervical dilation should be checked but only after the fetal heart rate pattern is assessed.

3. 1. Oligohydramnios, or a decrease in the volume of amniotic fluid, is associated with variable fetal heart rate decelerations due to cord compression. Maintenance of an adequate amniotic fluid volume during labor provides protective cushioning of the umbilical cord and minimizes cord compression. Cord compression can result in fetal metabolic acidosis, not alkalosis. Amnioinfusion is used to minimize cord compression, not to increase the fetal heart rate accelerations during a contraction. The goal is to maintain the amniotic fluid index at 8 cm. This can be determined by ultrasound.

4. 1, 2, 3, 4. Having the fetus at a negative station places the client at risk for cord prolapse. With a negative station, there is room between the fetal head and the maternal pelvis for the cord to slip through. A small (low-birth-weight) infant is more mobile within the uterus and the cord can rest between the fetus and the inside of the uterus or below the fetal head. With a large infant, the head is usually in a vertex presentation and occludes the lower portion of the uterus, preventing the cord from slipping by. When membranes rupture, the cord can be swept through with the amniotic fluid. In a breech presentation the fetal head is in the fundus, and smaller portions of the fetus settle into the lower portion of the uterus, allowing the cord to lie beside the fetus. Prior abortion and a low-lying placenta are not related to cord prolapse.

5. 3. A neonate with cold stress must produce heat through increased metabolism, causing oxygen use to increase and glycogen stores to be quickly depleted leading to hypoglycemia. Hyperactivity and twitching are signs of hypoglycemia. Yellowish undercast to the skin color suggests jaundice related to excessive bilirubin levels, not cold stress. Increased abdominal girth suggests abdominal distention, possibly indicating necrotizing enterocolitis. It is unrelated to cold stress or possible hypoglycemia. Increased, not slowed, respirations are associated with neonatal cold stress and hypoglycemia.

CHAPTER 3

1. 2. For a lumbar puncture, the nurse should place the infant in an arched, side-lying position to maximize the space between the third and fifth lumbar vertebrae. The nurse's hands should rest on the back of the infant's shoulders to prevent neck flexion, which could block the airway and cause respiratory arrest. The infant should be placed at the edge of the table during the procedure, and the nurse should speak quietly to the infant. A mummy restraint would limit access to the lumbar area. It involves wrapping the child's trunk and extremities in a blanket or towel. A prone position isn't appropriate because it limits visualization of the vertebral spaces.

2. 4. A child with congenital hypothyroidism who is receiving thyroid replacement therapy should be regularly assessed for blood levels of thyroxine and triiodothyronine and also undergo frequent bone age surveys to ensure optimum growth. Results of bone age surveys should demonstrate growth, indicating that the medication was adequate and effective. Electrolyte levels measure elements, such as sodium, chloride, and potassium that are unrelated to medication therapy. Thus, electrolyte levels would provide no information about the effectiveness of therapy. Metabolic rate is not helpful in determining if treatment is effective. Muscular coordination is not an indicator of successful treatment for congenital hypothyroidism.

3. 2. Drain cleaner almost always contains lye, which can burn the mouth, pharynx, and esophagus on ingestion. The nurse would be prepared to assist with a tracheostomy, which may be necessary because of swelling around the area of the larynx. An emetic is contraindicated because, as the substance burns on ingestion, so too would it burn when vomiting. Additionally, the mucosa becomes necrotic and vomiting could lead to perforations. Gastric lavage is contraindicated because the mucosa is burned from the ingestion of the caustic lye, causing necrosis. Gastric lavage also could lead to perforation of the necrotic mucosa. Insertion of an indwelling urinary (Foley) catheter would be indicated after the measures to remove the caustic substance have been started.

4. 1. The reason that UTIs are a problem in children with vesicoureteral reflux is that urine flows back up the ureter, past the incompetent valve, and back into the bladder after the child has finished voiding. This incomplete emptying of the bladder results in stasis of urine, providing a good medium for bacterial growth and subsequent infection. Vesicoureteral reflux does not cause bladder spasms or painful urination. However, the child may experience painful urination with a urinary tract infection.

5. 3. Usually, the first clinical manifestations of Duchenne muscular dystrophy include difficulty with typical age-appropriate physical activities such as running, riding a bicycle, and climbing stairs. Contractures of the large joints typically occur much later in the disease process. Occasionally enlarged calves may be noted, but they are not typical findings in a child with Duchenne muscular dystrophy. Muscular atrophy and development of small, weak muscles are later signs.

CHAPTER 4

1. 3. Bipolar disorder is characterized by mood swings from profound depression to elation and euphoria. Delusions of grandeur accompanied by pressured speech are common symptoms of the manic phase of bipolar disorder. Schizophrenia does not manifest as mood swings from depression to euphoria. Paranoia is characterized by unrealistic suspiciousness and is usually accompanied by grandiosity. OCD is a preoccupation with rituals and rules.

2. 2. Telling the client that these are common side effects that will go away after 6 weeks is most appropriate. This statement acknowledges the client's concerns, gives the client some information, and provides support. Telling the client that a lithium blood level is needed is inappropriate; the client's reports reflect common adverse effects, not indicators of possible lithium toxicity. Telling the client that the symptoms are no cause for concern minimizes the client's feelings and ignores the concerns. Withholding the lithium dose until the client feels better is inappropriate because doing so ignores the client's concerns. In addition, withholding the lithium dose could lead to a decrease in serum lithium levels and, consequently, the drug's therapeutic effectiveness.

3. 2. Encourage the client with auditory hallucinations to reveal the content of the hallucinations to help prevent harm to the client and others. Exploring the content of the client's hallucinations will help the nurse understand his perspective on the current situation. The client shouldn't be touched, such as when taking vital signs, without being told exactly what is going to happen. Debating with the client about his emotions isn't therapeutic. When the client is calm, the nurse should engage him in reality-based activities.

4. 1. Selective serotonin reuptake inhibitors such as fluoxetine are the medications of choice for long-term treatment of panic disorder. Propranolol and diazepam are occasionally used for the short-term management of this disorder; however, these are not the preferred medications. Clozapine may trigger the development of an anxiety disorder.

5. 3. Rationalization is a defense mechanism used to justify actions or feelings with seemingly reasonable explanations. Insight is comprehension of one's own behavior, commonly followed by an attempt to change it. Repression is involuntary exclusion from awareness of painful and conflicting thoughts or feelings. Based on the information provided, the client doesn't seem to be manipulating those around her.

CHAPTER 5

1. 4. Infection is the greatest concern to the nurse. Infection occurs more frequently because of the number of procedures performed on clients who require this therapy and people they come in contact with in the hospital. Infection can be reduced if proper infection control techniques are used and human contact is reduced. Deficiencies and toxicities of nutrients are rare because of the use of standard protocols and orders for TPN formulas. Hyperglycemia can occur with TPN administration; however, all clients receiving TPN have their serum glucose concentration monitored frequently, and the hyperglycemia can easily be managed by adding insulin to the TPN solution. An infection is a much more serious complication.

2. 2. Common adverse effects of lidocaine hydrochloride include dizziness, tinnitus, blurred vision, tremors, numbness and tingling of extremities, excessive perspiration, hypotension, seizures, and finally coma. Cardiac effects include slowed conduction and cardiac arrest. Palpitations, urinary frequency, and lethargy are not considered typical adverse reactions to lidocaine.

3. 3. The bronchodilator would be given first to open up the airways and alveoli. Prednisone is not correct because steroids are not used for the acute phase. The drug is to be held in the lungs for greater absorption. Two to three minutes is the incorrect length of time between puffs.

4. 4. Clozapine is associated with agranulocytosis. Therefore, the nurse must instruct the client about the need for weekly blood tests to monitor for this adverse effect. Akathisia and drug-induced parkinsonism are associated with high-potency antipsychotics. These effects are not common with this atypical antipsychotic agent. Constipation and sedation may occur with this drug.

5. 1. A client who complies with drug therapy is less likely to have a recurrence of cardiac failure. Client knowledge of how to check a radial pulse and actions to take if it is not within normal limits can prevent a toxic digoxin reaction. The other choices do not indicate the client's ability to monitor effectiveness of digoxin. Weight gain is possibly reflective of activity or diet; chest pain is angina and not reflective of digoxin use.

CHAPTER 6

1. 3. The nurse should validate the nursing assistant's ability to perform the fingerstick glucose procedure. The nursing assistant may not perform the procedure without having her skills validated by actually performing the procedure. Providing reading material about the procedure is not enough. If the nurse performs the procedure on her own, she forfeits the opportunity to validate the nursing assistant's skills, and therefore underutilizes the nursing assistant.

2. 1. Unlicensed assistive personnel (UAP) can be educated in correct lead placement for ECG monitoring. Assessment of clients and monitoring of unstable clients are not within the scope of practice for a UAP and should be done by the registered nurse. Client teaching must be completed by an RN, not by a UAP.

3. 2. Capital budgets generally include items valued at more than $500. Salaries and benefits are part of the personnel budget. Office supplies and client education materials are part of the operating budget.

4. 1. The participative leadership style reflects the team leader's value for freedom. The team leader supports the right of other team members to suggest alternatives to the plan of care. This situation does not reflect the values of justice, altruism, or equality. When the team leader reports incompetent nursing practice objectively and factually, these actions reflect the value for justice. When the team leader assists others in providing care when they are unable to do so, it reflects altruism or a concern for the welfare of others. When the team leader interacts with the staff nurses in a non-discriminatory manner, the team leader promotes the value of equality.

5. 4. If the client states that he doesn't want a feeding tube but doesn't explain that he outlined his wish in a legal document, the nurse should give the client information about an advance directive. Statements about his new brace or a sore are relevant to the client's condition and care plan; they don't require teaching about advance directives. The client expressing that he doesn't have anyone to make decisions on his behalf indicates a need for information about obtaining a health care power of attorney.

CHAPTER 7

1. **3.** Approved clinical guidelines take the existing evidence and evaluate it in order to develop standards of practice. Evidence-based research provides information that provides a basis for nursing care decisions. Outcome criteria are the expected behaviors or conditions that result from the implementation of approved standards.

2. **1.** As people age, the spine tends to flex forward, causing a shift in balance and an increased risk for falls. Decreased ability to adapt quickly is not a characteristic of aging. Inability to take responsibility has no application to the question. Increased reaction time is incorrect; it would be decreased.

3. **4.** Body surface area in relation to weight is the most reliable method for estimating proper medication dosage for a child. Body surface area is more accurate for dosage calculation than height or weight alone because height and weight vary widely. Developmental stage does not enter into dosage calculation.

4. **3.** When making rounds, nurses can note a variety of risks in the clients' rooms, in the hallways, and other areas where clients might be at risk. Using signs, color-coded armbands, and keeping the bed in a low position are also useful, but making rounds offers the opportunity for nurses to intervene immediately and teach the client, family, and staff when risks are noted.

5. **1.** At this time, the client's anger is not out of control, so empathy and talking are appropriate to diffuse the anger. Using time-out is appropriate when the client's anger is escalating and the client can no longer talk about the anger rationally. Restraints are appropriate only when there is imminent risk of harm to the client or others. Future strategies are discussed after the initial incident is resolved.

Appendix

Preparing for NCLEX Success

"Don't keep doing the same thing and expecting different results."
Said by somebody brilliant.

WHAT IS THE CAT?

Every NCLEX exam is different because of the unique way that the computer interacts with the test taker. The computer adaptive test "CAT" means that as you answer questions correctly, the computer adapts and gives you harder questions. The opposite is also true, if you answer incorrectly the next test question becomes easier. In a CAT, the test taker cannot go back and change answers because the computer has already adapted the test to fit the last answer choice.

It Seems Like Everyone Gets 75

NCLEX-RN test takers can have a minimum of 75 questions and up to a maximum of 265 questions. It may seem that everyone around you reports that they had the minimum amount of questions, but the average tester will land somewhere in the middle of the 75–265 question range. Every test taker should be physically and mentally prepared for 265 questions. To conserve mental energy and keep anxiety low, try not to focus on the question number or how hard the questions seem during the exam. Remember that the question may seem easy because you know the information! Instead focus on the question in front of you. While the computer is on you have a chance of passing!

Here are three do's during the CAT:

1. Do your best on each question without panic.
2. Do mentally move on after a hard question.
3. Do know that a majority of test takers will go over 75 questions.

Exam Day

On the exam day, arrive early to the testing center. Wear comfortable clothes in layers. Remember for security reasons a camera will be recording your actions during the exam. There are attendants who work at the testing center to help you through the process.

Duties of testing center attendants:

1. Check ID, take your picture, and complete security scans.
2. Give you a locker and seal up your mobile phone.

3. Replace your dry-erase board as you fill them up with writing (you are not allowed to erase).

4. Check you in and out for breaks.

You cannot bring any study materials with you to the testing center nor can you access your mobile phone to make calls or text. You have 6 hours to complete the exam with two built-in breaks (the first 2 hours into testing, the second after 3.5 hours). Know that you can take additional breaks at any time, and breaking may be necessary to prevent fatigue and decrease anxiety. Keep in mind, though, that during breaks the clock keeps running. Take short and strategic breaks. You can access your locker for food and drink during breaks so pack a snack. Earplugs are also available on request. As you add or remove clothing you will have to do so on breaks as well.

IDENTIFY TESTING HABITS

Tally Your Mistakes

Nursing students make mistakes on NCLEX style questions for many reasons. Some mistakes are due to not knowing information while others are due to testing habits. To be a stronger test taker, you must become aware of the reason for the errors you are making and make changes to improve! Until then, you could be in a cycle of making the same mistakes over and over and expecting different results.

To improve test-taking skills, reflect on the reasons you miss questions on practice tests and quizzes. Tally your missed questions like you see below and implement the following strategies to strengthen testing habits. All of these habits are amendable, but you have to be aware first.

Quiz 31	35/50 questions = 70%
Reason: Knowledge 卌	Reason: Read Wrong 卌
Reason: Reading in |||	Capture your own reason ||

Missing Questions Related to Knowledge

No nurse knows everything! However, there are topics that the generalist nurse should know when they sit for NCLEX. The purpose of this book is to give those major pieces of information to help you answer questions with success. Study your *Fast Facts*! Testing tricks and strategies can be helpful, but no trick can replace having the *FACTS* needed to answer the question.

Missing Questions Related to Reading a Question Wrong

There are many reasons a test taker reads a question incorrectly, but two main reasons are becoming fatigued and not managing stress and anxiety. Reading takes physical and mental energy. Fatigue, stress, and anxiety impact your energy to read and understand complex questions.

Fatigue

An athlete gains endurance by adding longer distances and more weight. Students should also increase endurance for the NCLEX-RN by taking longer and longer practice quizzes in preparation for a potential 265-question test. Students conditioned to sit for long practice quizzes will better tolerate a long NCLEX exam. Also, through reflection on practice quizzes and tests, you can evaluate if there is a pattern where you get tired and where you need to take breaks. Practice taking these breaks and see if this improves your score. Take the same breaks during the NCLEX.

Stress and Anxiety

No one likes to be judged on what they know, so it is normal to go into the NCLEX with anxiety. However, there are things that you can do that will decrease feelings of anxiety on test day. Take a trial run to the testing center the day before. Do self-care activities such as sleep and exercise in the days leading up to your test date. Try not to add pressure by taking the NCLEX before you feel ready, telling everyone you know that you are about to test, or convincing yourself that the world depends upon this one test. Wear your lucky test-taking t-shirt, know that you passed nursing school, and study to have the confidence to pass the NCLEX!

Missing Questions Related to Reading "Into" the Question

Reading NCLEX-style questions can be difficult, but some students mentally add to the question and change the question's meaning. This habit can change but first you must be aware that you have this habit. An example of this is a question involving a client with a tracheostomy. A student "reading in" would add that the client has an unstable airway. If the question did not give details about shortness of breath and increased mucus production with a weak cough it should not be assumed.

Carefully reflect on the reason you are missing questions. Remember that NCLEX writers put all the information you need in the question to answer correctly.

Capture Your Own Reason

A unique reason or pattern may become apparent as you review and reflect on the questions missed while preparing for the NCLEX exam. Be astute to this pattern, name it, and then track how many questions you have missed due to that reason. Then try to work on this reason and kick that habit!

APPROACHING NCLEX-STYLE QUESTIONS

Example Question

A 74-year-old client with a history of heart failure is admitted to the coronary care unit with pulmonary edema. The client is ordered an IV bolus of furosemide after the client is intubated and placed on a mechanical ventilator. Which parameter should the nurse monitor closely to assess the client's response to a bolus dose of furosemide?

1. Daily weight
2. Level of consciousness
3. Serum sodium levels
4. Hourly urine output

Identify the Subject

Read each question for the main subject. Put the subject in your own words. The subject may make more sense as you read the answer choices. Try to keep your anxiety in check as you read the question. It may not be as bad as you think! In the above example, the subject was the client's response to the IV bolus dose of furosemide. The subject was not about pulmonary edema and was definitely not about ventilator management. Practice reading NCLEX style questions and begin to figure out what the question is really asking.

Identify Important Information

In the example question, there is information that could impact the answer. For example, the setting and the age of the client may have an impact on the answer and should be kept in mind. There could also be distracting information that does not apply, such as the client is on a ventilator. It may not be initially apparent what the distractors could be as you read the question. Keep in mind the identified subject and build important supporting information.

Choose the Best Answer

Narrow down the answer choices that make sense for the identified subject and supporting information. In many instances, a test taker can eliminate one or two answer choices. To help you decide on a final answer, go back to the question's subject and reassess the main points.

Reading the answer choices can also help you better understand the question's subject. As you read the answer choices, it may dawn on you what the question is asking and how the subject can be narrowed down.

WAYS TO PRIORITIZE ANSWER CHOICES

Nursing Process

Use the nursing process to help with prioritization of answer choices. The first step in the nursing process is to assess. Nurses should always assess before they diagnose and implement a plan of care. The nurse should evaluate interventions performed. Some test takers are hesitant to select assessment answers after assessment data have already been given in the question's stem. Keep in mind that further assessment may be necessary to clarify a situation. The question's wording may also confuse a test taker by asking "What action should the nurse take?" The word "action" does not automatically mean an implementation answer choice. Performing an assessment is an action. Try to decipher if the question is asking the nurse to assess or implement.

Nursing Process Example 1

A client returns from an endoscopic procedure during which he was sedated. Before offering the client food, which action should the nurse take?

1. Assess the client's respiratory status.
2. Stimulate the client's gag reflex.
3. Place the client in a side-lying position.
4. Put the bed in a low and locked position.

Answer: 2
The question is asking the nurse to further assess. The test taker must recognize that the client not only had sedation but also had an endoscopic exam in which the throat was anesthetized. A positive gag reflex must be confirmed before the client can eat. Respiratory status is important after sedation, but protection of the client's airway before eating would be a higher priority. Placing the client side lying is not indicated. The client's safety with a bed in low and lock position would be important, but the subject is about offering the client food.

Nursing Process Example 2
The nurse enters the room of a client with an arterial line in their right femoral artery. The nurse notes that the client removed the dressing, and there is blood spurting from the puncture site. What action should the nurse take?

1. Assess the client's blood pressure and heart rate.
2. Apply gloves and apply pressure to the site.
3. Call the practitioner.
4. Apply a sterile dressing.

Answer: 2
The question's subject is the action after displacing an arterial line. Holding pressure will prevent further blood loss. Hemorrhage is a medical emergency, and no other assessment is necessary until the flow of blood is stopped. Calling the practitioner is necessary after pressure is held. A sterile dressing would not stop the flow of blood.

Maslow's Hierarchy of Needs
Knowledge of Maslow's Hierarchy of Needs can be a vital tool for establishing priorities on the NCLEX. Maslow theory states that physiologic needs are the most basic of human needs. Only after physiologic needs have been met can safety concerns be addressed. Only after safety concerns are met can concerns involving love and belonging be addressed. To help you prioritize using Maslow hierarchy, remember your ABCs—airway, breathing, circulation—or CABs—circulation, airway, breathing—depending on the situation.

Safety is also a priority concern in Maslow hierarchy. Once the physiologic needs have been met, focus on what action will keep the client the safest. Place the client's needs before any activity, charting, or machine. If an alarm sounds, check the client first. Assess laboratory values or vital signs before giving a medication. Assess a client's ability before having them perform an activity. Know the skill set of support staff member before making a staffing assignment. These are all examples of putting safety first.

Maslow Example 1
A client is admitted to a hospital coronary care unit with the admitting diagnosis of angina; rule out myocardial infarction. The client is due for a stress test in the morning. Which of the following action would the nurse do **first**?

1. Apply the telemetry monitor.
2. Obtain timed blood work.

3. Orient the client to room safety features.
4. Physically assess the client.

Answer: 1

The question's subject is the care of a client with a possible myocardial infarction. The physiologic priority with a client with angina would be to assess circulation through the cardiac rhythm. The nurse can then assess and carry out other prescriptions after the monitor has been applied and circulation is established. Safety is a priority, but only after physiologic needs have been met.

Maslow Example 2

An unlicensed assistive personnel (UAP) reports to the nurse about four clients. Which client should the nurse see **first**?

1. A client with a tracheostomy needing a dressing change on their right foot.
2. A client with acute onset of confusion trying to get out of bed.
3. A client newly diagnosed with diabetes needing insulin teaching.
4. A client's family who is concerned that the discharge is taking too long and is anxious to leave.

Answer: 2

A client with a status change such as acute confusion should be assessed first for safety concerns. The client with the tracheostomy and the client needing insulin teaching are stable and are not a priority. The client and family who are anxious to leave are the most stable of the group, and although their concerns may be valid, the client with the altered mental status should be seen first.

Therapeutic Communication

Some NCLEX questions focus on the nurse's ability to communicate effectively with the client. Therapeutic communication incorporates verbal or nonverbal responses and involves:

■ listening to the client
■ understanding the client's needs
■ promoting clarification and insight about the client's condition

Like other NCLEX questions, those dealing with therapeutic communication commonly require choosing the best response. First, eliminate options that indicate the use of poor therapeutic communication techniques, such as those in which the nurse:

■ tells the client what to do without regard to the client's feelings or desires (the "do this" response)
■ asks a question that can be answered "yes" or "no," or with another one-syllable response
■ seeks reasons for the client's behavior
■ implies disapproval of the client's behavior
■ offers false reassurances

- attempts to interpret the client's behavior rather than allow the client to verbalize his own feelings
- offers a response that focuses on the nurse, not the client.

When answering NCLEX questions, look for responses that:
- allow the client time to think and reflect
- encourage the client to talk
- encourage the client to describe a particular experience
- reflect that the nurse has listened to the client, such as through paraphrasing the client's response
- show empathy for the client's situation

Therapeutic Communication Example

During a dressing change, a client states "I don't know what to do. This wound will never close." What response by the nurse is **best**?

1. "You should think more positively. The wound will close."
2. "The medical staff is doing all they can to help you to heal."
3. "It seems that you are upset over your wound's progress."
4. "What do you think we should be doing to help you heal?"

Answer: 3

The therapeutic response to the client's statement is to explore the client's feelings through reflection of what the nurse understood. This strategy allows the client to feel heard and gather information about what the client is feeling. Explaining that the medical staff is doing all they can to help the client does not convey warmth and is chastising to the client. Asking the client what she feels the staff should be doing is also a nontherapeutic response by putting the responsibility back on the client based on the client's statement. It is also not therapeutic to tell the client to think positively.

Delegation

When making client assignments and delegating tasks, the registered nurse (RN) must first assess the skill level of the person taking on the assignment or task. A licensed practical/vocational nurse (LPN/VN) can take care of stable clients that have predictable outcomes. The LPN/VN can make observations that they report to the RN for analysis using the nursing process. Only an RN can complete on-going assessments in a complex or unstable client. Nursing judgment cannot be delegated. The RN also does admission assessments and discharge instructions. The RN completes the initial teaching to the client while the LPN/VN reinforces the teaching. The UAP completes unchanging procedures that they have been trained to complete.

Delegation Example

The registered nurse overhears two unlicensed assistive personnel (UAP) trade client care assignments. How should the nurse respond?

1. Do nothing, UAP assignments are interchangeable.
2. Explain to the UAP that the assignments cannot be traded.
3. Call the nurse manager about the overheard conversation.
4. Change the assignment on the assignment form to reflect the change.

Answer: 2

Assignments are made by the RN to reflect the skill set and safe workload of the team. The nurse should explain to the UAPs that the assignment cannot be changed except by the RN. To do nothing or to change the assignment on the assignment form does not correct the potentially unsafe situation the change may cause. Calling the nurse manager is "passing the buck" to the manager to deal with a situation the RN can handle.

UNDERSTANDING ALTERNATE-FORMAT QUESTIONS

Alternative Format Question Types

A majority of the NCLEX exam will be multiple-choice questions, including multiple-response questions (select all that apply). The NCSBN reserves the right to put charts, tables, or graphic images into multiple-choice questions. There are also alternative-format questions that you should be prepared to take. These include multiple-response, fill-in-the-blank, hot spot, chart/exhibit, ordered response, audio, and graphic options. There is no rule about how many alternative items a student must get per exam. Remember this is an adaptive test. The questions you get fit the level of question you are currently on.

Multiple-Response Questions—"Select All That Apply" (SATA)

Some students shudder at the thought of a SATA question but when prepared with *facts* you will feel better about answering SATA questions. To answer a SATA question, think of it as series of true or false questions. As you read the answer choices, mentally insert the words "true or false" and answer that best answers the question. With SATA questions, there will always be at least two correct answers. The moral of the story is read the question and choose the best answers for the question.

Sample SATA Question

Prior to a blood transfusion, which of the following nursing actions would be important? Select all that apply.

1. Listen to anterior and posterior lung sounds.
2. Obtain family history of transfusion reaction.
3. Obtain a full set of vital signs.
4. Assess skin of thorax and abdomen.
5. Assess color and clarity of urine.

SATA Answers Using the True or False Technique

Prior to a blood transfusion, which of the following nursing actions would be important? Select all that apply.

1. (True or False) Listen to anterior and posterior lung sounds. (True)
2. (True or False) Obtain family history of transfusion reaction. (False)
3. (True or False) Full set of vital signs. (True)

4. (True or False) Assess skin of thorax and abdomen. (True)

5. (True or False) Assess color and clarity of urine. (True)

Correct answers: 1, 3, 4, 5

Prior to a blood transfusion, the nurse should establish a baseline in case of a transfusion reactions. This baseline includes vital signs, skin of the thorax and abdomen where rash could form, urine color in case hematuria and decreased urine output occurs, and lung sounds in case pulmonary edema or bronchoconstriction begins. A family history of blood transfusion has no merit in the client's risk of a transfusion reaction.

Fill-in-the-Blank Questions

The name says it all! The NCLEX uses fill-in-the-blank questions to ask math problems. You will be provided an onscreen calculator, and will type in your answer in the box provided. You will be told how to round if necessary, and you will not have to give any units of measurements—just the number and the decimal if applicable.

Sample Fill-in-the-Blank Question

Order: Enoxaparin 45 mg subcutaneous twice/day. Enoxaparin available: 60 mg in 0.6 mL. How many milliliter(s) would equal one dose? Round you answer to the nearest hundredth of a milliliter.

_____mL

Correct answer: 0.45

45 mg ÷ 60 mg = 0.75 ÷ 0.6 mL = 0.45 mL

Ordered Response Questions—"Drag and Drop"

This one is also self-explanatory. You put the items in order using your mouse to drag and drop the ordered items. The directions will tell you how to rank the items greatest to least, least to greatest, by priority, or to sequence an order of steps.

Drag and drop question example

A nurse must complete an abdominal assessment on a client with right lower quadrant pain. Place the steps in order for the nurse to complete the exam.

Correct answer

Palpate the right lower quadrant.	Inspect the abdomen.
Palpate the nontender areas of the abdomen.	Auscultate the abdomen in four quadrants.
Auscultate the abdomen in four quadrants.	Percuss the abdomen.
Inspect the abdomen.	Palpate the nontender areas of the abdomen.
Percuss the abdomen.	Palpate the right lower quadrant.

The process for abdominal assessment is important so that the underlying organs are not disturbed during assessment. Inspection, followed by auscultation, then percussion, and finally palpation is the order with special attention to palpate the RLQ last due to the client's reports of pain in that area.

Hot Spot Questions

The hot spot question has the test taker choose an area on an anatomical illustration or graphic. You will be prompted by a question to use the cursor to "click" on an area that best answers the question. This is scored as correct or incorrect so you need to be *exact as possible* in the placement of your cursor.

Hot Spot Question Example

A client has a history of aortic stenosis. Identify the area where the nurse should place the stethoscope to **best** hear the murmur.

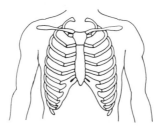

Correct answer

The nurse should place the stethoscope over the second intercostal space on the client's left side just to the left of the sternum.

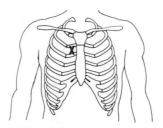

Chart/Exhibit (C/E) Questions

In the C/E questions, a client and clinical situation will be presented. You will then need to gather additional information provided under the "Exhibit" tab to answer the problem. This is similar to viewing sections of a client's chart. Gather the information necessary to best answer the question.

C/E Question Example

A 3-year-old client is being treated for severe status asthmaticus. After reviewing the progress notes, the nurse should determine that this client is being treated for which condition?

Progress notes	
8/1/15	Client was acutely restless, diaphoretic, and with SOB
0600	Sat 0530. Dr. T. Smith notified and ordered ABG
	analysis. ABG drawn from right radial artery. Stat
	results as follows: pH 7.28, Paco₂ 55 mm Hg (7.3 kPa),
	HCO₃⁻ 26 mEg/L (26 mmol/L). Dr. Smith with client now.
	————————————————— J. Collins, RN.

1. Metabolic acidosis
2. Respiratory alkalosis
3. Respiratory acidosis
4. Metabolic alkalosis

Correct answer: 3

Audio Item Questions

Audio questions present an audio clip using headphones provided by the testing center. After listening, you will select the answer that best fits the question. The question may ask what the nurse will do upon hearing the noise or to just identify what is going on with the client based upon the sound heard. It is a little tricky to present you with an audio question in a static book. Sorry there is no auditory example here, but this is what you may see:

Audio Question Example

Listen to the audio clip. What sound do you hear in the bases of this client with heart failure?

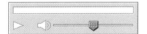

1. Crackles
2. Rhonchi
3. Wheezes
4. Pleural friction rub

Correct answer: 1

Graphic Option Questions

With graphic questions you will be shown a graphic or a series of graphics in addition to the text in the question. These are different than hot spot questions because these questions have you interpret the graphic, such as an ECG, to answer the question. The answer choices could also be graphic images.

Graphic Option Example

Which electrocardiogram strip should the nurse document as sinus tachycardia?

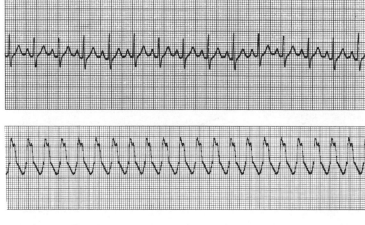

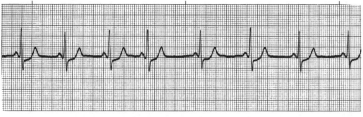

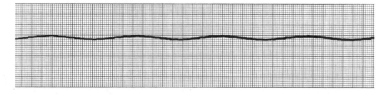

Correct answer: 1